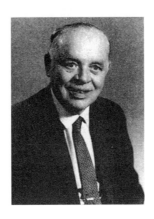

JOHN HARTLAND (1901–1977)

Most of the tributes to John Hartland on his death in 1977 bore witness to his personal qualities – warmth, energy and enthusiasms, ranging from classical music, photography, football, the detective novel to the wines of France – before describing his contribution in establishing the credentials of hypnotherapy as a branch of psychosomatic medicine and in rendering it more accessible to general medical and dental practitioners. Indeed, his personality had much to do with his own success as a therapist, together with his extraordinary care for verbal suggestion techniques: he took permanent delight in the richness and rhythms of the English language.

He thought later that he owed much to 30 years' experience in general medicine practice in West Bromwich, in the heart of the 'Black Country' of the English industrial Midlands, among a people for whom he felt great affection.

His commitment to psychiatry came, however, from frustration at being denied the opportunity to leave general medicine. This was in 1939 when at the outbreak of war he volunteered for the Royal Navy. He was told to stay where he was. The industrial Midlands were likely to be bombed. He turned his energies to the organization of an air raid post, to the raising of morale and money for military charities through the writing and production of musical revues, to the Red Cross, and – through curiosity in the phenomena of hypnosis – to psychiatry.

After the war he combined full-time general medicine with a hospital appointment as consultant psychiatrist and a growing private psychiatric practice. He began to lecture and demonstrate, first in Britain, then in the United States, France, Sweden, Australia and Singapore; was a driving force in the British Society of Medical and Dental Hypnosis; and edited the *British Journal of Medical Hypnosis*. The turning-point was the publication of his paper on "ego-strengthening technique" in the United States in the early 1960s. One of the greatest rewards of his travels to the United States was his friendship with Milton Erickson.

Nothing would have given him greater satisfaction today than to know that his book, which first appeared in 1966, is still valued and thought worthy of a fourth edition.

Hartland's Medical and Dental Hypnosis

The late David Waxman, editor of the third edition

Founder and First President of the section for Medical and Dental Hypnosis of the Royal Society of Medicine; Past President of the European Society for Hypnosis in Psychotherapy and Psychosomatic Medicine; Past President and Founder Fellow of the British Society of Medical and Dental Hypnosis; Past Vice President of the British Society of Experimental and Clinical Hypnosis; Past Affiliate of the Royal College of Psychiatrists; Founder Fellow of the International Society of Psychosomatic Obstetrics and Gynaecology; Formerly Associate Specialist in Psychiatry, Central Middlesex Hospital, London.

For Churchill Livingstone:

Publishing Manager, Health Professions: Inta Ozols
Project Development Manager: Karen Gilmour
Project Manager: Alison Ashmore
Design Direction: George Ajayi

Hartland's Medical and Dental Hypnosis

Michael Heap BSc MSc PhD
Clinical Psychologist, Wathwood Hospital, Rotherham, UK

Kottiyattil K. Aravind MBBS FRCS
General Medical Practitioner, Rotherham, UK

FOURTH EDITION

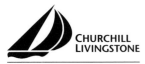
CHURCHILL
LIVINGSTONE

EDINBURGH LONDON NEW YORK PHILADELPHIA ST LOUIS SYDNEY TORONTO 2002

CHURCHILL LIVINGSTONE
An imprint of Elsevier Limited

Third edition 1989
Fourth edition 2002
    Reprinted 2007 (twice), 2008, 2009

ISBN: 978-0-443-07217-8

British Library Cataloguing in Publication Data
A catalogue record for this book is available from the British Library

Library of Congress Cataloging in Publication Data
A catalog record for this book is available from the Library of Congress

Note
Medical knowledge is constantly changing. As new information
becomes available, changes in treatment, procedures, equipment and
the use of drugs become necessary. The authors and the publishers
have taken care to ensure that the information given in this text is
accurate and up to date. However, readers are strongly advised to
confirm that the information, especially with regard to drug usage,
complies with the latest legislation and standards of practice.

Neither the publisher nor the author will be liable for any loss or
damage of any nature occasioned to or suffered by any person acting
of refraining from acting as a result of reliance on the material
contained in this publication.

Working together to grow
libraries in developing countries
www.elsevier.com | www.bookaid.org | www.sabre.org

ELSEVIER   BOOK AID International   Sabre Foundation

ELSEVIER
your source for books,
journals and multimedia
in the health sciences
www.elsevierhealth.com

Printed in China

The
publisher's
policy is to use
paper manufactured
from sustainable forests

Contents

SECTION 5 The professional practice of hypnosis

Extracts from the forewords to the second and third editions

SECOND EDITION

Each page makes clear that a long overlooked and seriously neglected need is being fulfilled, one of great importance in the furtherance of the scientific modality of hypnosis as an important adjunct in the healing arts. A methodology of the medical use of hypnosis of great value to the patient himself and to medicine as a whole is developed and adequately elucidated in this book. This is achieved by centring around a clear-cut well-ordered basic orientation which acquaints the medical practitioner with the varieties of hypnotic understandings pertinent to the clinical practice of medicine.

Milton H. Erickson

THIRD EDITION

The practice of hypnotherapy is both an art and a science. As an *art* it is often best communicated through an apprenticeship to an experienced expert. However, such an opportunity is not always provided for students in medical and dental study, and not easy for those already in practice who wish to become familiar with hypnotherapy. For both student and qualified practitioner this book is an attractive alternative because of the detail with which appropriate practices are presented. ... the intention is to present those in practice with what is positive that has been learned through successful hypnotherapy with patients. Welfare of the patient is what therapy is all about.

Ernest R. Hilgard

This work, which covers large areas of medicine and surgery, thus acquires great importance not only on account of the numerous and varied references to situations relieved by hypnosis, but also for the holistic vision permeating it and consequently the quality of approach for the patient, that important approach in diagnostic and therapeutic areas outside clinical hypnosis, we could call psychosomatistic. This orientation is a constant element which becomes more and more evident as one reads on. It concerns both the patient with his symptoms and the factors preceding and concurrent with the induction and deepening of the hypnosis responsible for these processes, as well as their spontaneous and induced phenomena, not to mention their therapeutic action. Here we should also note the importance given to the doctor figure, characterized by affective sensitivity, inner opening and a capacity for human contact, leading him to accept and use what the patient initially offers him, displaying trust, respect, empathy and sympathy, and forming together with the patient a unity made up of intimate responses.

A clear example of this is the studied attention devoted not only to words but also to pauses; in other words, the weighing up and interpretation of the possible significances behind the frequency, duration and quality of both utterances and silences, and an assessment of how and when they are inserted into the thread of sound.

It can therefore be especially recommended both for the valuable information concerning professional practice in many specialist areas and also because it may help to spread the understanding that it is possible to be therapeutic purely *as a person*, sometimes even without the need to resort to any other remedy.

Gualtiero Guantieri

Foreword to the fourth edition by Peter B. Bloom

My copy of the original edition of John Hartland's landmark text *Medical and Dental Hypnosis and its Clinical Applications* is dog-eared from my close study and underlining as I worked hard to add this clinical skill and experimental understanding to my work in medicine and psychiatry. As later editions became the standard text for succeeding generations of clinicians and researchers, the field of hypnosis grew with vigor and influence and entered a new period of acceptance and inevitable controversy. A few years after Dr David Waxman authored the third edition in 1989, it became apparent that we needed a further edition that leapt ahead of the previous volumes and which encompassed a clinically useful and scientifically rigorous integration of the enormous changes taking place in our field during the last decade. This is that book.

Michael Heap is a psychologist and Kottiyattil Aravind is a physician. They have each brought an exemplary level of scholarship and clinical experience to the rich traditions of clinical practice and experimental thought. Their differing backgrounds bring a freshness to this book that reflects the extensive contributions to our field by clinical psychology in the last forty years. But they do not depart from Hartland's own special stamp. The essence of Hartland's approach to hypnosis permeates the discussions on establishing a therapeutic alliance, making a sensible diagnosis, and planning treatment accordingly. In 1974, he stated to a gathering of clinicians in Australia that ego-building was the *sine qua non* of effective therapy. I am happy to see his original ego-strengthening routine is preserved in this edition; it still deserves our attention.

In the clinical section of this book, the use of hypnosis in an extensive variety of medical, dental, and psychological conditions is spelled out in learnable detail. Gentle are the interventions suggested for approaching patients dying of cancer or suffering disabling anxieties that limit their lives. Vigorous are the interventions that are brought to bear on relieving pain in obstetrics and dentistry. Those who seek a book on how to do hypnosis in these patients will not be disappointed. Similarly, those with a great deal of experience will be quickly surprised to find case examples that will help them find new ways to treat the most difficult patients we see in our offices throughout our careers. There is much in this volume for every clinician.

The most noticeable change in this edition is its increased reliance on good scientific thinking. The reader will find clear and logical descriptions of the evolution of what we know from the laboratory, and what we do not know. In recent years, the neurophysiological basis for response to hypnotic imagery for pain relief has become clearer, while the manner in which memory is stored and retrieved has become the basis of enormous controversy. Heap and Aravind describe the context in which these latter ideas have developed, and discuss the cultural soil which has allowed them to grow in some countries but not in others. Beginners reading this text will understand quickly what has evolved and be able to take their own position on these issues with intelligence and discernment. The advanced practitioner will find these discussions stimulating and challenging, and will recognize the new light they shed on what we know and believe.

I expect this edition will become dog-eared and underlined by many readers in the years to come as mine did in the past. For those who have awaited a definitive, comprehensive text, written by the consistent and even voices of only two authors, the wait is over. John Hartland would burst with pride that his tradition of excellence in patient care has been so well preserved and advanced. Ernest Hilgard, who wrote an earlier foreword, would compliment the authors on their grasp and respect for the science undergirding our work. Each would agree that the art of therapy is the fusion of scientific *and* clinical knowledge. I congratulate the authors on an extraordinary achievement.

Peter B. Bloom, M.D.
Past President,
International Society of Hypnosis;
Clinical Professor of Psychiatry,
University of Pennsylvania
School of Medicine

Swarthmore, PA, USA
June 2001

Preface

It is 35 years since the first edition of John Hartland's *Medical and Dental Hypnosis*. In that time, the book has proved immensely popular as an exposition of the principles and methods of clinical hypnosis in medical and dental practice, and as an adjunct to psychological therapy. Thirteen years have elapsed since the appearance of the third and most recent edition, authored by the late Dr David Waxman. Hence, if only for the sake of consistency, the fourth edition is now due. But what sort of book should it be? Our answer to this question has been to set ourselves several clear aims.

First, we have endeavoured to adhere to the original scope of each of the previous editions, namely to present a description, with case illustrations, of the major hypnotherapeutic procedures and techniques that are used in clinical practice. These are mainly, though not exclusively, confined to Sections 2 and 3 of the book and are sufficiently detailed, we hope, for the clinical hypnotist in training.

Second, in Section 1 of the book, we have endeavoured to present an account of hypnosis that is informed by mainstream psychology and its related disciplines, and draws upon the scientific evidence that has accumulated from over 50 years of laboratory investigations. In this task, we have tried to be descriptive rather than theoretical. However, we do not accept the traditional view, one that characterised the previous editions of this book, that hypnosis is a process whereby the hypnotist guides the subject into a state of trance characterised by hypersuggestibility and greater access to the unconscious mind. Rather, we consider that, during hypnosis, subjects actively deploy their skills in an endeavour to achieve the effects and experiences suggested by the hypnotist. Some subjects are apparently more successful than others (and we incline to the 'trait' school of thought) but people can be responsive for more than one reason; that is, more than one skill, aptitude or process is involved.

While the concept of 'trance' has lost much of its explanatory value, for clinical purposes at least, it is a useful description of the process of absorption and detachment from immediate realities that characterises everyday trance experiences. Some good hypnotic subjects may show a marked facility for this kind of experience, but we acknowledge that the relationship between measured hypnotic susceptibility and this characteristic (which we associate with absorption, although some would also refer to it as 'dissociation') is only a modest one.

We have made this distinction between suggestibility and absorption or trance an essential one in our presentation of clinical practices. For some purposes, an enhanced response to suggestion is an important focus of the therapy, whereas in others the achievement of a 'deep state of absorption' is the therapist's aim.

Throughout the book, we have attempted to present clinical practice in a way that is informed by a rational understanding of the nature of hypnosis and hypnotic phenomena. However, our rejection of the traditional understanding of hypnosis does not mean that practitioners who still adhere to that paradigm may not employ any of the procedures that we describe. To help the practitioner understand why this is so, in Section 3 we have developed the concept of the 'working model'. This is a set of assumptions about the patient's problem and how hypnosis may contribute to its alleviation or management. A working model may generate therapeutic procedures that are effective, yet the model itself need not be valid in a literal sense. In such cases, we can often say that the working model is a 'metaphorical representation' and we describe in Section 4 how metaphorical models may inform the effective application of hypnotic procedures to certain conditions and disorders.

Of metaphorical significance only, in our opinion, is the idea of the 'unconscious mind', and indeed we consider that it is an overvalued, limited and potentially misleading concept. In Section 3, we make the point that this has been the fate of a number of useful metaphorical constructs (including the hypnotic trance and, more recently, ego states) that have become reified and accorded explanatory powers that they do not possess.

We consider that this is one of the ways that hypnosis has come to be misused in 'recovered memory' therapy, an example of where a working model has been extended well beyond its range of useful application, with disastrous consequences. Likewise, we retain our British scepticism of the use of hypnosis to diagnose multiple personality disorder, or dissociative identity disorder, as we are now required to call it, a psychiatric classification rarely used in the UK.

Instead of the 'unconscious mind', we offer a dynamic (and certainly not original) working model involving a reciprocal process of unconscious-to-conscious expression of cognition and affect which is facilitated by the encouragement of overt communication ('talking therapy' being the most common method). On this working model, we base our presentation of what hitherto have been called 'hypnoanalytical techniques' but we avoid this term and prefer to speak about the psychodynamic application of hypnotic procedures.

In Section 3, we consider how hypnosis may be used within the major schools of psychotherapy. We use the term 'psychotherapy' in its broadest sense to include psychoanalytical and psychodynamic therapy, behaviour therapy, cognitive therapy and humanistic and existential therapy. We anticipate that many readers will be unclear about these distinctions and we have therefore presented brief summaries of the principles and practices that characterise each school. We have also attempted a short and critical account of the work and influence of Milton Erickson.

We must warn those readers who are familiar with any or all of the above schools of psychotherapy that they may find our accounts oversimplistic and at times idiosyncratic. Any idiosyncrasies probably arise first because we have presented our accounts with a view to describing how hypnotic procedures may be applied within each of the respective approaches and second because we set ourselves the task of developing a framework on which to base an eclectic or integrationist approach to hypnosis in psychotherapy.

There are two reasons for our emphasis on eclecticism. First, many practitioners of hypnosis are indeed eclectic in their application of psychotherapy, adopting a behavioural approach with one patient or client, a psychodynamic emphasis with another, a cognitive emphasis with another, and not uncommonly a combination of approaches with the same patient, even within the same session. Second, hypnotic procedures lend themselves very well to this way of working, allowing the therapist, guided by the client, to move fluently between the different levels as required. Our framework for this kind of work is presented in Section 3.

In Section 4, we present applications of hypnosis to specific conditions, disorders and problems that are commonly encountered in medical, dental and psychotherapeutic practice. Some problems are covered in greater depth than others and sometimes we have described non-hypnotic procedures. In the case of psychological disorders, we can only assume that the reader intending to use hypnosis for these is already accomplished in their treatment using non-hypnotic methods. As well as the procedures presented earlier in the book, we give readers some ideas for using hypnosis as an adjunct to a broader programme of therapy.

Throughout the book, we give, we hope, due acknowledgement to the minimisation of risk and to good ethical practice. In the appendices, we include rules for ethical practice as devised by the International Society of Hypnosis, and guidelines for using hypnosis for the resolution of early traumatic memories. Also, in Section 5, we address what we loosely term 'professional issues'. 'What is the evidence that hypnosis is effective?' is one question which we endeavour to answer by summarising the results of outcome studies. An impetus for our doing this is that the question is often asked of doctors, dentists and psychologists who are planning 'hypnotherapy' clinics or similar projects and have to make a good case when applying for funding and resources. In the same chapter, we address the question of whether hypnosis is effective as a method of interrogating witnesses to crime, and we adopt a critical perspective.

After we have explored the evidence for the benefits of hypnosis, we ask if the public are at risk from any adverse effects. We explore this question by considering lay hypnotherapists and stage hypnosis, and we adopt what we hope is a balanced perspective.

In our final chapter, we offer some advice to the serious practitioner of hypnosis who wishes to keep abreast of developments in the field and communicate with like-minded colleagues. In that chapter, we also return to the theme of the importance of representing and applying hypnosis in a manner that is consistent with existing knowledge and evidence, not only of hypnosis itself but of human psychology generally.

If there is only one criterion by which this book is to be evaluated, then let it be the extent to which we have adhered to the above precept. Of course, in many disciplines there is always some tension between, on the one hand, the academics, theorists and researchers and, on the other hand, those whose job it is to apply the knowledge to real-life problems. In the case of hypnosis, it is the ideas of the latter which have tended to predominate. Hence, the way hypnosis is presented and understood is often with disproportionate regard to the needs and expediencies of the clinical practitioner.

Even amongst those professionals trained in the exacting disciplines of medicine and psychology, it seems that an interest in hypnosis all too easily becomes a readiness to accept any fad or fashion that presents itself as a means of curing the ills of the age. Equally, there is a willingness to provide intellectual accommodation to the most outlandish notions about the workings of the human mind, brain and body. It still remains the case that any page turned at random in any book drawn at random from the hypnosis shelves of any bookshop will, more likely than not, provide readers with information that is unreliable, unsubstantiated, or plainly false.

It is regrettable that at the time of writing, in North America at least, where much of the progress in our understanding of hypnosis and the scope of its therapeutic applications has originated, the gulf between the theorists and the practitioners could hardly be wider. This state of affairs has arisen as a result of therapeutic practices that have been informed by, at the very best, some highly tenuous assumptions about human memory, which have little support in academic psychology and experimental hypnosis in particular.

It is our hope that, whoever the authors are by the time the next edition of this volume comes to be written, they will be able to report that this conflict was resolved in a manner consistent with existing scientific knowledge of human memory and mental processes. No other outcome can be considered as acceptable.

Note

In this book, we express many beliefs and opinions but it is unrealistic to suppose that we are always in complete agreement. We do not, however, consider it useful to readers to air our differences. Hence, statements beginning 'In our opinion' or 'In our experience' may be more representative of the opinions and experience of one of us rather than the other. Explicit references to the opinions or experience of just one of us (MH or KKA) does not imply disagreement; it is simply the case that the other author has not had sufficient experience to draw on to endorse what is being stated.

M.H.

K.K.A.

Sheffield 2001

Acknowledgements

We are wholly responsible for the accuracy of the information contained in this book and the quality of the instructions, advice and guidance we give to readers, likewise the opinions we express. We have, however, sought advice on certain topics and accordingly wish to thank the following colleagues: Dr Richard Brown, Mrs Valerie Heap, Mr Simon Houghton, Mrs Mary Lea, Professor Leslie Walker, and numerous international colleagues on the 'research list serve' email network organised by the Society for Clinical and Experimental Hypnosis.

Professor Paul Salkovskis has very kindly given us permission to present, in Chapter 21, a modified version of his diagram of the development of obsessive–compulsive disorder from his chapter 'Obsessions and compulsions' in *Cognitive Therapy in Practice: An Illustrative Casebook*, edited by J. Scott, J.M.G. Williams and A.T. Beck (Routledge, London, 1989).

We are grateful to the Springer Publishing Company, New York, for allowing us to reproduce, in Chapter 26, the 'Is it possible?' script that appeared in *Hypnosis and Behaviour Therapy: The Treatment of Anxiety and Phobias* by J.C. Clarke and J.A. Jackson (1983).

The British Society of Experimental and Clinical Hypnosis has kindly allowed us to reproduce, in Appendix 1 to this book, its guidelines on *Clinical Hypnosis and Memory*, compiled by Dr David Oakley and Mrs Marcia Degun-Mather.

We are grateful to the Central Office of the International Society of Hypnosis (ISH) for allowing us to reproduce, in Appendix 2, the Ethical Guidelines from the ISH Members' Directory.

We thank Mrs Gwyneth Parry (formerly Benson) for allowing us to reproduce in detail, in Chapters 14 and 19, her training handouts on using hypnosis with children and adolescents, and Mr Geoff Callow for providing us with details of the fantasy procedures that he has recently developed for children and adolescents, which we have described in Chapter 14.

Finally, we express our gratitude to Ms Inta Ozols, Ms Karen Gilmour and Ms Alison Ashmore of our publishers Harcourt Health Sciences for their advice, support and patience while we have been preparing this book.

M.H.
K.K.A.

The history and nature of hypnosis

In this section we address the question 'What is hypnosis?' We first do so from an historical perspective in Chapter 1. From our brief summary and the ensuing chapters on the nature and theories of hypnosis, it will be clear that hypnosis and its forerunner, mesmerism, are very much social constructs in which the behaviours and experiences of the participants (both hypnotists and subjects), and their understanding of these, are significantly determined by the expectations and demands of the context (the immediate situation and the wider social framework) in which the activity takes place.

Our approach to hypnosis is, however, not simply a social psychological one, and a review of the theories and several important research issues in Chapter 4 leads us to emphasise the importance of a range of cognitive skills that hypnotic subjects are able to deploy in their endeavour to have the experiences and respond in the manner suggested by the hypnotist. Some subjects appear to be better at this than others and we adhere to the more traditional view that hypnotic responsiveness is a stable trait (Chapter 3).

We consider that the pivotal concept in hypnosis is not 'trance' but 'suggestion' (and suggestibility). We explore both concepts in Chapter 2 and conclude that 'trance' in the sense of absorption on inner experiences is still of importance, although thus conceived it is of less explanatory significance than that assigned by earlier notions.

1

Overview of the history of hypnosis

INTRODUCTION

This chapter provides a brief and selective overview of the history of hypnosis. There are some very good comprehensive histories of hypnosis, but readers who are keen to explore this subject in depth can do no better than study *A History of Hypnotism* by Gauld (1992). Another good source is *Hypnosis in Europe* by Hawkins & Heap (1998).

COMMON THEMES AND PRACTICES

When one explores therapeutic or healing practices throughout history, across contemporary cultures, and even within our own culture, one discovers an almost limitless abundance of what are often extraordinary and bizarre ideas and practices, more so than in any other human enterprise, with the possible exception of religion. To understand why this is so would require a whole book in itself, and an interesting one at that. Suffice it to say that the explanation is emphatically not that the range of ideas and practices simply matches the enormous diversity of human illnesses and afflictions. We hope that readers may gain some insight into this interesting phenomenon from some of the later chapters in this book.

Healing or therapy involves a reciprocal role relationship. Two people – or it may be one person and a group of people – have a set of expectations about each other. The healer (and we mean by this term any kind of doctor

3

or therapist, orthodox and otherwise) is expected to undertake a series of actions, including (though not necessarily all of these) the taking of a history of the patient's problem, an examination of the patient, a diagnosis, some statement about the prognosis, the treatment itself, and monitoring and evaluation of treatment. Since many problems and illnesses naturally remit in time, and since the entire healing ritual itself may promote a healing reaction (usually labelled the 'placebo response'), healers may, enough of the time, appear to be successful with their patients, even when the practices adopted have no intrinsic healing properties themselves.

An important aspect of this interaction is that healers decide on behalf of the other, the patients, what is wrong with them, how they have come to have the problem, and what, therefore, is the solution to the problem. The healer is perceived by the patient as having the expertise to make these decisions. Thus the healer is always in a position of power vis-à-vis the person seeking to be healed. Even when the healing process itself is the responsibility of the patient, the solution to the problem is always in some way in the hands of the healer.

This may be literally so. The use of hands, with or without touch, is a common theme in the history of healing. In the Bible, one reads how Jesus healed by touching the person. British kings and queens were at one time said to have the gift of healing at their fingertips; they ruled by divine right and thereby had the power to heal by touch (hence the 'Royal Touch'), specifically the disease scrofula. We also have, of course, the 'laying on of the hands' of healers, and therapeutic procedures that formalise this, such as various massage techniques.

Another very common theme is the idea of fluids or humours, and invisible kinds of 'life forces' or energy. An early influential proponent of this was the physician Galen (AD 131–201). Along with this comes the idea that somehow these fluids or this vital energy become blocked and this causes problems, physical disease, illnesses of the mind, and so on. Healing occurs when the fluid or energy is re-channelled or unblocked. The healer has the power to do this. (Indeed, the obstruction of the flow of fluids and the alleviation of such is a common theme in modern medicine – viz. respiratory, cardiovascular, gastro-intestinal, genito-urinary, and, by analogy, certain neurological disorders.)

These forces or energies are essentially occult or magical in their conception. However, another process that occurs is the borrowing by healers of contemporary scientific discoveries and ideas. We shall see later that the ideas and practices of Franz Anton Mesmer in the 18th century were influenced by scientific discoveries and advances in the understanding of gravitational force and magnetism. For no good scientific reasons, energy fields (or 'vibrations') such as electromagnetic fields still form the hypothetical basis of some contemporary diagnostic and therapeutic practices (e.g. colour therapy, crystal healing, and Kirlian photography). Early in the

20th century, X-rays were popularised as having healing properties until it was discovered that they were actually dangerous.

With the rise of science over the last 300 years, the misappropriation of its hard-won gains by unconventional therapists has been a growing phenomenon, so that nowadays, much of what is labelled as 'complementary medicine' is an odd mixture of occultism, pseudo-science and blatant misinformation. Thus, we have the borrowing of ideas and discoveries, not only from the physical sciences, but also from the biological sciences and from conventional medicine itself. Examples are vitamins, minerals, biological rhythms, the immune system (as when, for instance, the claim is made that a therapy 'boosts the immune system'), and toxins (viz. 'detoxifying diets'). From psychology and neuropsychology, we have the alpha rhythm and the 'alpha state', subliminal perception, the unconscious mind, and cerebral laterality, the right side of the brain in particular being accredited with healing activity. The latest discovery to be accorded this dubious honour is endorphins, a common claim for a therapy now being that 'it causes the body to produce endorphins'. The neurotransmitter serotonin is currently showing signs of undergoing a similar initiation into the vocabulary of some unorthodox medical practitioners.

Yet another important theme is the idea of altered states of the mind or sleep-type experiences. Of interest here are the temples in ancient Greece that were devoted to Asklepios or Aesculapius, the Greek god of healing. One enormous temple, or Asklepieion, was constructed at Epidaurus in southern Greece. These temples were built in pleasant surroundings, usually near water. Priests attended to the patients, who were bathed regularly and put on diets, and when they were ready for healing they were taken to a special room, the abaton. They would be dressed in white robes and given soporific substances such as poppy seeds. There would be music, prayers and incantations, and it was believed that the gods would visit the sleeper. (The god of sleep is, of course, Hypnos; his son, Morpheus is the god of dreams.) There were similar temples in ancient Egypt.

Here we have an additional important theme, namely the use of prayer, incantations, magic spells or *suggestion*. The following is an incantation to be chanted by the patient prior to drinking a cure for an illness of the stomach. It was found on a papyrus scroll in an ancient Egyptian tomb.

Come, you who drive out evil things from my stomach and my limbs. He who drinks this shall be cured just as the gods above were cured.

(Hartley 1984, p 7)

The final theme is the idea of a crisis, some kind of violent reaction, which denotes that healing is taking place. In earlier times, this would be evidence of demons leaving the body. Later ideas were based on the notion of the release or unblocking of vital fluids or energy. More recently, but not dissimilar to the latter, we may speak of the release of pent-up emotions or an 'abreaction'. The idea of the crisis or abreaction is common in various cultures, as exemplified by tribal ceremonies in which people stand round in a circle, listening to the rhythmical beating of a drum, chanting, most likely hyperventilating, and finally falling over. This business of falling over is also evident in Christian healing ceremonies.

So, when we think about the history of hypnosis we may be tempted to make some kind of evolutionary link with very early practices, such as the healing activities in ancient sleep temples. However, it is probably more accurate to locate the origins of modern hypnosis in 18th century Europe, for it is the practice of mesmerism that is the true historical precursor of hypnosis.

MESMER AND THE RISE OF MESMERISM

Franz Anton Mesmer (1734–1815) was born in Iznang near Lake Constance in what was, at that time, the Austrian Empire. He graduated in medicine in Vienna at the age of 32. He was influenced by the writings of a number of people, notably the Swiss physician Paracelsus (1493–1541), who was Professor of Medicine at Basle. Paracelsus held that doctors should treat disorders of the mind as they would the body, and not leave it to the clergy with their ideas of demonic possession. He advocated the use of discoveries in chemistry for the treatment of illness, although, at that time, chemistry was not sufficiently developed to be of great use in this regard. He also emphasised the importance of natural healing and made use of magnets for 'drawing diseases out of the body' and healing broken bones.

A contemporary influence was Father Maximillian Hell (sometimes spelt Hehl) who lived from 1720 to 1792. He was a Jesuit priest and Professor of Anatomy at the University of Vienna and a follower of Paracelsus. He considered that the human body was the centre of magnetic influence. For treating patients, he constructed steel magnetic plates and attached them to the patient's body. He made some plates for Mesmer who experimented with them himself and concluded that the force at work was not true magnetism but something more universal.

Mesmer himself was interested in Newton's concept of universal gravitation and he attempted to apply this idea to human illness. In 1766, he wrote a dissertation on the influence of the moon and planets on the body. He proposed the existence of a universal force that he initially called 'animal gravity', but later he settled for 'animal magnetism'. He postulated that illness was associated with disturbances in the natural tidal flow of animal magnetism in the body and that he had the ability to restore this and thus heal the patient. He abandoned the use of magnets in favour of making slow passes with his hands over the patient's body from the head to the toe. He experimented on patients in Vienna and famously, in 1777, partially restored the sight of an accomplished pianist, a young lady of 18 years,

Marie-Thérèse Paradis, who had been blind since the age of 4 years. However, for some reason, her initially grateful parents quarrelled with him and their daughter's eyesight deteriorated. He also had some marital troubles at that time and so he left Vienna for Paris in 1778.

In Paris, he set up a practice and became very popular among those who could pay his fees. He devised group methods and these were conducted in salons in which there would be several large receptacles called 'baquets'. The baquet consisted of a tub filled with water and iron filings, 'magnetised' by Mesmer. From this protruded rods and the patients sat around and applied the rods to their afflicted parts. Some of the patients would have crises; they would swoon and go into convulsions, shaking, crying, laughing hysterically, and so on. Finally, they would appear to enter some kind of stupor with a glazed look in the eye – a sort of state of collapse. All of this indicated that the natural circulation of animal magnetism in the patient's body had been restored and the patient was presumably healed.

Mesmer had assistants who would tend to these people, and indeed he trained many students who set up their own magnetic practices throughout France. He also set up societies for animal magnetism, rather like masonic lodges. However, the government of the time did not like this; for one thing there was revolution in the air. Two enquiries were held, the most famous being the Franklin Inquiry in 1784, commissioned by King Louis XVI. Benjamin Franklin, who discovered the electrical nature of lightning and invented the lightning conductor, was at that time the American Ambassador in Paris.

The commissioners included the chemist Antoine Lavoisier and the physician Dr Joseph Ignace Guillotin, (whose eponymous invention, 10 years later, was to decapitate Dr Lavoisier). Mesmer would not cooperate, but his student, Charles Deslon, did. The commissioners performed many ingenious experiments into mesmerism and we recommend that the reader study their report, a translation of which appears in the magazine *Skeptic* (Franklin 1996). What the commissioners did, not only anticipates much of the scientific work on hypnosis that has been undertaken in the second half of the 20th century; it provides a model for the critical examination of any system of ideas and practices that makes extraordinary claims, of which, in our rational and enlightened age, there is no shortage.

For example, in one experiment, Deslon magnetised an apricot tree in a garden in Passy. A 12-year-old boy, who was susceptible to mesmeric procedures, was blindfolded and made to stand in front of four trees in succession and embrace each one. The prediction was that when he reached the magnetised tree, he would experience a crisis. What actually transpired was that he responded progressively to each tree by becoming more agitated and at the fourth tree he collapsed and appeared to lose consciousness. In fact, none of these trees had been magnetised and the boy was still 7.2 m (24 feet) away from the magnetised tree when he had his crisis.

In another experiment, a woman who was very susceptible to magnetism was, unbeknown to her, subjected to magnetic procedures by a trained physician who was hidden from her by a paper screen. She showed no inclination to respond, but when the physician performed the same manoeuvres in her view, and at the same distance, her crisis began within 3 minutes.

One of the important principles of the scientific method is Occam's razor – 'Non sunt multiplicanda entia praeter necessitatem' – named after the medieval priest and philosopher William of Occam (or Ockham) who died in 1349. 'Do not multiply entities beyond necessity.' Another way of saying this is that science attempts to explain things in terms that are already known and understood. The commissioners' results do not disprove the existence of animal magnetism; they only show that the various phenomena may be accounted for without reference to it. In the opinion of the commissioners, the critical factors in mesmeric practice were the patient's belief and imagination; there was no need to invent a new entity, animal magnetism, to explain what is observed. The reader will later see that this is paralleled by a similar debate today on whether the hypnotic trance exists as a phenomenon with explanatory properties, or whether hypnosis can be accounted for in terms such as expectation and the subject's repertoire of everyday cognitive skills.

The terms 'imagination' and 'belief' were used in a somewhat derogatory way by the Commission; a more constructive interpretation of their findings might be that something very interesting and useful was being discovered about the influence of these two psychological processes. (Nowadays some writers are doing something very similar when they dismiss hypnosis as, for example, 'just suggestion'.) However, the Commission was not concerned with evaluating the therapeutic effects of mesmerism.

THE MARQUIS DE CHASTENET DE PUYSÉGUR

So, mesmerism was discredited in medical and scientific circles. Mesmer faded from the scene, but he had a number of students. The most prominent one was the Marquis de Puységur (1751–1825) who, in 1784, received instruction from Mesmer. He was a benign French aristocrat and, unlike Mesmer, he treated rich and poor alike, including his peasants. He did not like the dramatic crises so he did not invoke them. Instead he preferred a relaxed, quiet state of mind. His most famous patient was a 23-year-old peasant, Victor Race, who suffered from inflammation of the lungs and bouts of feverishness. De Puységur mesmerised him on several occasions and encouraged in him a peaceful, calm state. Victor then talked about his domestic problems and any worries that he had, including his illness. In this state, his speech and intelligence seemed to improve and he also appeared to become clairvoyant and to have insight into the illnesses of others. Apparently, he was amnesic afterwards for this. De Puységur called this state 'artificial somnambulism' to distinguish it from the mesmeric crisis.

De Puységur also magnetised trees. For example, he had an elm tree, which he magnetised for group treatment. Ropes dangled from it and he would also touch the patients with an iron wand. Like Victor Race, the patients were rendered capable of insight into other people's illnesses. At the end of this group treatment, the patients would kiss the tree and awake from their artificial somnambulism, and they would be amnesic. Again, unlike Mesmer, de Puységur believed he could pass on his healing powers to his patients.

Although we should say that the Royal Commissioners identified the importance of psychological factors, de Puységur was one of the first practitioners to acknowledge the importance of these. In fact, from that time on, there was progressive recognition of psychological factors in mesmerism and hypnosis. Also, with de Puységur we see a more patient-centred approach, anticipating perhaps the method of free-association of psychoanalysis developed by Freud a century later.

THE ABBÉ DE FARIA

There are many important figures that we could mention but space limits us to a small handful. The next person on the scene to mention is the Abbé de Faria (1756–1819), a Portuguese priest who attended public demonstrations of mesmerism and then gave them himself. In 1819, he wrote a book (*De la Cause du Sommeil Lucide ou Étude sur la Nature de l'Homme*) rejecting the notion of animal magnetism and proposing something called 'lucid sleep'. His work is significant for three things in particular. First, he was the first person to document individual differences. He mesmerised 5000 people and found that one-fifth of them were capable of lucid sleep. This figure resembles the 10–20% of the population who are nowadays considered to be highly susceptible to hypnosis. Second, he proposed that the important factors in this process resided in the subject, not in the mesmerist. He said, 'We cannot induce concentration in individuals whenever we desire; rather we need to find people who are inherently susceptible' – just as we insist today. Third, his most radical departure was his induction technique. He replaced passes, magnets, trees, baquets and so on by verbal suggestion. He sat his patients on a chair and instructed them to focus all their attention on the concept of sleep, and this was the cue word. If susceptible, the person would eventually enter a state of lucid sleep.

JOHN ELLIOTSON

John Elliotson (1791–1868) was the leading figure of the mesmeric movement in Britain. He was a distinguished physician who promoted the use of the modern stethoscope. He was a forceful, larger-than-life character, despite being only 5 feet tall. He was Senior Physician at University College Hospital, London and Professor of the Practice of Medicine at the University of London. He advocated the use of mesmerism, including its application in surgery, and he lost his chair because of this. In 1843, he founded a journal called *The Zoist* and co-edited this for 13 years. The subtitle of *The Zoist* was 'A Journal of Cerebral Physiology and Mesmerism and their Application to Human Welfare' and it continued until the year 1856.

'Cerebral physiology' is more commonly known as phrenology, the location on the skull of 'organs' of human characteristics, abilities, aptitudes, and so on. Elliotson, like many people of his time, was very interested in and convinced by phrenological theory. Indeed, he combined the two procedures, mesmerising people and then demonstrating phrenological sites by pressing a finger on them and eliciting the predicted behaviours.

JAMES ESDAILE

Another important figure in this period is James Esdaile (1808–1859). He was a Scottish surgeon and employee of the East India Company. In 1845, he began experimenting with mesmerism as an anaesthetic, initially on convicts in Bengal. He eventually operated on hundreds of patients, notably about 200 with massive scrotal tumours. This was an endemic disease and was due to filariasis, transmitted by mosquitoes. These operations were well documented and it was observed that the patients showed little signs of experiencing any pain. Sometimes they would moan and groan, but not in the same way that one would expect if they were in severe pain. However, to mesmerise these patients took several hours a day for up to 12 days, so Esdaile had assistants working for him. His reported success rate was very high (Esdaile 1846). Some people attributed this to the malnourished and debilitated state of his patients and their submissiveness to their doctor, and he invoked much hostility from the medical profession. For sceptical discussions of Esdaile's methods, the reader is referred to Wagstaff (1981) and Chaves (1989).

JAMES BRAID

We now enter the post-mesmeric period in which the concept of sleep becomes more significant. The important landmark is what may be called a 'paradigm shift' and it comes with James Braid (1795–1860) who promoted the use of the term 'hypnotism', although he himself did not coin this word. He was a Scottish doctor practising in Manchester. In 1841, he witnessed an exhibition of mesmerism in a public demonstration by the French mesmerist La Fontaine and was very impressed, but he could not accept the theory that was being put forward.

There are, amongst others, three important contributions that Braid made. The first is his introduction of a new term. Originally, this was 'neurypnology' and in 1843 he wrote a book *Neurypnology or the Rationale of Nervous Sleep Considered in Relationship with Animal Magnetism*.

Second, he developed a new induction method. The subjects fixed their gaze on a point above eye level to produce strain. If the procedure was successful, the eyes would close and the subject would enter hypnosis. If unsuccessful, the subject was instructed to close the eyes and keep the gaze fixed. Later, the subject would be able to go into hypnosis just by imagining it. This new method became known as 'Braidism'.

Third, he developed new theoretical ideas that were rooted in physiology. He said that hypnosis was caused by visual fatigue but there were two stages. The first was the partial state. This involved excitement of all the sensors except sight, heightened awareness, passivity of the limbs, and full consciousness. In the second, the full state of hypnosis, the limbs would be rigid and immobile, respiration was slow, the person would be insensible, and then would be amnesic afterwards. Braid defined hypnosis as 'a derangement to the state of cerebral spinal centres by fixed stare, absolute repose of the body, immobility of the body, fixed attention on the words of the hypnotist, and suppressed respiration'.

Hence, hypnosis is a psychophysiological state. We shall see later that this can be thought of as the first serious 'special state' theory of hypnosis. Later on, however, in 1855, he changed his position about the nature of hypnosis to a more psychological stance: a state of mind induced primarily by suggestion. His new theoretical concept was 'monoideism': hypnosis is characterised by a state of heightened concentration on a single idea suggested by the hypnotist. In this state, imagination, belief and expectancy are more intense than in the normal waking state.

In this theory, we have the beginnings of the central role of suggestion in the elicitation of hypnotic phenomena, and the association of hypnosis with hypersuggestibility. However, the essential feature was still spontaneous amnesia. Without it, it was not true hypnosis. Amnesia became the defining characteristic of hypnosis for around 100 years and the mystery is that it is not characteristic of modern hypnosis now. What therefore has happened to this amnesia? One possibility is that the shared expectations of the hypnotist and the subject have altered.

JEAN MARTIN CHARCOT AND HIPPOLYTE BERNHEIM

Whatever the case, Braid made little impact at the time, and in England his ideas died with him. However, they were taken up on the continent and we now move to France and consider the ideas of Professor Jean Martin Charcot (1835–1893) and Professor Hippolyte Bernheim (1837–1919). Charcot was a leading neurologist and surgeon at the Salpêtrière Institute near Paris and he noted the similarity of hypnotic phenomena to neurotic symptoms in his hysterical patients who exhibited involuntary catalepsy, anaesthesia, amnesia, hallucinations, and so on. Thus, he established a putative link between hypnosis and mental illness. Bernheim was Professor of Medicine at Nancy. He was introduced to hypnosis by a medical practitioner, who practised nearby, called Dr Auguste Liébault, and he published a book in 1888 called *Hypnosis and Suggestion in Psychotherapy*, a very modern sounding title.

Now, a controversy evolved between Bernheim and Charcot and their associates, which continued for 20 years. Charcot insisted that hypnosis was an abnormal state of mind found in the mentally ill. However, Bernheim demonstrated that the entire range of hypnotic phenomena could be elicited in 15% of the normal population. Therefore, hypnosis was not confined to hysterics or neurotics. Charcot had a three-stage theory of hypnosis, namely lethargy, then catalepsy, then somnambulism. Bernheim was very critical of these stages and demonstrated that they were not representative of the usual response of subjects to hypnosis.

Bernheim saw hypnosis as a form of intensified suggestibility. For him, hypnotic phenomena are magnifications of everyday phenomena. Thus, rather than a special state, we have the emphasis on suggestibility, the idea that hypnosis has something to do with enhanced responsiveness to suggestion.

PIERRE JANET

Pierre Janet (1859–1947) was a French psychologist and psychotherapist who put forward a theory of hypnosis based on dissociation. Hypnosis produces a division of consciousness and eliminates conscious control of certain behaviours. Like Charcot, Janet's ideas were influenced by the behaviour of his patients. He and his collaborators were particularly interested in abnormal states of mind such as fugue states, multiple personality and automatism. He studied such phenomena as automatic writing, whereby a subject, under the instruction of the hypnotist, would write a message on paper, apparently without conscious awareness.

Janet's ideas on hypnosis lay dormant for 70 years and were revived by the American psychologist Ernest Hilgard, who formulated his neo-dissociation theory. Interestingly, this has been accompanied by a revival of interest in dissociative disorders. This theory will be described in the later chapter on modern theories of hypnosis.

THE DECLINE OF HYPNOSIS

The second half of the 19th century has been described by some as the heyday of hypnosis. Most of the eminent psychologists of the day were interested in it, whereas nowadays the opposite is the case. It then went into decline. There are a number of reasons for this. First, as we have seen, it became associated with phrenology and also with spiritualism. Phrenology, despite its popularity, was eventually discredited and replaced by more evidence-based neuropsychological theories.

Another reason for this decline was the advent of psychoanalysis. Sigmund Freud (1856–1939) worked with Charcot and used hypnosis, but he eventually abandoned it. Patients varied in their response to hypnotic procedures and direct symptom removal and hypnotic abreaction produced short-lived results. Patients were not necessarily truthful when questioned during hypnosis; thus, it was not a reliable method for gaining access to 'the unconscious'. Freud described his rejection of hypnosis in *Studies of Hysteria*, which he wrote with Josef Breuer in 1895.

Freud developed other methods, notably free-association. He also developed the very important idea of transference, the re-emergence of significant emotional conflicts that patients experienced in relation to significant figures in their early life. In analysis, these are manifested in the patient's feelings and fantasies about the therapist, hence the importance of the analyst's maintaining a more passive, neutral role that allows the transference to develop unhindered, a role inconsistent with that of the hypnotist.

Another reason for the decline of hypnosis was the rise of behaviourism. Science concerns itself with phenomena that are universally observable, or potentially so. Mental events such as thoughts, memories and feelings are privately experienced but behaviour is observed by all. Therapeutic methods based on this approach, namely behaviour therapy, gradually became popular amongst psychologists and psychiatrists. Paradoxically, a very well-known and influential behavioural psychologist, Clark Hull, *was* interested in hypnosis during the first half of the 20th century and he wrote a book called *Hypnosis and Suggestibility* in 1933 in which he described laboratory experiments on suggestion. He wished 'to divest hypnosis of its air of mystery, which surrounds it'. These aspirations were not seriously echoed for another 25 years.

THE MODERN SCIENTIFIC ERA

From 1950 onwards, we have the renaissance of hypnosis and we shall briefly examine these developments in the chapter on modern theories. One major controversy that has occupied psychologists who are interested in hypnosis has been whether, in order to explain the various phenomena, one needs to postulate a special state of consciousness, normally termed the hypnotic 'trance'. Many researchers and theorists have come to consider that this is unnecessary. This does not mean that 'there is no such thing as hypnosis'; in fact, the motivation to settle this controversy has resulted in much greater understanding of hypnosis.

One of the most important areas of activity has been the laboratory investigation of hypnotic phenomena and the development of explanatory theories grounded within mainstream psychology and neuroscience. A major achievement has been the development of scales for measuring responsiveness to suggestion and hypnosis. Another field of enquiry has been the attributes of people who are high in susceptibility. Most recently, we have seen investigators from a number of international medical and academic centres pursuing research on the neurophysiological and neuropsychological correlates of hypnotic phenomena and hypnotic susceptibility. There have been many laboratory studies investigating the alteration of pain perception by hypnotic suggestion and these have provided a vital grounding for one of the most important clinical contributions of hypnosis, namely pain management. A body of research literature is now accumulating on the evidence of the efficacy of hypnotic procedures for augmenting the treatment of a wide range of psychological and medical problems and conditions.

In 1955, the British Medical Association was sufficiently interested in hypnosis to set up an enquiry, the second one in its history (the first being in 1892), which reported favourably on hypnosis as a therapeutic medium, even recommending that hypnosis should be taught at medical schools and on courses for psychiatrists, and possibly anaesthetists and obstetricians. These recommendations were never taken up (Waxman 1986) but in the last 50 years there has been an acceleration in the establishment of hypnosis societies for medical doctors, dentists and psychologists in all continents. These organise their own training courses and scientific programmes for their members. We shall discuss these and the establishing of scientific journals of hypnosis in Chapter 34.

REFERENCES

British Medical Association 1893 Report of the Hypnotic Committee, 1892. British Journal of Medicine 2: 277
British Medical Association 1955 Medical uses of hypnotism. British Journal of Medicine 1(23 April): Supplement Appendix X
Chaves J F 1989 Hypnosis in the control of clinical pain. In: Spanos N P, Chaves J F (eds) Hypnosis: Cognitive-behavioral perspectives. Prometheus Books, Buffalo, ch 10, p 242
Esdaile J 1846 Mesmerism in India and its practical applications in surgery and medicine. Longmans, London
Franklin B 1996 Testing the claims of mesmerism. (Translated by C and D Salas, with Foreword by M Shermer.) Skeptic 4: 66–83
Gauld A 1992 A history of hypnotism. Cambridge University Press, Cambridge
Hartley L 1984 History of medicine. Basil Blackwell, Oxford
Hawkins P, Heap M 1998 Hypnosis in Europe. Whurr, London
Hull C 1933 Hypnosis and suggestibility. Appleton Century Crofts, New York
Wagstaff G F 1981 Hypnosis, compliance and belief. The Harvester Press, Brighton
Waxman D 1986 Hypnosis 1788–1986: Its history, development and status within the United Kingdom. Proceedings of the British Society of Medical and Dental Hypnosis 6: 3–8

2

The nature of hypnosis: suggestion and trance

INTRODUCTION

In this and the following chapter, we shall examine the nature of hypnosis from a descriptive rather than a theoretical perspective. We shall examine three pivotal concepts, namely suggestion, trance, and suggestibility or hypnotic susceptibility, and its measurement. The fourth component, the induction of hypnosis, will be presented in detail in Chapters 6 and 7.

EXAMPLES OF SUGGESTION

Of the various starting points for a discussion of the nature of modern hypnosis, perhaps the most logical and fundamental is 'suggestion'. Consider the following examples.

Ask a person or a group of people to imagine that they are sitting at a table on which is a bowl of fruit containing apples, oranges, grapes, bananas, lemons, and so on. By the side of the bowl of fruit is a paring knife. Ask them to imagine picking out from the bowl of fruit an orange or a lemon and holding it in their hand. Ask them to imagine the feel of the fruit on their hand, whether it is rough or smooth, whether it is cold or warm, whether it feels hard in the hand or soft and yielding. Suggest that maybe they can already smell the fruit. Then ask them to imagine taking the knife and cutting off a slice. Perhaps the smell is now stronger and some of the juice is on their fingers, making them feel sticky. Now ask them to imagine biting on the fruit and feeling it in their mouth, experiencing the taste of the fruit and whether it is ripe or sour. Further, ask them to imagine chewing on the fruit and feeling the juice in their mouth. Then, they are to imagine swallowing the fruit.

Having asked the participants to dismiss the image of the fruit from their minds, ask them to stretch out their arms at shoulder height with the palms facing inwards. Then ask them to imagine that in each hand they are holding a powerful magnet, with the north pole of one magnet facing the south pole of the other. There is thus a very strong attraction between the magnets and this is pulling their hands and arms closer together. Repeat the idea that the arms and hands are being pulled closer and closer together. Perhaps you can also ask them to imagine trying to resist the attraction of the magnets.

Again, ask the participants to dismiss that image from their mind and to relax their arms again. Now ask them to allow one of their arms to drop by their side. Then ask them to imagine that that hand is immersed in a bucket of ice-cold water. They can feel the wetness of the water on their hand and the coolness of the ice as they swirl their hand around in the bucket. Say that their hand is becoming colder and colder, and number and number. After a while, suggest that they take their hand out of the bucket, shake off the water, and press the back of their hand against the side of their face. Say that as they are doing so, they feel the cold and numbness in their hand now penetrating into their cheek. When they have spent enough time on this, they can then dismiss the image and relax once again and allow all the normal sensations to return to the hand and the face. (A positive response to these instructions is termed 'glove anaesthesia'.)

Each of these three examples is what is called a 'suggestion'. Suggestion gives rise to a range of measurable and replicable phenomena and observations that have the potential to be understood from within mainstream cognitive psychology. Suggestion is also central to an understanding of the process of hypnosis and it is therefore important to have an agreed definition of what constitutes a 'suggestion'.

DEFINING SUGGESTION

Before we attempt to define suggestion, we have to consider what exactly constitutes a definition. A definition of any object, phenomenon or process is a statement that gives its minimum essential properties, no more and no less. There should also be a consensus: we should all understand and accept the definition. It follows that the defining properties should be objectively observable, so that in any particular instance we can all agree that these properties are either present or absent. The definition then allows us to derive all other properties by the application of logic, mathematics or empirical investigation.

Impeccable examples of definitions are provided by Euclidean geometry. These illustrate the principle of strict parsimony in the choice of what the defining properties are to be. For example, a triangle may be defined as a three-sided plane figure. From this definition, we can derive other properties such as the fact that the angles of a triangle always add up to 180°. Hence, it is not necessary to define a triangle as a three-sided plane figure whose angles add up to 180°, since by the application of mathematics and logic we can deduce the last-mentioned property from the essential definition.

We consider that the best definition of suggestion is one that describes the activity of the person who administers the suggestion. Once we have agreed on what constitutes a suggestion in these terms, then we can investigate by empirical observation the additional properties and phenomena that are observed in response to a suggestion thus defined. As we shall see, however, it is in the nature of hypnosis, as with many psychological processes, that we can only speak of an *increased* probability that these additional phenomena will be observed.

A suggestion may be operationally defined as follows:

A communication, conveyed verbally by the hypnotist, that directs the subject's imagination in such a way as to elicit intended alterations in sensations, perceptions, feelings, thoughts and behaviour.

The three exercises earlier described are clearly examples of suggestions.

THE RESPONSE OF THE SUBJECT

Having defined suggestion operationally in terms of the communicative activity of the person giving the suggestion, all our interest now moves towards the experience and responses of the recipient. It is most often the case that when we investigate the effects elicited by a suggestion we do so through the subjective report of the recipient. However, we can also, as we shall see, make some reliable objective observations and measurements.

In the case of the first exercise, the participants may report, in varying degrees, that they had a visual image of the fruit and the knife, that they had a feeling of pleasurable anticipation as they picked up the fruit; that they felt the texture and temperature of the fruit in their hand; that they experienced some sense of the smell of the fruit; that they could taste the fruit and feel the juice trickling down their throat; and so on. Many participants also report increased salivation.

We could provide some measure of each of these by asking the subjects to rate the intensity and realistic nature of their experience on, say, a five-point scale. We could also provide an objective measure of the response by collecting and either weighing or taking the volume of the extra saliva produced as the subject imagines chewing on the fruit.

In the case of the second exercise, we could ask the subjects to rate how strongly the force of attraction felt between the two hands, or we could actually measure how close the hands came together after a fixed period of time.

In the third exercise, we could ask the subjects to rate how cold and numb the hand felt, likewise the cheek. We could also do some psychophysical ratings of the intensity of a tactile stimulus or even a potentially painful stimulus on the targeted hand, comparing these with the other hand.

For the moment, we are interested in examining those responses and experiences that we consider are *intended* by the suggestion. For example, suggesting to a person that a friend has just walked into the room may cause an increase in the person's heart rate. This change may be associated with an emotional reaction to seeing the friend, in which case it is a change that falls within the intention of the suggestion. On the other hand, for some people, the effort of creating an image of a friend (or any complex image for that matter) may itself lead to an increase in heart rate. In that case, this change is not one that is intended by the suggestion.

We should also note that the term 'suggestion' is also often used to describe the *response* of the subject. We shall discuss in further detail the various ways in which subjects may respond to suggestions but let us note that what we are interested in here is responding that has an automatic quality as reported by the subject. For example, the subjects for the 'magnets' suggestion will usually report that their arms seemed to come together with little or no conscious effort at movement on their part (although, of course, the exercise does require the conscious effort of concentrating on the ideas and images provided by the hypnotist).

TYPES OF SUGGESTION

Let us now examine a wider range of suggestions, some but not all of which are commonly used in clinical practice. We have classified the bulk of these according to the modality in which the suggestion is expressed, although, particularly in the case of ideosensory and ideomotor suggestions, more than one modality may be involved. We have also loosely classified most of the suggestions as either positive or negative. Positive suggestion communicates the idea that subjects will experience or do something, whereas a negative suggestion informs subjects that they will not experience or not be able to do something that normally they would. The latter are sometimes called 'challenge' suggestions for obvious reasons.

Ideosensory suggestions

Here we are restricting this term to changes in somatosensory experience. The term 'ideosensory' conveys the meaning that the sensory experience that the subject reports is in response to the idea communicated by the hypnotist and appears to the subject to have an automatic quality.

Positive

Relaxation. The hypnotist repeats suggestions that the subject's body is feeling heavy, warm and relaxed. This may be done systematically, asking the subject to think about each part of the body in turn, say from the forehead and then all the way down to the feet, with the suggestion that that part is feeling warm, heavy, relaxed, and so on.

Tickling. The hypnotist suggests that somebody is tickling the subject between the shoulder blades with a feather.

Negative

Glove anaesthesia. This was described in the third of the earlier exercises.

Ideomotor suggestions

The term 'ideomotor' conveys the meaning that a movement occurs *in response to the idea of that movement*; the subject does not merely move the limb or limbs in a deliberate manner. The following examples also contain ideosensory suggestions.

Positive

Postural sway. The hypnotist stands either in front of or behind the subject who is also standing. The hypnotist then repeats suggestions that the body is swaying backwards and forwards (as it will tend to do in order to maintain balance). It is then suggested that the body is swaying more in one direction (backwards or forwards). The idea that the wind is blowing against the body may be introduced and reassurances given that the hypnotist will support the subject should the subject actually fall in the suggested direction.

Chevreul's pendulum. The subject holds the string of a pendulum and fixates the bob, which initially is in the resting position. The hypnotist makes suggestions that when the subject thinks that the pendulum is moving in a particular direction, it will gradually start to do so, without any deliberate effort on the part of the subject.

Arm levitation. The hypnotist suggests that one of the subject's arms, which is resting either on the subject's lap or on the arm of the chair, is gradually feeling lighter and lighter (an ideosensory suggestion, see above). It will gradually come to feel so light that it will start to lift up and float in the air. A suitable image is offered, such as a large helium-filled balloon attached to a piece of string that is wrapped round the subject's wrist.

Arm lowering. One way to demonstrate this is to ask the subject to extend both arms forward with the hands at shoulder height and the palms facing upwards. It is then suggested that a heavy book is resting on one of the hands and it is forcing that arm down. Further suggestions are made of increasing heaviness and tiredness. The intended effect is for that arm to move down while the other arm remains in the same position.

Negative

Finger lock (or hand-clasp). The subject interlocks the fingers of the hands and the hypnotist suggests that the fingers are welded together or entangled like the roots of a tree and cannot be separated. At the count of 'three', the subject is to try to separate the hands and this will prove impossible.

Arm immobility or catalepsy. The hypnotist suggests that the subject's arm is so heavy that the subject is unable to lift it from the lap. Or, if the arm is in the raised position, it is now locked in that position and cannot be moved from it.

Eye catalepsy. The hypnotist instructs the subject to close the eyes (if they are not already closed) and then suggests that the eyes are glued tightly together. After repeating this suggestion a number of times, the hypnotist then suggests that, at the count of '3', the subject will be unable to open the eyes.

Arm rigidity. The subject makes a fist with one hand and raises the arm straight in the air. The hypnotist then suggests that the arm is now rigid and locked at the shoulder. One suitable image is that of the sword 'Excalibur' sticking out from a rock. The hypnotist suggests that the arm is impossible to bend or force down, and with one hand on the shoulder and the other hand grasping the subject's fist, the hypnotist endeavours to force the arm down (taking great care not to hurt the subject). The arm stubbornly resists the hypnotist's efforts.

The following four kinds of suggestion are termed 'hallucinations'. The reason for this is to convey the idea that the suggested experiences have a very real quality and the subject is able to interact with the images accordingly. (This theme will be discussed again later.) A good response tends to be observed only in a minority of subjects.

Auditory hallucinations

Positive

The fly. The hypnotist suggests to the subject, who usually has the eyes closed, that there is a fly buzzing round the subject's head. If the idea is experienced realistically, then the subject may be observed to show some adverse reaction such as jerking the head or flicking the imaginary fly away with the hand.

Negative

Deafness. The hypnotist suggests, for example, that the subject has lost the sense of hearing or can hear nothing else but the hypnotist's voice. Another suggestion is that the subject has lost the sense of hearing in one of the ears.

Visual hallucinations

Positive

Best friend. The hypnotist suggests that on opening the eyes, subjects will see their best friend sitting on the chair in front of them.

Negative

The chair. The hypnotist suggests that on opening the eyes, subjects will not see the chair that is presently in front of them.

Olfactory hallucinations

Positive

Bad smell. The hypnotist suggests that subjects are experiencing a foul smell, such as rotting cabbage, in their nostrils.

Negative

Anosmia. The hypnotist suggests that subjects have lost their sense of smell and tests this by holding a phial of ammonia solution under the nostrils.

Gustatory hallucinations

Positive

The orange. The hypnotist suggests that the subject is eating a delicious orange (see the earlier exercise).

Negative

The onion. The hypnotist suggests that subjects have lost their sense of taste and tests this by asking them to bite on a real onion. More commonly, the subject is simply informed that the onion is an apple.

Physiological changes

The intention of some suggestions is to alter directly certain physiological activities. This may be done at a general level, for example by suggesting relaxing imagery that may have the effect of reducing sympathetic arousal. Or a particular response may be targeted – earlier we gave the example of salivation. Another example, occasionally used in clinical hypnosis, is a suggestion aimed at altering blood flow. For example, using suitable imagery, the hypnotist suggests that the subject's hands are becoming very warm. Although the reported increase in hand temperature may not be accompanied by corresponding physiological changes (vasodilation), there is evidence that with practice, some subjects are able to alter blood flow in this manner (Barabasz & McGeorge 1978, Dikel & Olness 1980).

Complex suggestions

These suggestions are aimed at alterations in complex experiences rather than specific modalities.

Time distortion. The hypnotist suggests that time is slowing down and every second seems like a minute, every minute like an hour. Or it may be suggested that time is speeding up and every minute seems like a second.

Age regression. It is suggested that the subject is going back in time and becoming younger and younger. One method is to count backwards from the subject's present age to the targeted age.

Age progression. The suggestion is made that the subject is moving forward in time to some specified date or event.

Amnesia. The hypnotist suggests to the subject that, on alerting, the subject will remember nothing that happened during the hypnotic session until a cue is given, such as the hypnotist's tapping on the table. Instead, the material to be 'forgotten' may be selected by the hypnotist – for example, a piece of factual information that the subject would normally recall with ease.

Posthypnotic suggestion

Although we have yet to define what we actually mean by 'hypnosis', we can here take note of the fact that the subject's response in most of the above suggestions is intended to take place immediately, within the hypnotic session. The last example, however, illustrates a posthypnotic suggestion; the subject is to respond some time later, once the hypnotic session has been concluded.

FURTHER CONSIDERATIONS

In defining 'suggestion' in terms of what the hypnotist does, we are open to the criticism that whether or not hypnosis actually takes place depends on whether the subject responds in the intended manner. Let us explore this a little further by taking the example of glove anaesthesia. We can agree that the hypnotist has given a 'suggestion' and that the intention of that suggestion is for the subject to experience numbness of the hand and then the cheek. However, the subject may respond in a number of ways, some of which are not necessarily mutually exclusive.

1. The subject may totally ignore the suggestion.
2. The subject may attend to the suggestion, but make no attempt to go along with the ideas conveyed.
3. The subject may feel bored by the whole procedure, or become annoyed.
4. The subject may become anxious (and show increases in heart rate, sweating, respiration, etc.).
5. The subject may start giggling.
6. Subjects may try their best to go along with the ideas but not respond in any of the intended ways.
7. Subjects may not have any of the experiences suggested but, perhaps, in order to please the hypnotist, pretend that they are responding as intended. This is known as 'compliant' responding.
8. Subjects may respond as intended, to a greater or lesser degree, by means of some deliberate strategy, such as distracting themselves when tested for anaesthesia.
9. The subject may go along with the ideas and images and without being aware of using any conscious strategy, experience some degree of numbness.

Clearly only in 8 and 9 can the subject be said to be responding as intended. Traditionally 9 is considered to be a true hypnotic response – the so-called 'classic suggestion effect'. Some authorities (e.g., Spanos 1991, Wagstaff 1991) may question whether 8 and 9 are actually different.

It may seem obvious therefore that one should include in the definition of suggestion some reference to the fact that the subject responds in the manner of 9. We feel that this temptation should be resisted for the following reason. The distinction between responses that are described as conscious compliance (i.e. faking), goal-directed (or 'strategic') enactment, or automatic and unwilled, are not at all as clear and measurable as one might think. A definition is doomed to failure if it refers to properties that are themselves lacking clear definition or about which there is theoretical contention.

Whatever the case, in therapy at least, any of the above responses may be considered as saying something important about the patient or client and are therefore not to be dismissed as 'irrelevant'.

THE NATURE OF TRANCE

So far we have managed to describe the nature of hypnotic suggestion and how suggestions are administered without the need to refer to the idea that the subject is in any special state of the mind. That is, we have not referred to the subject as being 'in a trance'. Yet this is certainly what most people bring to mind when one mentions the word 'hypnosis'. Is it the case that when subjects respond in the intended way to the kinds of suggestions listed above (i.e. number 9 in the list), they are or have to be in a 'trance'? If so, what is a hypnotic trance and how is it induced in the subject?

The 'strong' interpretation of trance

The above question has been central to the history of hypnosis (and mesmerism). The traditional understanding of hypnosis is to consider that the hypnotist puts the subject into an altered state of consciousness and that this explains the phenomena, behaviour and experiences of the subject when these are different from those observed when he or she is not hypnotised. Thus subjects, in response to the hypnotist's instructions, move without conscious effort or are unable to move; see, hear and smell things that are not there; feel no pain when pricked with a needle; forget things they have just been told; think they are a child again; and so on. All this is explained by the subject's 'being in a trance'.

Let us call this a 'strong' interpretation of the trance concept. The term 'strong' is chosen because it seems that, used in this way, the idea of 'hypnotic trance' is similar to other altered states of consciousness such as sleep, concussion, epileptic seizure, alcoholic intoxication and drug intoxication. For example, we may observe that a person, normally alert, intelligent, well mannered and active, lies immobile and does not respond when we call the person's name or even when we give the person a nudge. We may explain this observation by saying that the person is in a state of sleep. Now, suppose that the same person is being very offensive and losing control of the emotions. This time our explanation is that the person is in a state of alcoholic intoxication. On yet another occasion, the person seems totally confused and does not know the time or place. We now explain this by saying that the person is in a state of concussion.

What do we observe when we use the explanation 'The person is in a hypnotic trance'? In former times, as well as hypersuggestibility, the hypnotic trance was associated with other unusual properties, such as spontaneous posthypnotic amnesia, awareness only of the hypnotist's voice, profound insensibility to pain, ability to perform superhuman or even supernatural feats, hypermnesia (the ability to remember accurate details of even remote events in one's life), and extreme literalism.

The 'weak' interpretation of trance

With more rigorous scientific investigation of hypnosis, these properties have been discounted or shown to be highly unreliable. In fact, it is very difficult to identify a person as 'being in a hypnotic trance' without reference to the phenomena we are trying to explain. For this and other reasons discussed in the later chapter on theories of hypnosis (Ch. 4), the usefulness of describing the 'hypnotic trance' as an 'altered state of consciousness' (akin to sleep, and so on) particularly as an *explanation* of hypnotic phenomena has progressively been eroded and some authorities do not use the concept at all.

Nevertheless, the concept of trance can still be very useful in the therapeutic application of hypnosis, if we adopt what may be called a 'weak' interpretation, namely:

A waking state in which the person's attention is focused away from his or her surroundings and absorbed by inner experiences such as feelings, cognitions and imagery.

Thus defined, trance is an everyday phenomenon, similar to daydreaming, meditation or absorption in a book, a television programme or music. The ability to become deeply engrossed in this way is termed 'absorption' and as a trait it can be measured by standardised questionnaires such as the Tellegen Absorption Scale (Tellegen & Atkinson 1974).

We shall see in Chapters 6 and 7 that when conducting hypnosis it is most often the case that we undertake some preliminary procedure intended to render the subject more responsive to the suggestions to follow. This procedure is termed the 'hypnotic induction' and the usual way of doing this is by a series of instructions and suggestions that encourage the subject to become very relaxed and absorbed in inner experiences, or in traditional terms, to 'enter a trance'.

Indeed, it may have occurred to the reader that, even without any such preliminaries, when one administers suggestions to subjects, one is encouraging them to put aside whatever is going on around them and to focus on the ideas and imagery being offered. Thus, suggestions encourage the experience of trance in the above 'weak' sense. Also, intuitively at least, it seems more likely that subjects will respond to the suggestions, particularly those that require profound changes in their experience (e.g. hallucinations or age regression) if they assume this kind of mental state. In fact, subjects often say that they did not respond as well as they might have to suggestions because they were distracted by external events or they were 'analysing what was happening', rather than 'going with the flow'.

Despite this, in laboratory studies, the correlation between measured hypnotic susceptibility and absorption is only modest and is rather unstable (Kirsch 1991). For example, Zachariae et al (2000) obtained correlations of only 0.27 (same context) and 0.38 (different contexts) between absorption and hypnotic susceptibility. We must concede, therefore, that absorption may not be of great significance so far as laboratory measurements of hypnotic susceptibility are concerned. However, absorption may be more important in the clinical context. We shall later argue that there are therapeutic applications in which one should try to maximise the patient's degree of absorption or trance experience.

'Depth' of trance

It has been the custom to use the expression 'depth' to refer to the extent to which the person is having a trance experience, and to distinguish 'light', 'medium' and 'deep trance' subjects. Traditionally, the deeper the trance, the more profound the subjective response to suggestions of changes in experience, such as hallucinations, analgesia, amnesia and age regression. 'Trance capacity' is not, however, a well-defined characteristic and may be related to absorption or to dissociation, which will be discussed in the next chapter. Crawford (1994) has presented some neurophysiological studies of individuals who have a marked capacity for absorption and may correspond to the traditional 'deep trance' subject. Barber (1999) also considers that this attribute pertains to a small minority of very susceptible individuals. He calls these 'amnesia-prone' subjects in preference to 'dissociation-prone'; the latter may be the preferred term of those writers with a state orientation to hypnosis.

Some further properties of trance

Further properties of trance, as defined above, have been determined by empirical research and include the following which, though not guaranteed, may be said to have an increased probability of occurrence as a result of trance. These properties may be observed in the everyday experience of trance and in the hypnotic trance experience:

1. Alteration in the experience of the passage of time, usually leading to underestimation (Von Kirchenheim & Persinger 1991).
2. Some amnesia for events that clearly registered because the subject responded overtly to them. An oft-quoted example is the 'highway trance' whereby, when driving, one realises that one has no memory of part of the journey, yet one was obviously wide awake, alert and responding to what was going on.
3. Attenuation of the experience of, and increased tolerance of, ongoing discomfort and pain.
4. When physically relaxed and tired, an enhanced predisposition to go to sleep.
5. With regular practice, the alleviation of the effects of stress (Benson 1975).

The aforementioned properties may all be exploited formally or informally for beneficial purposes. Property 1 we exploit on, say, a long train journey when, by absorbing oneself in a book or a daydream, time does not seem to drag so much. In clinical practice, it is used for the purposes of pain management, either where the pain results from some physical condition or where the patient is undergoing some uncomfortable medical intervention.

Property 2 is occasionally exploited in psychodynamic applications of hypnosis where some activity such as writing or other means of communication is outside of the patient's conscious awareness or 'dissociated'.

Again, we exploit property 3 in everyday life; we are all aware that being distracted from the discomfort of, for example, toothache by absorption in some pleasant activity makes the experience more bearable. Hypnotic pain management makes great use of this property.

The obvious application of property 4 is in the area of insomnia. Finally, the regular practice of self-hypnosis is a common component of clinical hypnosis (property 5).

A rather more contentious claim concerning the trance is that it facilitates access to unconscious material – memories, feelings, fantasies and even so-called 'inner resources' – which are normally below the level of conscious awareness but which may nevertheless exert an influence on the person's behaviour, thoughts and emotions. The contentiousness of the claim is related to the kind of theoretical rationale that is cited in its support. We shall, for example, argue in this book that the idea of 'the unconscious mind' is more a metaphorical construct than a psychological entity with a causative or explanatory function. Neither is it easy to demonstrate these claims empirically and the evidence tends to come from single case illustrations. However, it does not appear too contentious to assert that this process of inner absorption that we have identified by the term 'trance' has the property of facilitating greater self-awareness and self-understanding.

REFERENCES

Barabasz A F, McGeorge C M 1978 Biofeedback, mediated biofeedback and hypnosis in peripheral vasodilation training. American Journal of Clinical Hypnosis 21: 28–37
Barber T X 1999 A comprehensive three-dimensional theory of hypnosis. In: Kirsch I, Capafons A, Cardeña-Buelna E, Amigó S (eds) Clinical hypnosis and self-regulation: Cognitive-behavioural perspectives. American Psychological Association, Washington DC, ch 1, p 21
Benson H 1975 The relaxation response. William Morrow, New York
Crawford H 1994 Brain dynamics and hypnosis: Attentional and disattentional processes. International Journal of Clinical and Experimental Hypnosis 42: 204–232
Dikel W, Olness K 1980 Self-hypnosis, biofeedback, and voluntary peripheral temperature control in children. Pediatrics 66: 335–340
Kirsch I 1991 The social learning theory of hypnosis. In: Lynn S J, Rhue J W (eds) Theories of hypnosis: Current models and perspectives. Guilford Press, New York, ch 14, p 439
Spanos N P 1991 A sociocognitive approach to hypnosis. In: Lynn S J, Rhue J W (eds) Theories of hypnosis: Current models and perspectives. Guilford Press, New York, ch 11, p 324

Tellegen A, Atkinson G 1974 Openness to absorbing and self-altering experiences ('absorption'), a trait related to hypnotic susceptibility. Journal of Abnormal Psychology 83: 268–277

Von Kirchenheim C, Persinger M A 1991 Time distortion: A comparison of hypnotic induction and progressive relaxation procedures. International Journal of Clinical and Experimental Hypnosis 39: 63–66

Wagstaff G F 1991 Compliance, belief, and semantics in hypnosis: A nonstate, sociocognitive perspective. In: Lynn S J, Rhue J W (eds) Theories of hypnosis: Current models and perspectives. Guilford Press, New York, ch 12, p 362

Zachariae R, Jørgenson M M, Christensen S 2000 Hypnotizability and absorption in a Danish sample. International Journal of Clinical and Experimental Hypnosis 48: 306–314

3

Hypnotic susceptibility and its measurement

Chapter contents

INTRODUCTION

When one administers different suggestions to people, some will respond well, others not at all, and most somewhere in between. People who respond well to one kind of suggestion will, *on balance*, tend to respond better to another suggestion. Therefore, one may propose some kind of general trait that one may call, depending on one's theoretical position, 'suggestibility', 'hypnotic susceptibility' or 'hypnotic responsiveness'. However, the nature and variability of the inter-correlations are such as to suggest that this characteristic is itself composite in nature (Kumar et al 1999, Pekala 1991, Pekala et al 1995). This trait remains constant over long periods of time. For example, Piccione et al (1989) have followed up subjects over a period of 25 years and obtained high test–retest correlations. One study of monozygotic and dizygotic twins has indicated that the trait may be partly inherited (Morgan 1973). However, some authorities question the trait concept of hypnotic responsiveness. This controversy will be discussed in Chapter 4.

THE MEASUREMENT OF SUGGESTIBILITY OR HYPNOTIC SUSCEPTIBILITY

Standardised scales have been developed to measure suggestibility or hypnotic susceptibility. These scales have a high degree of reliability. Although most clinicians will probably rarely use them, it is important that they are familiar with the main ones that are referred to in the literature.

The most widely used scales are those developed in the 1950s and 1960s by André Weitzenhoffer and Ernest Hilgard, namely the Stanford Scales of

Hypnotic Susceptibility (SSHS) (Weitzenhoffer & Hilgard 1959, 1962). There are several of these, each consisting of a range of suggestions, and the subject's responsiveness to each is assessed. Collectively the scores attained for the suggestions yield a total score that, within the general population, has a broad distribution and a clear central tendency. Forms A (SHSS:A) and B (SHSS:B) are parallel versions, that is, the suggestions in Form B are nearly all different from those in Form A but the scales yield the same scores and distributions for the general population. The advantage of this is that they can be used for research purposes where the investigators are measuring susceptibility on two occasions and want to minimise learning and familiarity effects. The second item in these scales is a hypnotic induction. Form C samples a broader range of suggestions and discriminates among more highly susceptible subjects. It is now regarded as the 'gold standard' measure of susceptibility for the purposes of research. A version for group administration, the Waterloo–Stanford Group Scale of Hypnotic Susceptibility, Form C, has been developed (Bowers 1998).

The Harvard Group Scale of Hypnotic Susceptibility was developed by Ronald Shor and Emily Orne (Shor & Orne 1962). It is based on Form A of the Stanford Scale but the scoring is suitable for a group administration. This scale is often used as an initial screening measure when conducting research comparing the performances of high and low susceptible subjects. Very highly susceptible subjects can then be selected using Stanford Scale Form C.

These scales are very lengthy to administer and score (up to an hour or more). A quick method of measuring susceptibility is the Stanford Hypnotic Arm Levitation and Induction Test (the SHALIT). This is a standard arm levitation test (Hilgard et al 1979). It takes less than 10 minutes to administer and score and correlates with the SHSS:A at 0.63.

Also rather shorter than the standard forms is the Stanford Clinical Scale for Adults (Morgan & Hilgard 1978/1979a), which is designed to be more useful in the clinical context. There is also a version of this test for children (Morgan & Hilgard 1978/1979b). Another test of susceptibility for children is the Children's Hypnotic Susceptibility Scale (London 1963).

Rather different from these scales is the Hypnotic Induction Profile (HIP) developed by Herbert and David Spiegel (Spiegel & Spiegel 1987). This has the advantage of being briefer than the Stanford scales and it is itself a hypnotic induction procedure. In fact, the Spiegels and their colleagues use this procedure as their sole method of hypnotic induction and deepening. There are two main parts, an 'eye-roll' induction and an arm levitation routine with a posthypnotic suggestion for this. In the eye-roll test, subjects are asked to roll their eyes up towards their eyebrows and then lower their eyelids over their eyes while maintaining the upward gaze. A score is given for the amount of sclera that is visible between the iris and lower eyelids as the eyes are closing. An extra mark is also given for convergence of the eyes. The Spiegels consider that the eye-roll sign is a biological marker for hypnotic susceptibility. The arm levitation and posthypnotic suggestion yield a range of measures that need not concern us here.

The HIP score does correlate with the score for the Stanford Scales (Forms A and C) but not robustly (Orne et al 1978). In that study, the eye-roll sign alone did not correlate with the scores on Stanford scales. The HIP is grounded on a different theoretical basis and interpretation of hypnosis than the Stanford and Harvard Scales. It is more popular amongst clinicians than academic researchers, but it is by no means universally accepted.

There are a number of other scales but the only additional one that we shall discuss is the Creative Imagination Scale produced by Barber & Wilson (1978). This is based on a non-state interpretation of hypnosis and there is no hypnotic induction provided. Indeed, there is no mention of hypnosis; rather the idea is repeatedly conveyed that by using their imagination, subjects may create for themselves the experiences described as though they were really happening. The scale consists of ten items and, at the end of the test, subjects rate how realistic their response was to each suggestion, using a 5-point scale (0–4). Hence the lowest score for the entire scale is 0 and the highest is 40. This test takes about half-an-hour to administer and score. Because of differences in the composition of the tests, it does not measure exactly the same quality or qualities as the Stanford and Harvard scales (Hilgard 1982, Hilgard et al 1981, McConkey et al 1979). We therefore do not recommend it as a research instrument on hypnotic susceptibility. However, for clinical purposes it is easy to administer and can be used for individuals and groups. It may be modified for use with older children and adolescents (Myers 1983).

In the UK, Fellows (unpublished work, 1986) obtained an average score of around 19.5 for the Creative Imagination Scale (means and standard deviations for males, 18.6 and 6.9 respectively, and for females, 20.7 and 8.1). The sex difference was significant but it should be remembered that the samples were drawn from a student population.

Other scales

We have not included all scales in this discussion and we refer the reader to Council (1999) for a more in-depth account. Scales omitted from our discussion but worth mentioning here are the Barber Suggestibility Scale (Barber & Wilson 1978), relatively brief and based on a non-state interpretation; and the Carleton University Responsiveness to Suggestion Scale (Spanos et al 1983), an instrument mainly, though not exclusively, used for research purposes in the investigation of Spanos's ideas on hypnotic responsiveness (see Ch. 4).

APPLICATIONS OF HYPNOTIC SUSCEPTIBILITY SCALES

Hypnotic susceptibility scales are widely used in clinical and non-clinical research for the purposes of investigating differences between people of varying susceptibility (both in and out of the hypnotic context). Of interest in clinical research is whether higher susceptibility to hypnosis is predictive of a better outcome and, if so, for what kinds of problem. Most of the research suggests that any relationship tends to be weak and this is probably because there are many other factors influencing outcome that do not correlate with susceptibility. Also there are likely to be ingredients in any hypnotherapeutic procedure unrelated to hypnotic susceptibility. Wadden & Anderton (1982) in a review of clinical trials of hypnosis concluded that hypnotic susceptibility was more likely to be a factor in outcome for problems that they termed 'automatic' as opposed to 'self initiated'. The former kinds of problems seem to be those with a significant somatic component such as pain, asthma, skin complaints and possibly other psychosomatic problems. The latter include problems such as smoking and obesity.

These findings do not suggest that a susceptibility scale may be of great use as a screening instrument for determining whether or not to use a hypnotic-based treatment approach for any given problem. There are exceptions to this; for example, in later chapters we shall suggest that some formal assessment of hypnotic responsiveness can be useful in the treatment of pain and possibly psychosomatic problems. Wickramasekera (1993), in the treatment of somatisation disorders, includes a thorough assessment of hypnotic susceptibility in planning the type of treatment strategy adopted. Those who use the Hypnotic Induction Profile claim that it is useful diagnostically in differentiating, for example, psychotic patients from those with dissociative disorders (Spiegel & Greenleaf 1992, Spiegel & Spiegel 1987).

The administering of a scale prior to treatment may give very useful indications of the types of suggestion to which the patient is more likely to respond in treatment. We (Heap et al 1994) have used the Creative Imagination Scale in our work with psychosomatic patients. One impression that we had was that with a patient who scores low on this scale, one has to spend more time customising the kinds of images used in treatment, whereas high scorers may respond well to standard images. The same may be true in pain patients.

A scale such as the Creative Imagination Scale can be a good way of introducing hypnosis to a patient. It is a useful way for the budding practitioner to become experienced at administering suggestions, as it is read from a script. It is also useful for teaching purposes as a practical exercise. One problem with using any scale in clinical practice is that if the patient is not very responsive, then he or she may have less confidence in the therapy and a lowered expectation of success, and this can be a problem in its own right.

In North America, the question of whether one is using hypnosis with a patient or not has assumed more legal significance than elsewhere. For this reason, the matter of whether a patient is of high or low hypnotic susceptibility may prove important if, at some future date, the practitioner is involved in legal issues concerning the patient.

One criticism of all of these scales has been that they do not really measure susceptibility to hypnosis! The rationale of this criticism is that if one wants to measure the person's susceptibility to hypnosis, then the correct procedure would be to assess the person's responsiveness with and without a hypnotic induction. The results would then indicate how profoundly the person responded to the hypnotic induction that is presumed to enhance the person's responsiveness to suggestion (Hilgard 1981, Weitzenhoffer 1980). This research has in fact been done in the laboratory by Kirsch & Braffman (1999). This report indicates that the increase in suggestibility that is effected by a hypnotic induction and deepening routine is actually quite modest, and an appreciable proportion of people had no increase at all.

CORRELATES OF SUSCEPTIBILITY

One of the enigmas of hypnosis is that although people appear to vary widely in their susceptibility, and although susceptibility itself is such a stable characteristic, it does not correlate robustly with any major dimension of personality or cognitive style. One reason for this, as we have already mentioned, may be that there are a number of reasons why a person is highly responsive to hypnotic procedures, so that two people may obtain the same high score for different reasons.

Some traditional ideas

Traditionally, it is considered that people who tend to be logical, scientific and reality-oriented tend to be lower than average in susceptibility, whereas those who are intuitive, creative and artistic tend to be higher in susceptibility. However, one constantly comes across glaring exceptions to the prediction.

Age

Hypnotic susceptibility peaks between the years of 9 and 13 and shows a very slow decline thereafter (Gardner & Olness 1981).

Sex

By and large, there is no significant major difference between the sexes in terms of their hypnotic susceptibility. However, when differences have been found, albeit marginal in magnitude, the trend is for females to be more responsive (De Pascalis et al 2000; see Gibson & Heap 1991, p 42–44, for a further discussion of this).

Expectation

Two definite predictors of susceptibility are known to be, first, a positive attitude to hypnosis and, second, the expectation that one is a responsive subject (Kirsch & Braffman 1999, Spanos 1991). Related to this is the observation that people who have anxieties about 'losing control' and therefore find it difficult to 'go with the flow' while attending to hypnotic suggestions, tend, on balance, to be less responsive (Barber 1999).

Absorption

People who habitually find that they can become easily engrossed in a daydream, a book, a piece of music, and so on, to the exclusion of whatever is going on around them, also tend to score higher on susceptibility scales. We have noted in the last chapter that this characteristic is known as 'absorption'. We have, however, also noted that the relationship is not a strong one, indicating that absorption is by no means a key defining property of hypnosis.

Fantasy proneness

Related to the previous attribute is a characteristic known as 'fantasy proneness'. This refers to the extent that a person develops a fantasy life separate from the reality of the person's existence. Some people do this to a remarkable degree, Walter Mitty and Billy Liar being two fictitious caricatures. People with this tendency may appear to be, say, mixing and interacting with a group of people yet their private experience is that of engaging in some kind of elaborate fantasy, far removed from what is going on around them. By no means is this a pathological trait, although it can, of course, give rise to problems. Such a person may be immensely creative – for example, a great writer of stories. However, there is evidence that some people develop this characteristic as a way of coping with extremely harsh and brutal circumstances in their childhood. More positively, a person may do this through the encouragement of parents – for example, in writing stories or playing creatively (Rhue & Lynn 1987, 1989).

Vividness of imagery

It might be thought that people with particularly good visual imagery would be high scorers on susceptibility scales. The relationship between the ability to produce vivid imagery and hypnotisability is, however, rather weak and not very reliable (de Groh 1989), although there is some indication that people with no capacity at all for visual imagery tend to make poor subjects. This finding can be understood by bearing in mind that hypnosis is not just imagining the situations described by the hypnotist; the subject must *interact* with those images. So, it is not uncommon to have a subject who says something like, 'Well, I got a vivid image of a bucket of ice and water, but I couldn't feel any numbness at all', whereas another subject might say, 'When you said, "Think of a bucket of ice and water", I could not see that very clearly, but when you said, "Put your hand in the bucket", it felt cold right away'.

Dissociative ability

'Dissociation' is a rather ill-defined concept that has become more diffuse and amorphous the more it has been required to do and explain. When we dissociate, we displace from conscious awareness experience that would normally be available to consciousness.

The concept of dissociation was originally a clinical or psychopathological concept introduced by Pierre Janet (see Ch. 1) in his accounts of hysterical disorders and hypnotic phenomena. However, it may be extended to cover more everyday phenomena; an example is the highway trance that was discussed earlier.

People with good dissociative capacity may, for example, have the ability to displace from consciousness their awareness of a painful stimulus or some other ongoing stimulation, yet still respond to it in some way. More pathological instances of dissociation include feelings of depersonalisation and unreality and, in extreme cases, fugue states in which people are amnesic of their identity and personal circumstances. We shall see in the chapter on theories of hypnosis that Hilgard (1986) developed a theory based on the broader concept of dissociation, as have Woody & Bowers (1994).

Dissociative capacity can be measured by a questionnaire called the Dissociative Experiences Scale (Bernstein & Putnam 1986). Scores on this correlate positively but rather marginally with hypnotic susceptibility (Frischholz et al 1992), although Spanos & Burgess (1994) consider that this may be due to expectation on the subject's part. Whatever the case, it does not appear that highly susceptible subjects are necessarily always high on dissociative capacity (see also Barber 1999).

Cognitive flexibility

There is an attribute termed 'cognitive flexibility' which is the ability to switch from one mental activity or state of mind to another with ease.

Evans (1991) has summarised evidence that this is positively related to hypnotic susceptibility. Cognitive flexibility is thought to be related to 'sleep control' (Evans 1991). People with good sleep control fall asleep easily and are able to take a nap anywhere where it is convenient. They can also take a nap when they are not sleepy, in anticipation of their having to remain awake for a longer than usual period. They tend to be more susceptible to hypnosis (Evans 1991).

Clinical correlates

In terms of clinical conditions, there is disputed evidence (Spanos & Burgess 1994) that patients with dissociative disorders are higher than average in hypnotic susceptibility (Bliss 1986). Patients with eating disorders who control their weight by purging and vomiting are higher than average in susceptibility in contrast to those who do so by severe dietary restraint (Pettanati et al 1990). There is some evidence, although this has not been consistent, that people with anxiety disorders such as phobias are also higher than average in their susceptibility (see Evans 1991). Patients with post-traumatic stress disorder are suspected of being more susceptible than average (Cardeña 2000), while those with obsessive–compulsive disorder tend to have lower than average scores, even when successfully treated (Hoogduin & de Jong 1986). The findings on patients with psychotic disorders are somewhat mixed and probably depend on the mental state of the patient (see Evans 1991).

TYPES OF SUGGESTIBILITY

There is an unfortunate tendency in some of the hypnosis literature to fail to acknowledge that there are different types of suggestibility and that not all are related to hypnotic responsiveness. Even Waxman (1989) in the previous edition of this book falls into this trap by defining suggestibility as 'the degree to which an individual is inclined towards the uncritical acceptance of ideas and propositions' (p 20). This may be true but it is not a statement about hypnotic suggestibility.

In a study in 1945, Eysenck & Furneaux distinguished between primary and secondary suggestibility. Primary suggestibility is typified by ideomotor responses and is related to measured hypnotic susceptibility. Secondary suggestibility is more complex and concerned with direct or implied changes in sensory modalities and has been linked to ease of persuasion and gullibility. It is unrelated to hypnotic responsiveness.

Gudjonsson (1992) has identified a trait known as 'interrogative suggestibility'. This is the extent to which individuals are prone to change their account of events as a result of interrogative pressures such as leading questions and adverse feedback. In such circumstances, some individuals actually come to believe the (false) account of events that the interrogators are insisting is the truth, with disastrous consequences when the interrogators are police officers investigating a crime. Interrogative suggestibility is not related to hypnotic susceptibility (Register & Kihlstrom 1988). Gudjonsson (1992) also identifies 'compliant' interviewees who are eager to please their interrogators and wish to avoid conflict. Thus they may *knowingly* make false statements that comply with the demands of their interrogators. Again, compliance is generally not regarded as typical of hypnotic responding, although Wagstaff (1981, 1991) considers it to be an essential feature.

Finally, we must not forget the placebo effect. This is associated with the expectation of physiological and experiential changes, usually contingent on the administration of a supposed remedy for a complaint that is known in fact to have no actual properties to cause such changes. We must not overlook subjects' needs for alleviation of their symptoms when considering the mode of action of a placebo.

POSTSCRIPT

In this and the previous chapter, we have studied three pivotal aspects of hypnosis, namely suggestion, trance, and suggestibility or hypnotic susceptibility. Chapters 6 and 7 will be devoted in detail to the fourth component, namely the hypnotic induction.

REFERENCES

Barber T X 1999 A comprehensive three-dimensional theory of hypnosis. In: Kirsch I, Capafons A, Cardeña-Buelna E, Amigó S (eds) Clinical hypnosis and self-regulation: Cognitive-behavioral perspectives. American Psychological Association, Washington DC, ch 1, p 21

Barber T X, Wilson S C 1978 The Barber Suggestibility Scale and the Creative Imagination Scale: Experimental and clinical applications. American Journal of Clinical Hypnosis 21: 84–108

Bernstein E, Putnam F W 1986 Development, reliability, and validity of a dissociation scale. Journal of Nervous and Mental Diseases 174: 727–734

Bliss E L 1986 Multiple personality disorder, allied disorders and hypnosis. Oxford University Press, New York

Bowers K S 1998 Waterloo–Stanford Group Scale of Hypnotic Susceptibility, Form C: Manual and response booklet. International Journal of Clinical and Experimental Hypnosis 46: 250–268

Cardeña E 2000 Hypnosis in the treatment of trauma. International Journal of Clinical and Experimental Hypnosis 48:225–238

Council J R 1999 Measures of hypnotic responding. In: Kirsch I, Capafons A, Cardeña-Buelna E, Amigó S (eds) Clinical hypnosis and self-regulation: Cognitive-behavioral perspectives. American Psychological Association, Washington DC, ch 5, p 119

de Groh M 1989 Correlates of hypnotic susceptibility. In: Spanos N P, Chaves J F (eds) Hypnosis: The cognitive behavioral perspective. Prometheus Books, Buffalo, ch 2, p 32

De Pascalis V, Russo P, Marucci F S 2000 Italian norms for the Harvard Group Scale of Hypnotic Susceptibility. International Journal of Clinical and Experimental Hypnosis 48: 44–55

Evans F J 1991 Hypnotisability: Individual differences in dissociation and the flexible control of psychological processes. In: Lynn S J, Rhue J W (eds) Theories of hypnosis: Current models and perspectives. Guilford Press, New York, ch 5, p 144

Eysenck H J, Furneaux W D 1945 Primary and secondary suggestibility: An experimental and statistical study. Journal of Experimental Psychology 35: 485–503

Frischholz E J, Braun B G, Sachs R G et al 1992 Construct validity of the Dissociative Experiences Scale: II. Its relationship with hypnotisability. American Journal of Clinical Hypnosis 35: 145–152

Gardner G G, Olness K 1981 Hypnosis and hypnotherapy with children. Grune and Stratton, New York

Gibson H B, Heap M 1991 Hypnosis in therapy. Erlbaum, Chichester

Gudjonsson G H 1992 The psychology of interrogations, confessions and testimony. Wiley, Chichester

Heap M, Aravind K K, Power-Smith P 1994 A psychosomatic research clinic. Hypnos: Swedish Journal of Hypnosis in Psychotherapy and Psychosomatic Medicine 21: 171–175

Hilgard E R 1981 Hypnotic susceptibility scales under attack: An examination of Weitzenhoffer's criticisms. International Journal of Clinical and Experimental Hypnosis 22: 258–259

Hilgard E R 1982 Hypnotic susceptibility and implications for measurement. International Journal of Clinical and Experimental Hypnosis 30: 394–403

Hilgard E R 1986 Divided consciousness: Multiple controls in human thought and action (expanded edition). Wiley, New York

Hilgard E R, Crawford H, Wert A 1979 The Stanford Hypnotic Arm Levitation and Induction Test: (SHALIT): A six-minute hypnotic induction and measurement scale. International Journal of Clinical and Experimental Hypnosis 27: 111–124

Hilgard E R, Sheehan P W, Monteiro K P et al 1981 Factorial structure of the Creative Imagination Scale as a measure of hypnotic responsiveness: An international comparative study. International Journal of Clinical and Experimental Hypnosis 29: 66–76

Hoogduin C A L, de Jong P 1986 Hypnosis and hypnotisability in obsessive–compulsive disorders. Hypnos: Swedish Journal for Hypnosis in Psychotherapy and Psychosomatic Disorders 13: 3–7

Kirsch I, Braffman W 1999 Correlates of hypnotisability: The first empirical study. Contemporary Hypnosis 16: 224–230

Kumar V K, Pekala R J, McCloskey M 1999 Phenomenological state effects during hypnosis: A cross-validation of findings. Contemporary Hypnosis 16: 9–21

London P 1963 Children's Hypnotic Susceptibility Scale. Consulting Psychologists Press, Palo Alto

McConkey K M, Sheehan P W, White K D 1979 Comparison of the Creative Imagination Scale and the Harvard Group Scale of Hypnotic Susceptibility, Form A. International Journal of Clinical and Experimental Hypnosis 27: 265–277

Morgan A H 1973 The heritability of hypnotic susceptibility in twins. Journal of Abnormal Psychology 82: 55–61

Morgan A H, Hilgard E R 1978/1979a The Stanford Hypnotic Clinical Scale for Adults. American Journal of Clinical Hypnosis 21: 134–147

Morgan A H, Hilgard E R 1978/1979b The Stanford Hypnotic Clinical Scale for Children. American Journal of Clinical Hypnosis 21: 148–155

Myers S A 1983 The Creative Imagination Scale: Group norms for children and adolescents. International Journal of Clinical and Experimental Hypnosis 31: 28–36

Orne M T, Hilgard E R, Spiegel H et al 1978 The relation between the Hypnotic Induction Profile and the Stanford Hypnotic Susceptibility Scales, Forms A and C. International Journal of Clinical and Experimental Hypnosis 27: 85–102

Pekala R J 1991 Hypnotic types: Evidence of a cluster analysis of phenomenal experience. Contemporary Hypnosis 8: 95–104

Pekala R J, Kumar V K, Marcano G 1995 Hypnotic types: A partial replication concerning phenomenal experience. Contemporary Hypnosis 12: 194–200

Pettanati H M, Horne L R, Staats J S 1990 Hypnotisability in patients with anorexia and bulimia. Archives of General Psychiatry 147: 1014–1016

Piccione C, Hilgard E R, Zimbardo P G 1989 On the degree of stability of measured hypnotizability over a 25-year period. Journal of Personality and Social Psychology 56: 289–295

Register P A, Kihlstrom J F 1988 Hypnosis and interrogative suggestibility. Personality and Individual Differences 9: 549–558

Rhue J W, Lynn S J 1987 Fantasy proneness: The ability to hallucinate 'as real as real'. British Journal of Experimental and Clinical Hypnosis 4: 173–180

Rhue J W, Lynn S J 1989 Fantasy proneness, hypnotisability and absorption: A re-examination. International Journal of Clinical and Experimental Hypnosis 37: 100–106

Shor R E, Orne E C 1962 Harvard Group Scale of Hypnotic Susceptibility Scale: Forms A. Consulting Psychologists Press, Palo Alto

Spanos N 1991 A sociocognitive approach to hypnosis. In: Lynn S J, Rhue J W (eds) Theories of hypnosis: Current models and perspectives. Guilford Press, New York, ch 11, p 324

Spanos N P, Burgess C 1994 Hypnosis and multiple personality disorder. In: Lynn S J, Rhue J W (eds) Dissociation: Clinical and theoretical perspectives. Guilford Press, New York, ch 7, p 136

Spanos N, Radke H L, Hodgins D C et al 1983 The Carleton University Responsiveness to Suggestion Scale: Normative data and psychometric properties. Psychological Reports 53: 555–563

Spiegel H S, Greenleaf M 1992 Personality style and hypnotizability: The fix-flex continuum. Psychiatric Medicine 10: 13–24

Spiegel H S, Spiegel D 1987 Trance and treatment. Basic Books, New York

Wadden T A, Anderton C H 1982 The clinical use of hypnosis. Psychological Bulletin 91: 215–243

Wagstaff G F 1981 Hypnosis, compliance and belief. Harvester Press, Brighton

Wagstaff G F 1991 Compliance, belief, and semantics. In: Lynn S J, Rhue J W (eds) Theories of hypnosis: Current models and perspectives. Guilford Press, New York, ch 12, p 362

Waxman D 1989 Hartland's medical and dental hypnosis. Baillière Tindall, London

Weitzenhoffer A M 1980 Hypnotic susceptibility revisited. American Journal of Clinical Hypnosis 22: 130–146

Weitzenhoffer A M, Hilgard E R 1959 Stanford Hypnotic Susceptibility Scale: Forms A and B. Consulting Psychologists Press, Palo Alto

Weitzenhoffer A M, Hilgard E R 1962 Stanford Hypnotic Susceptibility Scale: Form C (SHSS: C). Consulting Psychologists Press, Palo Alto

Wickramasekera I 1993 Assessment and treatment of somatisation disorders: The high risk model of threat perception. In: Rhue J W, Lynn S J, Kirsch I (eds) Handbook of clinical hypnosis. American Psychological Association, Washington DC, ch 27, p 587

Woody E Z, Bowers K S 1994 A frontal assault on dissociative control. In: Lynn S J, Rhue J W (eds) Dissociation: Clinical and theoretical perspectives. Guilford Press, New York, ch 3, p 52

4

Theories of hypnosis

INTRODUCTION

In this chapter, we shall not attempt a review of all the major theories of hypnosis. We shall focus on the division between theories that postulate special or unique mechanisms to account for hypnotic phenomena, and those that offer explanations in terms of cognitive and social psychological factors that are common to non-hypnotic contexts. We shall not present an historical review although we have noted in Chapter 1 how certain historical figures in the field endeavoured to understand the processes underlying hypnosis.

It is also worth mentioning here that the great Russian physiologist Ivan Pavlov developed a theory of hypnosis in animals, the principal underlying mechanism being inhibition of cortical and then subcortical activity. This is summarised in a book by the American psychologist William Edmonston (1981). A modern approach to understanding hypnosis that has been influenced by Pavlov's ideas is that described by Edmonston in his book (and in Edmonston 1991). He has postulated that 'neutral hypnosis' (hypnosis limited to a standard induction and deepening routine) is equivalent to relaxation and that phenomena that are labelled 'hypnotic' are merely facilitated by relaxation. Edmonston proposed that we use the word 'anesis' as a more appropriate term, but this has not proved a popular idea and the theory has not generated much research activity.

In the 1960s in the UK, the physician Barry Wyke (1957, 1960) put forward a neurophysiological theory not dissimilar to Pavlov's and based on the activity of the reticular activating system, a neural network that regulates arousal and wakefulness. This was influential amongst a number of medical doctors in the UK, but there appears to have been little interest beyond that.

WHAT SHOULD A THEORY EXPLAIN?

Before examining some modern psychological theories, it ought to be asked what should be the purpose of any theory of hypnosis. It appears that the answer to this has something to do with accounting for what some term 'counter-expectational observations'. However, as the expectations of the hypnotic subjects themselves are an important factor, we shall avoid the ambiguity of this term by speaking of 'out-of-the-ordinary' observations. A theory of hypnosis should also explain individual differences in hypnotic susceptibility and any correlations between hypnotic susceptibility and other personality factors and dimensions of cognitive style. Let us first, however, explore what we mean by 'out-of-the-ordinary observations'.

When we observe the behaviour of hypnotic subjects and hear their accounts of what they experience, we only seek an explanation when what we have observed or heard from the subject is out of the ordinary, that is, when it is different from what one normally observes out of the hypnotic context. For example, suppose a hypnotic subject moves an arm in response to an arm levitation suggestion. Normally when people are thinking about their arm and it moves upwards, they report that they are doing this voluntarily, with conscious effort. So, if hypnotic subjects simply report that they moved the arm voluntarily, then no special explanation is required. However, if the subject reports that the arm lifted automatically, without the subject consciously moving it, then an explanation is called for.

We can argue likewise when, to the appropriate suggestions, subjects appear to be less sensitive to pain; to be unable to open their eyes, move their arm, or utter their name; be unable to recall something that they have just heard; report extremely vivid experiences when they are asked to imagine being a child again; believe that somebody is standing in front of them when such is not the case; report that they are unable to see something that is in front of them; are unable to hear a sound, such as their own voice; and carry out an instruction, given some time previously, in an apparently automatic and compulsive manner.

SPECIAL-STATE OR SPECIAL-PROCESS THEORIES

Although we require explanations for all of these observations, it does not immediately follow that we need special processes or mechanisms that are different from those we use to explain observations that are not 'out of the ordinary'. However, special-state or special-process theories do just this by hypothesising that when people are subjected to a hypnotic induction, they are in some special state of consciousness, different from the ordinary 'waking' state, and which we may call the 'hypnotic trance'. The properties of the trance are such as to explain all of the above phenomena.

In Chapter 2, we listed several other known altered states of consciousness, namely sleep, alcoholic intoxication, epilepsy and concussion. We said that each of these states is associated with certain reliably observed behaviours and experiences on the person's part and it is commonplace to explain these by saying that they occur because the person is in a state of sleep, in a state of intoxication, in a state of concussion, and so on. Of course we still have to investigate what actually constitutes the state in question in order eventually to fully explain what we are observing. Therefore, it is important to investigate the nature of this state of hypnotic trance before we can fully explain the subject's responses and experiences.

The theory of dissociated control

The modern theory that possibly corresponds most with the 'state' or 'special process' approach to hypnosis is a relative newcomer, namely the 'dissociated control' model associated with Erik Woody and the late Kenneth Bowers of the University of Waterloo, Ontario. This approach (Woody & Bowers 1994) has the advantage of being based on an existing neuropsychological model of the voluntary and involuntary regulation of behaviour, created by Norman & Shallice (1986). This model envisages two systems that regulate everyday behaviour. The lower-level, 'decentralised' system consists of units or schemas that govern particular actions. When a schema is activated at a certain threshold, the corresponding action is executed. Schemas are activated or inhibited by other schemas or by environmental triggers. This process is termed 'contention scheduling' and for well-learned habits this proceeds automatically with little centralised control.

Often we have to execute a complex or unfamiliar sequence of actions, or sometimes strong habitual tendencies need to be inhibited. For instance, with a well-learned activity such as driving a car we can rely a great deal on contention scheduling. However, sometimes the activity has to be executed in a different way – for example, when driving the car on the side of the road opposite to that which is customary. Relying on contention scheduling here would have disastrous consequences. Now, a higher-level system, known as the 'supervisory attention system', is able to intervene in order to control the activation of the schemas, biasing the distribution of activation according to the requirements of the task. This constitutes the basis of willed, as opposed to automatic, action.

Woody & Bowers (1994) postulate that hypnosis disengages the supervisory system from its influence on the lower-level system, and the behaviour and experiences of the hypnotised subject are more automatically triggered by the hypnotist's suggestions.

According to Norman & Shallice (1986), the supervisory system is a function of the frontal lobe. Damage to the frontal lobe will interfere with this function and is associated with problems in the planning and regulation of behaviour and in the inhibition of automatic responses. Hence, a hypnotised subject behaves like a patient with frontal lobe damage, responding in a genuine automatic and involuntary manner to the suggestions and instructions of the hypnotist.

In support of this is some neurophysiological and neuropsychological evidence consistent with the idea that during hypnosis, in highly susceptible subjects, the activity of the frontal lobe, notably on the left side, is attenuated (see Gruzelier 2000 for a summary of this). A problem for this theory, however, is explaining self-hypnosis and self-suggestion and it fails to account for a range of observations that will be shortly described.

Neo-dissociation theory

Woody & Bowers (1994) contrast their dissociated control model of hypnosis with the neo-dissociation model of Ernest Hilgard (1986). Hilgard adopted a broader definition of dissociation than Janet (see Ch. 1), one that underlies a whole range of everyday phenomena. Unlike the theory of dissociated control, Hilgard's model assumes that the actions of the hypnotised subject are controlled in the normal way; it is the subject's *awareness* of this that is dissociated.

Let us first give further consideration to the regulation of behaviour. Imagine that you are driving to a meeting at which you will be expected to give a presentation. Unfortunately you have not yet prepared what you are going to say and you are spending much of the time rehearsing this in your mind. At the same time, you are having to execute a perceptual–motor skill of the highest order, namely drive your car. Somehow you manage to focus on the cognitive rehearsal of your talk sufficiently, even though you also successfully operate the car and negotiate the traffic. Indeed, you are doing this so well that you cannot even recall certain parts of your journey. Suppose, moreover, you are giving a lift to a colleague who insists on telling you about his holiday. Somehow you are managing to process the information he is giving you sufficiently to be able to make the right sorts of comments, such as 'How nice!' when he tells you how friendly the people were and, 'Oh dear!' when he tells you that his wife fell over and hurt her knee. While all this is going on, from time to time you notice you have a headache, while, at other times, although the headache does not exactly disappear, you somehow 'forget it'.

We can imagine that all this is possible because there is a part of your mind that controls what requires your attention at any particular time and yet this does not mean that all the other activities that you engage in have to stop. Like Hilgard, we can call this part of your mind the 'executive ego' and all the other units of activity 'cognitive control structures'.

Now, the executive ego is limited in the priority it is able to assign to any particular activity. In the example of your driving to the meeting, there may be parts of your journey that are unfamiliar to you, or the driving conditions become very difficult, and it is impossible for you not to give your attentional priority to your driving and ignore the other activities mentioned. Thus, Hilgard talks about 'constraints on ego autonomy'.

To simplify his theory, hypnosis and hypnotic suggestions are ways in which the hypnotist can influence the subject's executive ego in the assignment of attentional priority to various activities and experiences. Thus, through hypnosis, experiences and activities that would normally be represented in consciousness may become dissociated from awareness. Hilgard uses the concept of 'amnesic barrier' to describe the mechanism whereby this is achieved. Amnesic barriers have the quality of permeability so that some processes, experiences or activities may be considered to be highly autonomous, separated from the rest of the system by an impermeable amnesic barrier. Others are considerably less so.

This account of dissociated cognitive control structures that are separated by amnesic barriers of varying permeability forms the basis of a psychodynamic model of personality structure that has been very influential in the field of hypnosis. The idea of 'parts' of a personality or 'ego states', will be discussed in Chapter 16.

The hidden observer

The most famous laboratory demonstrations of Hilgard's neo-dissociation theory involved the elicitation of profound analgesia in highly susceptible subjects (Hilgard et al 1975). Subjects are required to keep their hand in a bucket of ice-cold water and rate the degree of pain experienced on a scale from, say, 0 to 10. Without suggestions of analgesia, the ratings, given orally, are towards the upper end of the scale. In response to suggestions of analgesia, these ratings may come down to the lower end of the scale. In accordance with the neo-dissociation model, the experimenter then suggests that there is a hidden, 'unhypnotised' part of the person that is still experiencing the pain in the usual manner. This 'hidden observer' is asked to rate the pain experienced on the 0–10 scale in writing, using the free hand. Typically, these ratings correspond to the pain ratings given without suggestions of analgesia but still during hypnosis. These experiments have been repeated using suggested deafness (Crawford et al 1979).

Some writers, for reasons that we will see later, consider that the hidden observer effect is an artefact created by the experimenter, with the subject duly complying. Other people have taken it more seriously. For example, Watkins & Watkins (1990) consider that when hypnosis is used for pain relief, and indeed when patients undergo any analgesic procedure, there is a hidden part that is feeling the pain that would normally be present at a conscious level. Watkins & Watkins (1990) consider that this is not without adverse consequences for the patient. In the present authors' opinion, however, this is an example of an idea taken beyond its useful sphere of application. Indeed, it is not clear where the hidden observer effect fits in the alleviation of clinical pain through hypnosis (see Ch. 26).

It is worth mentioning here the work of the late Professor Martin Orne at Harvard University. Like Hilgard, Orne has been one of the commanding figures in the field of modern hypnosis. Although it seems that he tended to adopt a state orientation, he nevertheless conducted some influential research on the role of contextual demands and social pressures in hypnotic phenomena. Orne (1959, 1962) considered that there were observable differences between the behaviour of susceptible subjects during hypnosis and those instructed to simulate hypnosis. The differences hinge on a concept that he termed 'trance logic'. For example, he demonstrated that genuine hypnotic subjects, when asked to hallucinate a person sitting in a chair in front of them, would also describe objects that would ordinarily be obscured by the person's body. This is of course illogical. Simulators tended to deny being able to see the objects because the hallucinated person was in the way. Orne also reported that true hypnotic subjects, as they traversed the room, avoided colliding with a chair for which they had been given a negative hallucination suggestion. Simulators tended to bump into the chair, as one would logically expect. In another demonstration of trance logic, Orne (1972) regressed a student to a time when he was unable to speak English. Orne conversed with him in his native tongue (German) and then suddenly asked him 'Do you speak English?' Variations of this question were given and each time the student replied 'Nein'. Again this is illogical. (This effect can also be demonstrated by regressing subjects to their early years and asking them questions in a vocabulary that they would not at that time understand; they still tend to respond to the questions.)

'Trance logic' is the ability to hold two contradictory beliefs or pieces of information in mind without experiencing the usual sense of conflict, and this may be understood in dissociative terms. Needless to say this concept has its detractors. For example, in the positive hallucination test, it may simply be that hypnotic subjects create a transparent image of the person.

Although it may be debated whether the neo-dissociation theory is actually positing a 'special state', Hilgard is clear that some important change is happening when a person is subjected to a traditional hypnotic induction. He says:

Looked at in other ways, we find that hypnotic procedures are designed to produce a readiness for dissociative experiences by disrupting the ordinary continuities of memories and by distorting or concealing reality orientation through the power that words exert by direct suggestion, through selective attention or inattention and through stimulating the imagination appropriately.

(Hilgard 1986, p 226)

PROBLEMS WITH SPECIAL-STATE THEORIES

The major theoretical controversy in the field of hypnosis over the last 50 years has been whether special processes (such as, although not exclusively, a trance state) are required to explain hypnotic phenomena, notably the kind of out-of-the-ordinary observations listed earlier.

A longstanding criticism of the 'special-state' way of understanding hypnosis runs as follows. Suppose we say 'John is slurring his speech because he is in a state of intoxication', or 'Mary is not responding to us because she is in a state of sleep'. We can answer the questions 'How do you know that John is intoxicated?' and 'How do you know that Mary is asleep?' by reference to some defining property of the state in question that is independent from the observations we have made. That is, we can say that John is slurring his speech because he is intoxicated and we know that he is intoxicated because we have just done a breathalyser or blood test. Likewise we can say that Mary is not responding to us because she is asleep and we know that she is asleep because we have tested this by observing her EEG.

Unfortunately, we cannot do this with our explanation that a subject's behaviour and experiences occur because the subject is in a hypnotic trance. We cannot test our explanation by referring to some independent objective marker that reliably indicates that a trance state is present. It is true that, particularly in recent years, neurophysiological correlates of responses to specific hypnotic suggestions have been identified in certain highly responsive subjects and these differ from those observed in subjects of low susceptibility. However, there is no known physiological marker that identifies the 'state of hypnosis' across the range of out-of-the-ordinary phenomena such as is provided by the examples given earlier. However, this is not to say that one day an objective marker that distinguishes the 'hypnotised' from the 'non-hypnotised' subject will not be found.

In Chapter 1, we referred to an important principle that underlies rational thinking and the scientific method, namely Occam's razor. This states that we should try to explain things in terms of what we already know and understand, before we resort to hypothesising the existence of special entities, forces, energies, and so on. The implication of this is that those who do invent a special construct to explain a set of phenomena are the ones on whose shoulders the burden of evidence rests in demonstrating that such an entity exists or is required to exist by the available evidence.

In fact, in contradiction to this, it is not unusual for much scientific enquiry to be invested in attempting to refute the existence of some hypothesised construct or entity. In Chapter 1, we saw how the Royal Commissioners investigated Mesmer's practices and concluded that there was no evidence to support the existence of animal magnetism.

NON-STATE OR SOCIAL AND COGNITIVE THEORIES OF HYPNOSIS

Over the last 50 years, an increasing number of investigators have come to acknowledge the central importance of normal psychological processes in accounting for the behaviour and experiences of the hypnotic subject. Indeed, many respected authorities go so far as to assert that the only unusual characteristics of hypnosis are the expectations and beliefs held by both the hypnotist and the subject.

Nobody, in fact, would seriously contest that everyday psychological processes are involved in responding to hypnotic procedures. Clearly one ingredient is selective and sustained attention, and, as we previously noted, absorption. At least with regard to neutral hypnosis, mental and physical relaxation is normally a major feature. Also, much of hypnosis requires subjects to deploy their imagination. Indeed, one of the major figures in the 'non-state' approach to hypnosis over the last half-century, the American psychologist T. X. Barber, made imagination (or the ability to fantasise realistically) one of the central features of his understanding of hypnosis (see Barber et al 1974). In support of this is the higher-than-average hypnotisability of individuals who have a propensity for vivid fantasy (see Ch. 3). Also, Barber and his colleagues (see Ch. 7) demonstrated the equivalence of 'task-motivating' instructions to traditional trance-inducing procedures in enhancing suggestibility.

Another ingredient of hypnosis is expectancy. The hypnotist creates the expectancy in subjects that they will have certain experiences and responses and, in a motivated subject, some would assert that this is sufficient for those experiences to occur. Although others would argue that expectancy effects are only a by-product of hypnosis, at least one authority, Irving Kirsch, a psychologist at the University of Connecticut, considers that response expectancy is the essence of hypnosis (Kirsch 1991). He and others have demonstrated experimentally how responsiveness to hypnotic suggestion can be modified by manipulating expectancy on the subject's part.

In these accounts of hypnosis, therefore, no special processes are required to explain the observed phenomena. But how does one account for the out-of-the-ordinary effects of hypnosis outlined earlier? All of these appear to be radically different from one's everyday experience.

Compliance

If readers examine again the list of out-of-the-ordinary phenomena, one important consideration may present itself. The authenticity of each one relies on one crucial condition, namely that the subjects' behaviour and verbal accounts accurately represent their private experience. For example, if subjects say they cannot see something in front of them, then it is assumed that they are being truthful, likewise if they say they cannot remember something they have just been told. Similarly, if subjects do not show evidence of discomfort when a painful stimulus is applied, we assume that it is because they are not in pain, not that they are consciously suppressing the reaction.

Now, one characteristic of good hypnotic subjects that experts are agreed on is that they are very vigilant and sensitive to whatever the hypnotist is expecting of them. Therefore, how can we be sure that the subject is not just being compliant? 'Compliant' here means that subjects give the overt response that the hypnotist appears to be expecting, but this conflicts with their subjective experience.

The answer is that it is very difficult to tell. Indeed, this fact is exploited in experiments on hypnosis that require non-hypnotised control subjects to be placed under the same demands as the hypnotised subjects. These 'simulators', as they are called, are instructed to do their best to fool the experimenter, so that the experimenter cannot detect that they are not hypnotised. Setting aside Orne's experiments described above, invariably they succeed.

The obvious answer to our earlier question would seem to be that simulators know that they are simply complying and genuine hypnotic subjects know that they are really experiencing the suggested effects. Hence, all one has to do to find out who is who is to ask them. Unfortunately, this is not as simple as it seems. Let us explore why this is so.

Probably for all non-state theorists, it is not possible to explain hypnotic phenomena without reference to the subject's efforts to satisfy the demands and expectations that are created by the hypnotic context, that is the situation in which it is conducted and the actions and communications of the hypnotist. Indeed, it needs always to be acknowledged that in most contexts in which hypnotic subjects find themselves – the laboratory, the clinic, in front of an audience, in a forensic interview – there are social forces independent of hypnosis that exert a powerful influence on the individual's behaviour. Hence, there will be a marked tendency for people in such situations not only to be coerced into doing whatever is required of them, but also to exhibit compliance, that is to engage in deception, in order to meet the contextual demands.

At least one theorist, the British psychologist Graham Wagstaff at the University of Liverpool considers that compliance is a major component of hypnotic responding (Wagstaff 1981, 1991). Coming from the standpoint of role theory, two American psychologists, Theodore Sarbin and William Coe (Coe & Sarbin 1991, Sarbin & Coe 1972) have come to a similar conclusion. For them, hypnotic subjects, to a greater or lesser degree, are so motivated to play the role of the good hypnotic subject that they will, where necessary, engage in deception to comply with that role.

What evidence informs us that these explanations require serious consideration? First, consider this experiment. Highly hypnotisable subjects were each given the suggestion that they were selectively deaf to their own voice. Those subjects who indicated that they could not hear their voice were asked to speak under a condition called delayed authority feedback (DAF) where the subject's voice is played back to the subject over earphones with a slight delay. It is very difficult to speak normally under such conditions; voice pitch and volume rise and speech become dysfluent. What happened in the case of those subjects who responded positively to the selective deafness suggestion? DAF had the usual effects on their speech (Barber & Calverley 1964, Scheibe et al 1968).

Now consider these experiments. Highly hypnotisable subjects responded positively to the suggestion of posthypnotic amnesia for some material presented during hypnosis. The suggestion had specified that the amnesia would immediately lift when the hypnotist gave a certain signal, but instead of giving the signal, the experimenters put increasing pressure on the subjects to be honest. One procedure involved connecting subjects to a 'lie detector'; in another condition, 'amnesic' subjects were informed that good hypnotic subjects would, in fact, be able to recall the material at that stage. What happened? Nearly all subjects exposed to such pressures breached their amnesia, whereas those who were not, did not do so (Coe & Sluis 1989, Coe & Yashinski 1985, Howard & Coe 1980).

Now consider this interesting experiment. After testing, 15 out of 45 highly hypnotisable subjects professed that they saw nothing on a piece of paper on which was clearly written the number '8'. They had all previously been given the hypnotic suggestion that on opening their eyes they would see a piece of paper that was entirely blank. Here is a striking demonstration of a negative hallucination. However, the 15 subjects were then interviewed by a different experimenter who asked them to draw what they had seen. Before they did so, she informed them that people who are faking hypnosis always say that they see nothing, whereas genuine hypnotic subjects initially see something written on the paper which then fades from view. What happened next? Fourteen of the 15 subjects drew the number '8' (Spanos et al 1989).

Finally, consider this experiment. A group of highly hypnotisable subjects were informed, in the manner of Hilgard's hidden observer paradigm, that a hidden part of them was experiencing the actual pain as they were responding to suggestions of analgesia. As in Hilgard et al (1975), the hidden observer responded with realistic ratings of the level of pain, in contrast to the low levels reported overtly by the subjects. In another condition, subjects were again told that they possessed a hidden observer, but were not informed of the level of pain that it was supposed to experience. Finally, in a third condition, subjects were told that the hidden observer experienced even less pain than the 'hypnotised part' during the hypnoanalgesia test. What were the ratings of the hidden observer in the second and third conditions?

The answers are that in the second condition the hidden observer's pain ratings did not differ from the rating of the 'hypnotised part', and in the third condition they were lower than those ratings (Spanos & Hewitt 1980, Spanos et al 1983).

What are these experiments telling us? One interpretation could be that individuals who are reported to be highly hypnotisable are complying, or less charitably, faking, in order to keep up the pretence of being a deeply hypnotised person.

Strategic enactment

The foregoing is a selective and deliberately one-sided account of certain experimental work that challenges some basic assumptions about hypnosis that often go unquestioned by clinicians and by the public at large. There are, however, processes at work in the hypnotic interaction, in addition to these, that do not imply that the subject is having no experience at all related to the suggestions.

For example, an important process is 'strategic enactment', an idea promoted by the late Professor Nicholas Spanos, a psychologist from Carleton University, Ottawa, and the most prolific figure in academic hypnosis in the latter part of the 20th century. Professor Spanos was tragically killed in 1994 when the plane he was piloting crashed.

Spanos adopted a strong, non-state, sociocognitive position on hypnosis (Spanos 1991). He acknowledged the role of compliance in hypnotic responding, but developed the theme of strategic enactment. He considered that, in contrast to special-state formulations of hypnosis, hypnotic responding is goal-directed activity on the subject's part. That is, unlike accounts provided by dissociation theories, the subject is not passively 'letting things happen' but actively 'making things happen'. For example, when attending to the arm levitation suggestion, the responsive subject does not wait for the arm to rise but lifts the arm, attempting to create, through imagination, the feeling that it is being pulled up. When given suggestions of analgesia, the subject adopts a cognitive strategy (e.g. self-distraction) instead of simply waiting for the suggestion to take effect. When tested for suggested posthypnotic amnesia, the subject is not struggling to recall the lost information, but adopting a strategy, such as attention switching, that disrupts recall.

Now, what implications does this have for our understanding of individual variations in hypnotic susceptibility and its apparent stability over time? One possibility is that at least some people who respond poorly to hypnotic suggestions may have the wrong attitude. For one reason or another, they do not allow themselves to be actively engaged in utilising their cognitive skills to make the suggested responses happen, as is the case with more 'hypnotisable' people. Is it possible, then, that we could train them to adopt the correct approach and thus increase their hypnotic susceptibility? And would this training have a permanent effect?

These questions define a major project that Spanos and his colleagues and students engaged in from the early 1980s onwards. They developed a training programme called the Carleton Skill Training Program (CSTP). This is now available in published form (Gorassini & Spanos 1999). The aims of the programme are to instil in subjects a positive attitude to hypnosis (by dispelling misconceptions, and so on); to encourage the belief in subjects that they too can be responsive hypnotic subjects; and to educate the participants in the idea that to be a good hypnotic subject one has to be actively involved in creating the suggested experiences and responses, rather than to passively wait for them just to happen. The latter aim is achieved by taking the subjects through a range of suggestions (e.g. arm levitation, finger lock, book hallucination) and coaching them in the 'strategic enactment' of each one. Advocates of this approach claim that it leads to a permanent increase in hypnotic suggestibility (Spanos et al 1988). Others remain unconvinced (Bowers & Davidson 1991).

The position of the authors on this tends to be with the latter group. We acknowledge that no single process underpins hypnotic responding, and 'strategic enactment', as described by Spanos, is likely to be involved in a significant way. However, it seems probable that the CSTP is training individuals in just one way of responding to hypnotic suggestions, but not necessarily the way of all untrained, highly responsive subjects. Also, we are not satisfied that the results adequately account for the individual differences and the stability of susceptibility that both occur naturally. There is now evidence that at least some susceptible individuals are different from unsusceptible subjects on cognitive tests involving attention, and on neuropsychological and neurophysiological measures, both in and out of the hypnotic context (Crawford 1994, Gruzelier 1998). Neurophysiological studies (Barabasz et al 1999, De Pascalis 1999) have revealed that some highly susceptible subjects are having genuine experiences (e.g. profound analgesia and reduced perceptual responses when imagining visual and auditory blocking stimuli) rather than responding compliantly.

Attribution

One problem for sociocognitive theories is that, to a significant degree, subjects report that the effects of suggestions tend to operate in an automatic fashion and that, for the most part, they are not deliberately enacting them. Good hypnotic subjects regularly insist that they are, or have been, hypnotised. How do we account for this?

It is not uncommon in certain contexts for hypnotic subjects to be surprised by their behaviour during hypnosis. To them it is 'unusual' and thus, unlike 'usual' behaviour, requires an explanation. This is especially so in the case of stage hypnosis, when participants may find it difficult to account for why they did the things they did and seemed to be under the control of the hypnotist. A ready explanation is available to them, namely that they were 'hypnotised' or 'in a trance' and this is the one they will often adopt. (If, instead, they had received an appreciable fee for their performances, probably their explanation would be 'I did it because I was paid to'.) A laboratory equivalent of this is the study of the behaviour of hypnotic subjects who respond positively to suggestions that require them to engage in a dangerous or anti-social activity (Coe et al 1972, Levitt et al 1975, O'Brian & Rabuck 1976, Orne & Evans 1965). The validity of the attribution 'I did this because I was hypnotised' or 'I was in a trance' can then be tested by studying the behaviour of non-hypnotic subjects who are placed in the same conditions and subjected to the same contextual demands, and who have the same degree of commitment to participating. The differences between hypnotised and non-hypnotised subjects are, in fact, non-existent or, if anything, there is greater compliance by *non-hypnotised* subjects. Hence the attribution 'I behaved like this because I was hypnotised' is not supported. The factors determining the behaviour in question appear to be non-hypnotic – role demands, expectations, and so on.

Can we apply the same analysis to subjective experience as opposed to overt behaviour? There is no reason why not. We seek to make sense of our internal experiences – sensations, feelings, ideas, emotions – particularly when we observe out-of-the-ordinary changes in them. Obvious everyday examples are pain and uncomfortable physical symptoms, tense feelings, mood changes, and so on. We tend to look for external cues, causative factors and confirmation (as when we seek our doctor's opinion on the reason for our pain and discomfort) to make sense of these private experiences.

So, consider the hypnotic subjects who, by actively deploying their repertoire of cognitive skills, successfully reduce their experience of a painful stimulus, disrupt their recall of a set of words they have only just heard, allow their arm to lift seemingly without effort or vividly relive a childhood memory. They may attribute these changes as a product of their own goal-directed activity, but they may also refer to important external cues and information that are telling them that what they are experiencing is 'happening to them', is involuntary, and is the result of their 'being hypnotised'. Evidence that the interpretation 'voluntary' or 'involuntary' is influenced by context is discussed by Lynn et al (1990).

Self-deception

We can go even further than the idea of modification of attribution by context. To what extent are we ourselves able to control the way we interpret our own experiences and behaviour? One idea that Coe & Sarbin (1991) have drawn on is 'self-deception'. For example, not all hypnotised subjects breach posthypnotic amnesia under pressure, or modify their accounts of their hypnotic experience when the demands are changed. Perhaps these subjects are deceiving *themselves* as well as the hypnotist and other observers. That is, they are required to behave 'as if' they are amnesic and they come to believe it.

At first sight, 'self-deception' may appear to be no more than a convenient label for those residual observations that do not accord with the theory – the pieces of the jigsaw that don't fit. But let us give this idea the benefit of some further thought.

In order to be consistent with any valued role that we are occupying at any time, we often have to engage in varying degrees of deception. That is, we deceive those who expect us to behave in accordance with that role. This deception is conveyed by our behaviour, both verbal and non-verbal. For example, patients will expect their doctor to care about them and to be knowledgeable about their medical condition. Yet doctors may be so exasperated by what they regard as the unreasonable demands of particular patients that they feel unable to care about them at all. Moreover, they may have little idea what the patient's medical problem is or what can be done about it. However, to maintain the role of a good doctor, a role that the doctor highly values, the doctor's overt behaviour and speech will communicate care, concern and competence.

So we deceive others, but can we deceive ourselves in a similar way? The answer has to be 'Yes', if we bear in mind that deception, and our awareness that we are engaging in deception, are not all-or-none matters, but are a matter of degree. In Coe & Sarbin's (1991) terms, we have the ability to conceal things – that is, to 'keep secrets' – from ourselves in order to maintain consistency with our 'self-narrative', the story we tell of ourselves to others and *to ourselves.*

For instance, as required, 'amnesic' hypnotic subjects behave as if they have no control over their memory processes. When asked to report directly on this, under greater pressure, most will eventually change their story and thus demonstrate that they do have control over their memory. But others may conceal this from their own self-awareness, and continue to play the role of the amnesic subject.

What readers must decide

What do readers make of all this? Have the traditionalists successfully demonstrated that special processes are required to account for hypnotic phenomena? Are the sociocognitive theories 'specious' as one authority has lately called them? Or have they enriched our understanding of what goes on during this peculiar interaction handed down by history? Do their explanations amount to no more than simply putting what for them are more acceptable labels on what is observed? Is the special process–sociocognitive debate merely a conflict of semantics?

One conclusion that readers may come to is that perhaps all the theorists we have mentioned are like the proverbial group of blind people trying to discover what an elephant is, each only feeling just one part. Indeed, some authorities have provided explanations of hypnotic phenomena that integrate information and ideas from a wide range of viewpoints. The work of the Australian psychologists Peter Sheehan and Kevin McConkey exemplifies this; their research has been of particular value as it emphasises the importance of analysing the subject's experiences of hypnotic phenomena and the importance of the subject's aptitudes and cognitive skills (Sheehan & McConkey 1982).

Readers must decide for themselves on these matters, but must not rely on this one chapter. Further study of the literature combined with experience of using hypnosis is necessary to appreciate the complexities of this phenomenon.

OUR DEFINITION AND WORKING MODEL OF HYPNOSIS

We ourselves have no new theory to propose but we would like to provide a full definition and working model of hypnosis that are useful for clinical purposes and integrate ideas and observations from laboratory investigations.

Definition of hypnosis

Putting together our previous definitions of suggestion and trance, and our brief description of hypnotic induction, we can define hypnosis as follows:

The term 'hypnosis' is used to denote an interaction between two people (or one person and a group) in which one of them, the hypnotist, by means of verbal communication, encourages the other, the subject or subjects, to focus their attention away from their immediate realities and concerns and on inner experiences such as thoughts, feelings and imagery. The hypnotist further attempts to create alterations in the subjects' sensations, perceptions, feelings, thoughts and behaviour by directing them to imagine various events or situations that, were they to occur in reality, would evoke the intended changes.

Working model of hypnosis

Hypnosis involves the coming together of a number of psychological processes and skills, including attention (selective and sustained), absorption, expectancy, imagination and very often, though not always, relaxation. Good hypnotic subjects are able to manipulate their conscious experiences – perceptions, thoughts, images, memories, feelings – under the direction of the hypnotist to attempt to achieve the suggested effects.

Subjects vary in this ability, which is relatively stable. All subjects come under pressure to fulfil the role of the good hypnotic subject and the observed behaviours are markedly influenced by the context. Compliance or deception is likely to be a significant factor underlying the behaviour of a significant number of subjects. Those subjects who have the ability to create, at least to some degree, the suggested effects, may, because of the context, interpret their experience as the result of their 'being hypnotised'. They may thus deny their own agency in creating the experiences.

Hypnotic phenomena are not explained by reference to an altered state of consciousness. However, one dimension of the experience of hypnosis for which the term 'trance' may be apposite is the extent to which subjects are absorbed in the suggested experiences, to the exclusion of their immediate surroundings and concerns. Some individuals may have a marked capacity to do this and thus resemble what are traditionally described as 'deep trance' subjects. The role of the hypnotic induction can be construed either as encouraging this internal absorption or as increasing responsiveness to suggestions by enhancing motivation, commitment and expectancy.

A NOTE ON LANGUAGE

It is clear that according to this working model, hypnosis is something that the person *does* (or more correctly, two people do). Despite this, we are still saddled with a vocabulary and phraseology based on the traditional interpretation of hypnosis. Thus we say that we 'induce' hypnosis and 'deepen' it, that people are 'in' or 'under' hypnosis, or indeed they are 'hypnotised', ('deeply', 'lightly', etc.), that they 'come out of it', and so on. Unfortunately it is often difficult to change long-established habits of expression.

REFERENCES

Barabasz A, Barabasz M, Jensen S et al 1999 Cortical event-related potentials show the structure of hypnotic suggestions is crucial. International Journal of Clinical and Experimental Hypnosis 47: 5–22

Barber T X, Calverley D S 1964 Experimental studies in 'hypnotic' behaviour: Suggested deafness evaluated by delayed auditory feedback. British Journal of Psychology 55: 439–446

Barber T X, Spanos N P, Chaves J F 1974 Hypnosis: Imagination and human potentialities. Pergamon, New York

Bowers K S, Davidson T M 1991 A neodissociative critique of Spanos's social-psychological model of hypnosis. In: Lynn S J, Rhue J W (eds) Theories of hypnosis: Current models and perspectives. Guilford Press, New York, ch 4, p 105

Coe W C, Sarbin T R 1991 Role theory: Hypnosis from a dramaturgical and narrational perspective. In: Lynn S J, Rhue J W (eds) Theories of hypnosis: Current models and perspectives. Guilford Press, New York, ch 10, p 303

Coe W C, Sluis A 1989 Increasing contextual pressures to breach posthypnotic amnesia. Journal of Personality and Social Psychology 57: 885–894

Coe W C, Yashinski E 1985 Volitional experiences associated with breaching posthypnotic amnesia. Journal of Personality and Social Psychology 48: 716–722

Coe W C, Kobayashi K, Moward M L 1972 An approach toward isolating factors that influence antisocial conduct in hypnosis. International Journal of Clinical and Experimental Hypnosis 20: 118–131

Crawford H J 1994 Brain dynamics and hypnosis: Attentional and disattentional processes. International Journal of Clinical and Experimental Hypnosis 42: 204–232

Crawford H J, Macdonald H, Hilgard E R 1979 Hypnotic deafness: A psychophysical study of responses to tone intensity as modified by hypnosis. American Journal of Psychology 92: 193–214

De Pascalis V 1999 Psychophysiological correlates of hypnosis and hypnotic susceptibility. International Journal of Clinical and Experimental Hypnosis 47: 117–143

Edmonston W E 1981 Hypnosis and relaxation: Modern verification of an old equation. Wiley, New York

Edmonston W E 1991 Anesis. In: Lynn S J, Rhue J W (eds) Theories of hypnosis: Current models and perspectives. Guilford Press, New York, ch 7, p 197

Gorassini D R, Spanos N P 1999 The Carleton Skill Training Program for Modifying Hypnotic Suggestibility: Original version and variations. In: Kirsch I, Capafons A, Cardeña-Buelna E, Amigó S (eds) Clinical hypnosis and self-regulation: Cognitive-behavioral perspectives. American Psychological Association, Washington DC, ch 6, p 141

Gruzelier J 1998 A working model of the neurophysiology of hypnosis. Contemporary Hypnosis 15: 3–21

Gruzelier J 2000 Redefining hypnosis: Theory, methods and integration. Contemporary Hypnosis 17: 51–70

Hilgard E R 1986 Divided consciousness: Multiple controls in human thought and action. Wiley, New York

Hilgard E R, Morgan A H, Macdonald H 1975 Pain and dissociation in the cold pressor test: A study of hypnotic analgesia with 'hidden reports' through automatic key-pressing and automatic talking. Journal of Abnormal Psychology 190: 280–289

Howard M L, Coe W C 1980 The effects of context and subjects' perceived control in breaching posthypnotic amnesia. Journal of Personality 48: 342–359

Kirsch I 1991 The social learning theory of hypnosis. In: Lynn S J, Rhue J W (eds) Theories of hypnosis: Current models and perspectives. Guilford Press, New York, ch 14, p 439

Levitt R E, Aronoff G, Morgan C D et al 1975 Testing the coercive power of hypnosis: Committing objectionable acts. International Journal of Clinical and Experimental Hypnosis 23: 59–67

Lynn S J, Rhue J W, Weekes J 1990 An integrative model of hypnotic involuntariness. (Is hypnotic behavior truly involuntary?) In: Van Dyck R, Spinhoven Ph, Van der Does A J W, Van Rood Y R, De Moor W (eds) Hypnosis: Current theory, research and clinical practice. VU University Press, Amsterdam, p 17

Norman D A, Shallice T 1986 Attention to action: Willed and automatic control of behavior. In: Davidson R J, Schwartz G E, Shapiro D (eds) Consciousness and self-regulation, vol 4. Plenum Press, New York, p 1–18

O'Brian R M, Rabuck S J 1976 Experimentally produced self-repugnant behavior as a function of hypnosis and waking suggestion: A pilot study. American Journal of Clinical Hypnosis 18: 272–276

Orne M T 1959 The nature of hypnosis: Artifact and essence. Journal of Abnormal and Social Psychology 58: 277–299

Orne M T 1962 Hypnotically induced hallucinations. In: West L J (ed) Hallucinations. Grune and Stratton, New York, p 211–219

Orne M T 1972 On the simulating subject as a quasi-control in hypnosis research: What, why and how? In: Fromm E, Shor R E (eds) Hypnosis: Research developments and perspectives. Aldine–Atherton, Chicago, p 399–443

Orne M T, Evans F J 1965 Social control in the psychological experiment: antisocial behavior and hypnosis. Journal of Personality and Social Psychology 1: 189–200

Sarbin T R, Coe W C 1972 Hypnosis: A social psychological analysis of influence communication. Holt, Rhinehart and Winston, New York

Scheibe K E, Gray A L, Keim C S 1968 Hypnotically induced deafness and delayed auditory feedback: A comparison of real and stimulating subjects. International Journal of Clinical and Experimental Hypnosis 16: 158–164

Sheehan P W, McConkey K M 1982 Hypnosis and experience: The explanation of phenomena and process. Erlbaum, Hillsdale

Spanos N 1991 A sociocognitive approach to hypnosis. In: Lynn S J, Rhue J W (eds) Theories of hypnosis: Current models and perspectives. Guilford Press, New York, ch 11, p 324

Spanos N P, Hewitt E C 1980 The hidden observer in hypnotic analgesia: Discovery or experimental creation? Journal of Personality and Social Psychology 39: 189–200

Spanos N P, Gwynn M I, Stam H J 1983 Instructional demands and ratings of overt and hidden pain during hypnotic analgesia. Journal of Abnormal Psychology 92: 479–488

Spanos N P, Cross W P, Menary E P et al 1988 Long-term effects of cognitive skill training for the enhancement of hypnotic susceptibility. British Journal of Experimental and Clinical Hypnosis 5: 73–78

Spanos N P, Flynn D M, Gabora N J 1989 Suggested negative visual hallucinations in hypnotic subjects: When no means yes. British Journal of Experimental and Clinical Hypnosis 6: 63–67

Wagstaff G F 1981 Hypnosis, compliance and belief. Harvester Press, Brighton

Wagstaff G F 1991 Compliance, belief, and semantics in hypnosis: A nonstate, sociocognitive perspective. In: Lynn S J, Rhue J W (eds) Theories of hypnosis: Current models and perspectives. Guilford Press, New York, ch 12, p 362

Watkins J G, Watkins H H 1990 Dissociation and displacement: Where goes the 'ouch'? American Journal of Clinical Hypnosis 13: 1–10

Woody E Z, Bower K S 1994 A frontal assault on dissociative control. In: Lynn S J, Rhue J W (eds) Dissociation: clinical and theoretical perspectives. Guilford Press, New York, ch 3, p 52

Wyke B D 1957 Neurological aspects of hypnosis. Proceedings of the Dental and Medical Society for the Study of Hypnosis. Royal Society of Medicine, London

Wyke B D 1960 Neurological mechanisms in hypnosis: Some recent advances in the study of hypnotic phenomena. Proceedings of the Dental and Medical Society for the Study of Hypnosis. Royal Society of Medicine, London

Basic procedures in clinical hypnosis

In the previous section we developed the concepts of suggestion and trance. The key distinction between these two plays a role in determining how hypnosis is applied clinically. After considering how one prepares a subject for hypnosis in Chapter 5, we describe a range of induction and deepening procedures in the following two chapters. Procedures that are designed directly to encourage the trance experience are described in Chapter 6, and in Chapter 7 we describe those that are aimed at enhancing the patient's responsiveness to the suggestions and therapy to follow. We include discussion of the theoretical rationale for this distinction, which we interpret not as a dichotomy but as one of emphasis.

Matters of immediate concern to safe and ethical practice are presented in Chapter 8, a theme to which we shall return in later sections. Chapter 9 covers methods and applications of self-hypnosis; these are consistent with an emphasis on the trance experience. Chapters 10, 11 and 13 are very much concerned with broadening the concept of 'therapeutic suggestion' and its application in clinical practice, while Chapter 12 details a number of common and very useful suggestive techniques for the control of tension, anxiety and anger. Finally, Chapter 14 acknowledges that while children are very good candidates for clinical hypnosis, the methods so far discussed need to be adapted to suit characteristics such as their personal interests, variable attentiveness, and level of maturation.

5

Preparation for clinical hypnosis

INTRODUCTION

In this chapter, we shall consider the structure of a session of clinical hypnosis and the process of preparing patients for their initial session of hypnosis.

THE STRUCTURE OF THE CLINICAL HYPNOSIS SESSION

The orthodox approach to therapeutic hypnosis is centred on the notion that hypnosis is a special state that is achieved by the hypnotist's guiding the patient through a sequence of overlapping stages as follows:

1. Preparing the patient.
2. The induction of the hypnotic state or trance.
3. Deepening of the above.
4. Therapy, namely suggestions, imagery-based techniques and posthypnotic suggestions. The assumption is that in the 'trance state' the patient is more responsive to these.
5. Alerting.
6. Posthypnosis discussion.
7. The use of self-hypnosis by the patient between sessions.

This structure, in fact, requires no modification to accommodate the understanding of hypnosis that we have outlined in Section 1 of this book.

PREPARATION

The setting

It makes sense to recommend that hypnosis should be conducted in a quiet and comfortable setting where no interruptions are likely. In reality, this may not be possible, first because of the type of problem being treated (e.g. dental anxiety, in which case the setting will be the dental surgery) and second because the facilities available to practitioners may be the same as those that they use for their routine professional work (e.g. a doctor's office in a noisy and hectic health centre). In point of fact, there is not too much of a problem with all this. Patients can cope with a great deal of noise and bustle if this is expected in the environment in which they are being seen. When undertaking therapy for psychological problems, the recommended conditions are those that one would advocate were hypnosis not being used (privacy, a minimum of interruptions, etc.). So far as the seating offered to the patient is concerned, a reasonably comfortable chair will suffice. Some patients are prone to aching in the back and shoulders if there is no support for the head but often the latter can be improvised if necessary. A cold temperature can be very distracting, and too warm and stuffy an atmosphere can cause the patient to develop a headache and to feel unduly drowsy during and after the session. Other than this, no special conditions are necessary.

Introducing hypnosis

When introducing the idea of using hypnosis with your patient, two initial possibilities arise. In some cases, your patient may have requested hypnosis or has come to you in the expectation of having hypnosis. In other cases, you will yourself introduce the idea of using hypnosis as a means of helping patients with their problems. In the latter instance, the question may arise as to whether or not you describe what you intend to do as 'hypnosis'. This is a rather more complex matter than at first it may seem and, as it involves ethical matters, we shall defer discussion of this until Chapter 8.

Once there is an explicit understanding between you and your patient that hypnosis is to be a treatment modality, it is important that your patient has a clear understanding of hypnosis and a positive expectation about its real nature. An early question to ask patients is whether they have experienced hypnosis before. One possibility is that they have had some treatment involving hypnosis and that it was a beneficial experience. Clearly this bodes well and it makes sense to find out what particular procedures were used so that they may be considered again for the patient's current problem. On the other hand, the previous experience may not have had a successful outcome. This need not be much of a problem: people can usually accept that no treatment is guaranteed to work 100% of the time. However, further enquiry may disclose misconceptions that need to be corrected before you proceed. For example, the patient may complain, 'I wasn't hypnotised because I knew what was happening/ was still in control/ remembered everything when I opened my eyes...etc.' These misconceptions will be explored shortly.

Finally, it is unfortunately the case that the most common experience of hypnosis by many patients is as a means of entertainment. In recent years, this may have been through the medium of television, but your patient may also have attended a live show and indeed may have actually participated. If anything were calculated to convey an entirely false expectation of the nature of therapeutic hypnosis, then it would be stage hypnosis. Some patients who have witnessed a stage hypnosis show will be concerned that hypnosis places them under the control of the therapist who may, if the therapist wishes, make the patient behave in ridiculous ways. Contrariwise, some patients may have unrealistic expectations of the power of the therapist to relieve them of whatever is the difficulty or affliction for which they are seeking help. This is typified by the remark of one patient, John, who said: 'If hypnosis can make my mates behave like that, then it should be able to cure my stammer'.

Of course, one can argue that this faith on the patient's part may be a therapeutic asset. More likely, however, the disparity between the patient's expectations and the therapist's ability to deliver on these will prove too great a schism for patients to be actively engaged in the resolution of their problems. (In John's case, hypnosis *did* help him to improve his speech, though not without considerable effort on his part.)

Even without the contaminating influence of stage hypnosis, patients do occasionally ask for hypnosis with the idea that it provides a magical solution to their problems. In such instances, the belief is commonly held that during hypnosis subjects are 'put under' in a manner similar to somebody who is being 'put under an anaesthetic', and their mind may be then reprogrammed to eliminate the problem. Another expectation of some patients is that hypnosis will reveal the reason for their having the problem, and they will thus be cured.

These assumptions about how hypnosis may effect a cure or improvement illustrate the concept of 'a working model'. As will be noted later in this book, a treatment based on either of these assumptions may sometimes be effective. Generally, however, these working models belie the complexities of the problems for which people seek help.

One of the objections that practitioners raise in the face of these simplified ideas is that patients or clients are assuming that they will be passive recipients of the ministrations of the therapist who is thereby expected to do all of the work. 'Some patients just want a magic cure' is a not uncommon lament amongst practitioners of hypnosis. (It is probably not just in the field of hypnosis that this complaint is voiced, but it may be that people's conception of hypnosis encourages the idea of passivity under the magic curative influence of the hypnotist.)

It is important, therefore, that while you make clear to patients that hypnotic procedures are of proven effectiveness and that you are confident that they will benefit from your treatment, hypnosis is not magic but has a proper scientific basis and the patient is always an active participant in the treatment.

Describing hypnosis

One good way of describing hypnosis to the patient is by reference to the two components, suggestion and absorption or trance. You may say something like this:

Hypnosis is a way of helping people to feel very relaxed and to respond to suggestions and ideas that are going to help them. However, it's not the same as being asleep. When you're asleep, you aren't aware of what's going on around you. During hypnosis, people usually say that they are still aware of what is going on around them but it doesn't seem to matter. It goes into the background. In fact, it's rather like when you are absorbed in a book or some music or a daydream; you know that things are going on around you but you just don't need to take any notice. But it's important, when I'm talking to you, not to put *me* in the background! Stay in touch with my voice and the meaning of my words.

Many patients will be concerned that they are not going to prove responsive to hypnosis. Therefore, say something like this:

I shall be suggesting ideas and asking you to imagine various scenes that are going to help you overcome your problems. Don't worry if I suggest something and you don't experience anything – only a few people respond to *all* the suggestions.

Some people erroneously believe that during hypnosis you cannot or must not move; also that you are controlled by the hypnotist. Therefore, say something like this:

It's important that at any time during hypnosis you do anything at all to help yourself feel more comfortable – say if you need to cough or change position. Just go ahead. Also remember this. You are always in control. The idea is for you to just go along with whatever I am suggesting, but, in the end, if there is something you do not want to think about or imagine, you don't have to do so at all.

Occasionally, patients may have a fear that they will 'get stuck' in hypnosis. Therefore, say something like this:

At the end of the hypnosis session, I'll ask you to open your eyes and be fully alert again. This is something you actually do for yourself, so really, at any time, you will be able to open your eyes and end the session of hypnosis. There is no way you can 'get stuck' in hypnosis.

It is not uncommon for people to believe that following hypnosis they will not remember what happened. Therefore, say something like this:

People usually remember most, if not all, of what they experience during hypnosis.

Each individual patient may have personal questions to ask and may need further reassurance on various points, so it is a good idea to ask if the patient has any questions before proceeding.

Physical contact

One important point concerns the matter of physical contact with your patient or client during hypnosis.

Deliberate physical contact between doctor (or dentist) and patient, or therapist and client, always conveys some meaning. For doctors or dentists in their everyday work, the implicit message is usually something like 'I'm getting on with the job of helping you with your physical/dental health' and patients usually interpret the practitioner's proximity and physical contact in this way. However, touch is also a way of communicating feelings and emotions – care, sympathy, affection, physical and sexual attraction, and so on. The language of interpersonal distance and physical contact is a very subtle one and misunderstandings may easily arise. This may be more the case in a situation such as hypnosis, about which the patient may have some uncertainties as to what constitutes authentic conduct on the practitioner's part. (This issue has come up in our experiences in cases in which the hypnotist very clearly behaved in an unethical manner.) Moreover, during hypnosis, subjects have their eyes closed and therefore have no access to visual cues that are an important component of the communication. Thus, uncertainties around the meaning of touch may easily arise and cause anxiety on the patient's part.

Some hypnotic procedures do require the hypnotist to touch the subject and we recommend that the practitioner seeks the patient's permission beforehand, saying exactly what physical contact will occur. For example: 'At some point I may take hold of your wrist and lift your arm up. Is this OK? I don't *have* to do it if you'd rather not'. You might, instead, ask permission *during* hypnosis in the same way.

When you ask permission from your patients or clients in the above way, they will also receive, as it were, the meta-communication 'I have respect for you and care about your feelings'. Should patients refuse, you must abide by their wishes without any further exploration of the reasons for this. So far as the conduct of hypnosis is concerned, you are not permitted to make any interpretation as to why patients are uncomfortable about physical contact from you, or to perceive it as your goal to enable them to accept this.

Some readers will feel it is unnecessary to ask permission to touch when they are engaged in some intervention with a patient which of necessity entails physical contact. They already have the patient's permission. Indeed, they have a huge advantage over psychologists and psychotherapists because physical proximity and touch may greatly reinforce any kind of therapeutic communication.

We wish to stress that in no way are we saying that it is unethical to touch a patient or client during a session of psychotherapy. Different schools of psychotherapy have different rules concerning what constitutes *good practice* in terms of their particular theoretical framework.

In the next chapter, we shall discuss the preliminaries to the actual induction of hypnosis and then present a number of induction and deepening routines.

6

Hypnotic induction and deepening procedures: first approach

INTRODUCTION

In this and the next chapter, we shall discuss what a hypnotic induction and deepening routine is in theory and in reality. Arising from these deliberations are two approaches to the induction of hypnosis, one based on *the concept of trance* the second on *the concept of suggestion and suggestibility*. These two approaches lead to somewhat different preliminary procedures and induction and deepening routines. They overlap considerably, however, and only differ in terms of the degree of emphasis given to the two aforementioned aspects of hypnosis. We shall discuss the situations in which one approach may be more preferable than the other.

DEFINITION OF THE INDUCTION PROCESS IN THE FIRST APPROACH

For the purposes of this approach, we can adopt the 'weak' or 'naturalistic' trance interpretation – namely 'the experience of detachment from immediate surroundings and absorption in inner experiences'. The effectiveness of the induction and deepening may then be evaluated in terms of the extent to which the patient engages in the process of inner absorption. So let us formally define hypnotic induction (and deepening) as follows:

A series of instructions and suggestions aimed at encouraging the subject to have a trance experience (as defined in Ch. 2).

Note that, as in the earlier discussion of suggestion, we have defined the induction according to the intention of the process.

Before undertaking any set of induction and deepening procedures, we suggest that you always ask yourself this question: 'What purposes are the induction and deepening methods intended to serve?' We have defined the intention as encouraging the subject to have a trance experience according to our previous definition, but we still have to ask, 'What purpose is this intended to serve in helping patients with their problem?' The answer to the question depends on your 'working model' that determines the treatment you are undertaking at any particular moment. This concept will be discussed in depth in Chapter 15; it comprises the assumptions you are making about the causative or predisposing factors that underlie the patient's problem and how your treatment addresses these. Some common purposes of induction and deepening methods based on this approach are as follows (see also Ch. 2 on the properties of the trance).

You may wish to help your patient undergo uncomfortable or anxiety-provoking dental or medical procedures by the use of distracting and relaxing imagery, likewise to tolerate acute pain caused by a medical condition or injury. You may have patients who are experiencing occupational stress and you wish to teach a daily self-hypnosis procedure to enable them to take time out from the immediate pressures of work. In a similar vein, you may have a patient who suffers from insomnia, made worse by the annoyance and frustration of not sleeping or the constant 'churning over' of minor worries. Finally, you may be intending to help your patient confront and resolve a traumatic memory. You want your patient to relive this memory in some way, but you may also want to guard against your patient becoming so distressed that the patient will be further traumatised. Accordingly, you teach a method whereby the patient switches in imagination to a 'safe place' to relax again.

There are many more applications – for example, in psychodynamic therapy – but let us now look at some common methods based on this general approach.

We do not consider physical relaxation to be a defining property of hypnosis (although one therapist, Edmondston (1981), has equated the two) and frequently, at any point in a session of hypnosis, your patient will not be relaxed. However, for present purposes, relaxation methods are the most practical and commonly used procedures for hypnotic induction. They need not be unduly lengthy and may be shortened according to the demands of the situation.

With the exception of the first method described (the Spiegel eye-roll), these methods emphasise absorption on inner experiences to the relative exclusion of whatever is going on in the patient's surroundings and the patient's immediate concerns. In other words, they emphasise the trance experience.

PRELIMINARIES TO THE FIRST APPROACH

The following is a good method to begin with as it helps the patient become accustomed to the idea of sitting in a chair listening to your voice while having the eyes closed. We call it 'sensory focusing' (not to be confused with 'sensate focusing', a procedure used in sex therapy). Say to the patient the following:

Close your eyes now and just get used to sitting in the chair with your eyes closed listening to my voice. Remember that at any time you can do anything that you need to do to make yourself feel more comfortable. Right now be aware of anything that is going on around you, for example, the sounds of the traffic in the distance, the sound of birds, and so on. You may also hear noises in the room such as the ticking of the clock. Gradually, your awareness of everything that is going on around you can go into the background where it doesn't matter so much. As you do this, you become aware of things that are going on *within* you, such as physical feelings. You may be aware of the way your body feels as you sit comfortably in the chair ... feelings such as warmth or coolness, heaviness or lightness. You may notice the pressure of the different parts of the chair on your body. Some parts of you may not be as relaxed as other parts, but that doesn't matter right now. You may notice the movements of your breathing. Just allow your breathing to be comfortable and steady. You may be aware of thoughts passing through your mind. You don't have to think about anything special right now and you don't have to keep anything out. Whatever wants to come to mind just let it come. Or your mind may be quiet right now. In your own time, just let me know how that feels.

When you are talking to the patient like this and whenever you are using the present approach to hypnotic induction, use a calm and soothing voice, but it is not necessary, nor particularly helpful, to be overly monotonous. Mark out certain key words and phrases, either by being a little firmer in tone or softening the tone, as with words such as 'relaxed', 'comfortable' and 'calm'. You can pace your delivery with the patient's breathing by timing your suggestions of relaxation with the patient's outward breath.

With experience, you can use this preliminary routine to gain an idea about how patients may respond to your induction. Do they appear comfortable and calm, or tense and on guard? Are they fidgety or still? Very occasionally, a patient will have a problem with maintaining eye-closure, say through some anxiety about losing control. Later in this book we shall present elaborations of this method that assist the therapist and patient in addressing what might be important issues that come to the fore at the beginning of a first session of hypnosis.

During the above and the subsequent induction and deepening procedures, do not fall into the habit of 'drifting off' yourself so that you end up staring at the wall or floor; you need to be constantly observing your patient for non-verbal cues to pace your delivery. Use plenty of pauses to allow the patient time to observe the experiences you are suggesting. Make liberal use of phrases such as 'That's fine', 'Good!', and 'Well done!' Your patient is allowed to speak! However, patients may also need your permission. From time to time you can say 'How does that feel?', 'Is that OK?', 'Tell me if there is anything particular you notice right now', and so on.

INDUCTION AND DEEPENING METHODS OF THE FIRST APPROACH

The eye-roll method

There is a tradition in the history of hypnosis, at least from the time of Braid, for associating the induction of hypnosis with visual fixation and ocular fatigue. Spiegel & Spiegel (1987) begin their Hypnotic Induction Profile (see Ch. 3) with the following procedure (which does not actually require fatigue of the eye muscles as such). If nothing else, it serves as a starting point for the formal induction of hypnosis and involves the creation and then the release of tension in the eyes and forehead. You would only use this method as an induction, rather than a deepening method, as it involves the opening of the eyes. Say the following:

In a few moments, I am going to ask you to open your eyes and to roll your eyes up as though you are trying to look at your eyebrows. After a little while I shall ask you to take in a deep breath and as you are breathing out, you lower your eyelids over your eyes whilst still keeping them in the upward gaze. On the second outward breath, you relax your eyes.

The patient then opens the eyes and goes through this procedure. As the eyes are closing on the outward breath, say:

That's fine. Feel that sense of relaxation ... Now you just allow yourself to carry on relaxing.

You then proceed with one or more of the deepening methods below.

An elaboration of the above method is to lift one of the patient's arms by the wrist just as the patient is rolling the eyes upwards. Some practitioners lift the whole arm all the way up to the vertical position but it is more practical to raise just the forearm so the arm is comfortably flexed at the elbow, with your hand taking the weight of the arm. The idea is to very gently let go of the arm as the eyelids are closing. If the arm falls, say that as it is falling the patient is becoming more and more relaxed. Some regard it as a sign of dissociative capacity if the arm remains in the raised position. In that case, you may eventually suggest that it is becoming heavy and gradually falling to the patient's lap or, if you intend using ideomotor signals (see Ch. 19), you can allow the arm to remain in that position.

Breathing methods

A short breathing technique is as follows.

In a few moments, I am going to ask you to take in three deep breaths and, as you breathe out, you will feel a sense of deepening relaxation on each outward breath. Now, *one* ... take a deep breath and now let go of that breath and feel your whole body relaxing. And *two* ... and *three* ...

Make liberal use of the suggestions 'very relaxed', 'very heavy', 'going deeper and deeper', and so on. After the third breath say:

Breathe normally now, and notice how you are continuing to become more relaxed each time you let go of your breath.

A more protracted method is as follows:

One way of coming to feel very relaxed is to think about your breathing. You don't have to do anything special with your breathing, but as you breathe out, just give some emphasis to that outward breath, as though you are *letting go* of anything that you don't want at the moment ... physical tension ... worrying thoughts ... difficult feelings .... And, as you breathe out, just prolong that outward breath a little, so you breathe down near the bottom of your breath, whilst still breathing in a comfortable way.

As you breathe out, your whole body relaxes. You lose tension in lots of muscles in your body, your heart rate slows down quite naturally, and you actually sweat less as you are breathing out, all the things that are to do with being relaxed and are the opposite of being tense. So just by thinking of this happening on the outward breath, you can help it happen even more. You don't have to try to make this happen, it will just happen automatically.

Now, as you breathe in, imagine holding that relaxation steady, so that as you breathe out, you add a little bit more relaxation, as though you are accumulating relaxation on each outward breath. Now, with each breath, as you let go of that breath, just allow a word, a thought, an image, or an idea, to come to mind that you associate with being relaxed. It might be a word like 'relax' or 'calm', something that you hear spoken in your head, or see in your mind's eye, or both. It might be a picture of something, a symbol that you associate with being relaxed. As you are letting go of each breath and as you are breathing out, bring that to mind and by doing that you will automatically relax a little bit more without trying, without *making* things happen.

Progressive relaxation

The progressive muscular relaxation method was popularised by Jacobson (1938) and originally involved working through the body, tensing and then relaxing each group of muscles. It is a rather lengthy procedure, and for the purposes of hypnotic induction or deepening, one can dispense with the method of tensing the muscles. You may also combine the procedure with the 'relaxing on the outward breath' technique. Some practitioners like to start with the feet and work upwards, or with the forehead and work downwards. One reason for choosing the latter sequence is that the upper part of the body experiences tension and relaxation more noticeably than the lower limbs. Say to the patient:

Now I would like you to think about each part of your body in turn starting with your forehead, and imagine that as you breathe out, that part of your body is relaxing. So just think of your forehead now and as you are thinking of your forehead and as you are breathing out, imagine your forehead relaxing and any tension draining away, so your forehead feels comfortable and relaxed and your head feels clear.

In a similar fashion, move to the eyes. Then the muscles of the cheeks, mouth, jaw and lips, using words such as 'letting go', 'relaxing', 'feeling nice and heavy' and 'warm and comfortable'.

Then focus on the back of the head and the neck and shoulders. One method is to talk about a 'wave of relaxation' that goes down the head with each outward breath, then down the neck and down the shoulders, all the way down the back and into the chair.

Then focus on the arms and say:

As you breathe out, imagine a wave of relaxation all the way down your arms, from your shoulders down to your elbows, from your elbows down to your wrists, and all the way down to your fingers and out at your fingertips. Feel your arms now ... comfortable, warm and heavy.

Then move on to the front of the body and say:

As you breathe out, imagine that wave of relaxation all the way down the front of your body, from your chest down to your stomach and to your waist, a nice, warm, comfortable feeling with each breath.

Next describe:

A wave of relaxation all the way down your legs from your waist to your knees, from your knees down to your ankles, down to your toes and out into the floor, leaving your legs comfortable and heavy.

Then very briefly recapitulate the procedure by saying:

Now think of your body as one. From the top of your head all the way down your head and face, a wave of relaxation with each breath; from your neck, down your shoulders, all the way down your arms to the tips of your fingers, a wave of relaxation with each outward breath. Down your body to your waist and all the way down your legs to the floor, with each breath, a wave of relaxation, driving the tension completely out of your body.

Arm heaviness from the resting position

Patients rest their arm on the lap. Ask them to focus their attention on the arm (left or right) and to imagine that the arm is becoming heavier and heavier. Repeat these suggestions and then say that in a few moments you will lift the arm by the wrist, then let it go, and the patient will feel how heavy it has become when it drops onto the lap. Say that when it drops down heavily the patient will experience a sense of deepening relaxation.

Lift the arm gently by the wrist a little way, then say, 'Very heavy … ' and, letting the arm go, ' … and relax'. Do this several (e.g. three) times with greater emphasis each time.

Then say, 'And now the other arm'. Lift that arm by the wrist and drop it in the same manner as above, about three times.

One interesting thing you will notice using this method is that individuals differ in the degree to which they are willing to 'let go' and give you the whole weight of their arm. So when you lift the arm, there is little weight to it, and when you let go of the arm it glides down rather than drops heavily. Perhaps this is evidence of some anxiety on the patient's part about experiencing hypnosis (or possibly the patient feels tense about being physically touched by you – you will already have heeded our earlier advice about this and obtained permission from your patient to make the kind of contact required by this method). When this happens, you need to spend some time holding the wrist up and gently encouraging the patient to allow you to support the entire weight of the arm and to allow it to drop naturally when you release it.

Imagery described by the therapist

It is very useful to end a sequence of induction and deepening methods with some imagery. Not everyone has good visual imagery so we incorporate in our suggestions all possible modalities. You may either construct the imagery for the patient, or invite the patient to provide a personal image or preferred scene.

One common method is to ask patients to imagine going down a series of, say, 20 steps to a beach or a garden. You can either ask patients which image they prefer, or you can allow for both possibilities in your instructions by suggesting to patients that they can choose the scene and making your suggestions more general. If you do specify the scene, you need to establish that this is an acceptable one since very occasionally patients may have had an unpleasant experience in that situation or it may simply be that it is not their idea of a relaxing place.

There now follows a summary of the routine for a beach scene, which you can modify for any other scene such as a garden.

Suggest to the patient that the patient is standing at the top of 20 steps leading down to a sandy beach. Describe the scene in all modalities: the sights (the sandy beach, the clear blue sky, the deep blue of the sea, the bright golden sun); the sounds (the sea, sea gulls, a gentle breeze); feelings (the warmth of the sun, the gentle breeze on the face); and other modalities (e.g. the tang of the sea). Then say that the patient is about to walk down the steps to the beach and you will count the steps as the patient is going down:

As I am counting, with each step you will become more deeply relaxed and at the twentieth step you will be very deeply relaxed indeed.

Begin counting the patient down the steps. Pace each count with the patient's outward breath and intersperse appropriate suggestions – 'going deeper and deeper', 'very heavy', 'very relaxed', 'feeling very safe just to let go', etc.

After the twentieth step, take the patient for a stroll around the beach, again describing the scene in all modalities and using suggestions of relaxation, warmth, and so on. Suggest, for example that:

As you look down on the sand, you see lots of interesting things – pebbles, shells, seaweed, debris. Perhaps one of the pebbles attracts your attention. You pick it up and hold it in your hand. Perhaps it feels smooth in your hand. Or rough. Is it cold or does it feel warm? And is it just one colour or different colours? Perhaps you want to put it down now or you feel it's somehow special and you want to keep it.

Eventually, you may suggest that the patient has come to a special part of the beach:

… your own special part of the beach where you can sit or lie down. Maybe in the sun or in the shade. Somewhere where you can be on your own for a while and feel absolutely safe. As you sit or lie down, just allow your eyes to close in imagination and feel surrounded by your special place. Completely safe. And you can just let your thoughts wander and allow what wants to come to mind to come to mind. You don't need to think of anything in particular if you don't want to and you don't have to keep anything out.

While you are relaxing in your special place, time doesn't seem to matter. Time can seem to extend in all directions, so that one second can be a minute and one minute can be an hour. You can have all the time you need to be in this special place and get all you want from the experience.

The 'safe place' or 'special place' method

This is a very commonly used procedure in the final stages of the induction and deepening routine. Say to the patient:

While you are relaxing like this, it is nice to take yourself in your imagination to somewhere where you know you feel safe and relaxed. A very special place where you can go to in your imagination whenever you want to. Take all the time you need for you to choose this special place. It may be a place you've only been to once, maybe on a holiday. Or a place you go to regularly. It can be outdoors, or indoors. You might be on your own or with others. You might be doing something active, or just sitting or lying down. It doesn't have to be a *real* place. It can be just a fantasy, or a combination of both.

Imagine being there in any way that comes easy for you. Some people imagine in moving pictures, like a video. Others see still pictures like photographs. You may just have a strong feeling of being there, surrounded by that place. Maybe there are sounds and even smells as well.

Take all the time you need and when you are in that special place just let me know by nodding your head.

It is important that the patient does not feel rushed, so allow plenty of time for this and continue to use comments such as 'That's fine... take all the time you need ... continuing to relax ... '. When the patient signals, you can then continue as follows:

That's fine. Now, you don't have to listen too hard to my voice because my meaning will get through. You can stay in your special place now, but if at any time you find your thoughts wandering and you want to return to your special place and all the good feelings that go with it, just give the place a name – the name of the place or a name you associate with it. And whenever you think of that word, immediately that place will come to mind and all those good feelings. So you can use your special place as a kind of base to return to whenever you want to cut short a chain of thoughts that you don't want.

The last suggestion illustrates the use of a cue or anchor, a ploy that will be presented in Chapter 11.

Now you can either administer some general positive suggestions or an ego-strengthening routine (see Ch. 11) or count from, say, 1 to 20, in which case say:

I am just going to count from I to 20 so that you can stay in touch with my voice but remain in your special place. You can use my counting in any way you wish, perhaps by allowing yourself to become more deeply relaxed and more deeply absorbed, with each count.

Again, pace your counting with the patient's outward breath and intersperse with suggestions of relaxation, comfort, safety, and so on. (You can, incidentally, use this counting method on its own as a deepening technique.)

Notice that patients do not have to inform you of their special place. Some will do so afterwards. Patients may choose a scene that they often think about in everyday life. This is fine, but a bonus is when the patient says something like, 'I wasn't sure what to choose when suddenly I found myself thinking about a place I went to years ago. I haven't thought much about it since, and I was really surprised when it came to mind'. Or a patient who has chosen an oft-remembered scene sometimes says something like, 'Suddenly a friend I haven't thought about in ages popped up from nowhere'. The bonus is that such patients go away from the session with something they didn't have when they came – a sort of discovery or, more correctly, a re-discovery that adds something extra and special to their experience.

The fractionation technique

Some practitioners adopt this method because they believe it may lead to a more profound experience of hypnosis, perhaps for patients who need a great deal of time to 'let go' and have the full experience. The technique involves taking patients a little way along an induction method, then stopping and telling them to open their eyes and starting the whole thing again. The second time round, you take them further, but once again stop, alert them, and start all over again. You may do this four or five times. It is obviously a very lengthy procedure, but it may be worthwhile with patients who do need to experience hypnosis at a very gradual pace.

ALERTING THE PATIENT

If you are intending to conduct further sessions of hypnosis with the patient then, prior to alerting, it is a good idea to say something such as the following:

Now that you have experienced relaxing in this way, you will find that in the future, each and every time you experience these procedures you will become more *easily* relaxed, more *quickly* and more *deeply*. More *easily* relaxed, more *quickly* and more *deeply*.

When the time is coming for the patient to be alerted say:

In a minute or so, I shall be asking you to alert yourself to your surroundings once again and to open your eyes. Before I do this, I shall count down from 5 to I so you can be getting ready to open your eyes at the count of I. When you open your eyes, you will be fully alert, fully oriented to your surroundings, and ready to carry on with the rest of the day. Any normal feelings, such as a bit of stiffness or tiredness, will quickly pass once you have taken a deep breath and had a good stretch, and you will find that you will feel the benefits of relaxing like this for the rest of the day, feeling alert, relaxed and refreshed.
So, I'll now count down: 5 … 4 … 3 … 2 … I … alert, wide awake and refreshed.

As you are counting down, allow your voice to become firmer and more 'matter of fact', in keeping with the patient's gradual re-orientation to the surroundings. If, incidentally, you have used a deepening method that involves counting *down*, it makes sense to count *upwards* when you alert the patient.

Very occasionally, some patients do not open their eyes. The most obvious reason for this is that patients have become so absorbed with the experience that they have stopped attending to you. The possibility of sleep should not be overlooked either. Repeat the alerting instructions more forcibly. Sometimes patients may be reluctant to leave behind such a pleasant experience and to return to the grim realities of their everyday life; or possibly some important thoughts or feelings have come to mind that are now occupying their attention. If you suspect that this is so (you cannot intuitively know everything that is happening with your patients), you may wish to ask patients to give a signal that they are still in touch with your voice and then simply say, 'In your own time, just let me know what is happening now'.

At the conclusion of the entire therapeutic session, patients may be somewhat drowsy. Should you notice this, suggest that they spend some time having a walk in the fresh air, particularly if they are driving away from the session.

'SIGNS OF TRANCE'

While administering an induction and deepening routine, you will be keen to know if the patient is responding in the desired way, namely 'going with the flow' and becoming relaxed and absorbed by inner experiences. You can never be sure either way about this until you ask the patient afterwards. Some useful pointers are as follows.

As in everyday trance experiences, patients will tend to be quite still and there will also be a reduction in reflexes such as swallowing. When movements do occur, they will be slow rather than brisk and purposeful. Generally, it is not a good sign if the patient is unduly fidgety; should you notice this, then your suggestions should be targeted on physical relaxation in the first place. The facial musculature is smooth and the expression fixed. If the forehead is furrowed, this may indicate that the patient is not comfortable about something. In that case, remember that you can always say something like, 'Just tell me if that feels OK now'. Initially, the respiration may increase but gradually it will tend to become slow and shallow, with the occasional deep sighing breath. All the cues that indicate that the person is physically relaxed should be present. Of course, once you start therapy, all this may change if, for example, you are asking the patient to imagine some problematic situations.

After alerting the patient, ask how long the patient thinks that the hypnosis session lasted. A good sign is if the estimate is half or less of the actual time that elapsed.

COMPLICATIONS

We shall discuss the matter of risks and precautions in later chapters. For the moment, it is only necessary to deal with two possible complications.

When the patient loses touch with you

It is inevitable that from time to time a patient loses touch with your voice and 'drifts off'. Up to a point, because of repetition and the pace of your delivery, this need not be a serious problem. Also, with some applications of hypnosis, such as in dentistry and in the case of uncomfortable medical procedures, it does not matter at all. However, as a general rule, any therapeutic effect of the practitioner's communications is lost if the patient has ceased attending. We know that some practitioners will claim that the patient's 'unconscious mind' is still receptive to the messages, and on this basis some have claimed that people can even learn things while they are asleep. This has not, at the very least, been our own personal experience.

There is also the possibility that patients may fall asleep, especially if they are already very tired. In such cases, a change to a slower and deeper respiratory pattern may be observed.

As was earlier suggested, should it be suspected that the patient has lost contact with the therapist, a simple request for the patient to give a signal may be the most useful action, and in our experience there is usually a positive response. If the signal is not given, then this can be repeated more forcefully until the patient responds. It is very rare, in our experience, for this to be necessary.

Signs of distress

Certain individuals refuse to have hypnosis because of the fear of 'losing control', or during hypnosis they start to feel panicky. Similar problems occasionally arise using other relaxation methods such as progressive muscular relaxation and autogenic training. Indeed, there are well-documented phenomena termed 'relaxation-induced anxiety (and panic)' and 'autogenic discharges' in the autogenic training literature (see Lehrer & Woolfolk (1993) for a review and discussion of these phenomena) whereby the patient responds to the procedures by becoming tense and anxious. There may be a number of reasons why this happens: a fear of loss of control has been cited amongst them, as has an inadvertent tendency to hyperventilate.

If it is simply a question of calling the procedure 'hypnosis' that is causing the patient to feel anxious, then one could replace this label with a more commonplace term such as 'relaxation'. However, as we shall discuss later, there are problems with this.

Patients who express such anxieties about hypnosis may be reassured by being explicitly informed that at any time during the session they will be able to call a halt to the proceedings. A useful method is to suggest that if at any time they wish this to happen, then all that they have to do is raise their hand and the therapist will immediately stop and gently alert the patient.

Occasionally, a subject may become distressed for no apparent reason. This may happen paradoxically when the patient has been asked to imagine a pleasant scene.

Case example

Clare was happily reliving playing with a family pet as a child when she suddenly began crying. It transpired that she was reminded of when the pet died and she experienced some of the feelings of sadness that she felt at the time. This was not something she had thought about for a long time and she was taken by surprise. She could not understand how she could suddenly become so upset over something that had happened so long ago – 'This is just not *me*!' she said.

What should one do when this happens? If one is undertaking psychotherapy, then clearly the feelings and material elicited may be important to explore and resolve, and later in this book we shall discuss ways of helping the patient do this. Even in a context such as the dental surgery this sort of thing may happen and it is important to be sensitive and empathic but one does not have to feel that there is some very special and skilful manoeuvre one has to do. However, one should not simply insist on alerting the patient. Experience suggests that suddenly 'pulling someone out' of an upsetting memory can be very unsettling. Empathise and offer the patient a choice – for example, 'Do you want to stay with that or shall we leave it now?' Ask permission in this way as much as possible. If the patient wants to share the experience with you, allow plenty of time. If the patient wants to 'put it away', you might suggest going in imagination to another 'safe place'. Don't rush the patient. If time is pressing and you need to close the session soon, when alerting, ask the patient to picture where he or she is now, what day and date it is, what he or she will be doing for the rest of the day, and so on. Ask for a signal to indicate when the patient feels fully oriented and ready for the eyes to open. If it is possible, allow time after re-alerting for the patient to talk about the experience.

It is not easy to close such a session satisfactorily when you are pressed for time and have a queue of patients waiting. You must, however, make sure that the patient does not go away feeling 'ashamed' or 'weak' for having 'broken down'. Reassure the patient that such worries are completely unfounded and that the reactions and experiences are natural and understandable in this kind of work.

When somebody shares an upsetting emotional experience with you and you assume, as it were, the role of a caring friend or parental figure, a special bond is established between the two of you, particularly when the other person is rarely able to express these feelings to anyone else. This is obviously a good thing in many therapist–patient relationships but it is not without its difficulties. For example, dentists cannot act in the role of counsellor or psychotherapist in their patients' lives, yet expectations of this kind may be created when a patient has an emotional reaction of the sort we are discussing. In Chapter 34, we discuss the importance of adhering to one's own professional domain when using hypnosis.

THE FIRST AND LATER SESSIONS

The first hypnotic session will consist of a series of induction and deepening routines. For example, you may start with the eye-roll method, followed by a breathing technique, then progressive relaxation and finally, an imagery method. In some contexts, such as dental treatment, the induction does not need to be so prolonged.

It is useful to ask the patient, after alerting, what aspects of the induction and deepening were most helpful, and whether there was anything you did that was not useful. Any concerns and difficulties that the patient had may also be voiced. The information will be very useful in subsequent sessions and in the process of teaching the patient a self-hypnosis routine (see Ch. 9).

In any event, as the patient becomes familiar with the experience of hypnosis, subsequent inductions may be abridged with no loss of effect. For example, patients may focus on a relaxing image chosen by themselves, while you count and offer suggestions of increasing comfort and relaxation. Or very proficient subjects may be able to use a self-hypnosis routine, indicating to you when they are ready to proceed with the rest of the therapy.

GROUP HYPNOSIS

Occasionally, you may use hypnosis on a group of people, either for demonstration purposes or for therapy, as in the case of a group treatment for smoking cessation. Although it may be useful to introduce the idea of hypnosis with some tests of suggestibility, as in the approach to be discussed in the next chapter, it makes sense to use the hypnotic induction and deepening procedures described here since these do not require the careful monitoring and pacing required by the second kind. With a group you obviously cannot customise your imagery to each subject's personal preferences; hence, you will make greater use of open-ended suggestions and those that allow some choice on the part of the subjects – for example, the 'safe place' technique rather than the 'steps to the beach' scene.

It is also important to make sure at the alerting stage that everyone follows your instructions. Some members of the group may have fallen asleep, while others may have 'blanked you out' and are absorbed in their own thoughts. With a group, therefore, a more prolonged and forceful delivery of alerting instructions may be warranted (e.g. a countdown from 10 with plenty of reorienting suggestions). Then check whether any individual members require your further attention.

We shall discuss further safeguards concerning group work in Chapter 23.

REFERENCES

Edmondston W E 1981 Hypnosis and relaxation: Modern verification of an old equation. Wiley, New York
Jacobson E 1938 Progressive relaxation. University of Chicago Press, Chicago
Lehrer P M, Woolfolk R L 1993 Specific effects of stress management techniques. In: Lehrer P M, Woolfolk R L (eds) Principles and practice of stress management, 2nd edn. Guilford Press, London, ch 5, p 139
Spiegel H S, Spiegel D 1987 Trance and treatment. Basic Books, New York

Hypnotic induction and deepening procedures: second approach

INTRODUCTION

Thus far we have focused on procedures and ploys whereby the central purpose is to help the patient or client engage in the experience we have identified as 'trance', and when, for the purpose of therapy, this is an end in itself and less of a means to an end. We are still conceiving of trance in terms of our earlier 'weak' or naturalistic definition and not as a unique altered state of consciousness.

There are many applications of hypnosis in which this experience of inner absorption is, if anything, more a means to an end than an end in itself. In such applications, the principal therapeutic tool is suggestion. That is, the intention is to directly change the patient's problematic behaviours, cognitions, feelings, and so on by the use of suggestion and appropriate accompanying imagery. Moreover, this change has to be permanent and not just for the duration of the hypnotic session, hence the use of such techniques as posthypnotic suggestion, to be described in later chapters. What, then, is the purpose of the induction and deepening procedures?

MAXIMISING THE IMPACT OF SUGGESTION

Consider these suggestions, which might be used during hypnosis for therapeutic purposes:

1. Every time you put a cigarette to your lips you will think of this picture of a diseased lung.
2. Gradually, you are feeling the pain in your arm easing and it is becoming more and more comfortable.

3. As soon as you see the examination paper, you will be as calm as you are feeling now.
4. After your operation, you will feel stronger each day; any discomfort you feel will not really bother you, and you will have little bleeding.
5. From now on, whenever you are standing at the tee, you will execute a perfect swing.

Clearly to maximise the chances of a successful outcome of therapy, we need to maximise the impact and influence of these suggestions. How can this be done? Obviously there are various means. For example, in case 1, the patient's much revered family doctor could 'put the fear of God' in the patient by banging on the table and yelling the command at the top of his voice! Suggestion 2 might be more effective if we simultaneously ask the client to swallow a 'painkilling drug' (actually a placebo). In case 3, the suggestion may be more likely to work at the end of a confidential chat between tutor and student in which the former reassures the latter about progress being made. Suggestion 4 will be particularly effective when delivered by surgeons or anaesthetists in their best bedside manner. Finally, suggestion 5 can be reinforced by a slap on the back by a much-respected coach at the end of a successful training session. Why, then, use hypnosis at all with any of these patients or clients?

The hypnotic induction and hypersuggestibility

The answer to the above question is as follows. According to convention, when you hypnotise a subject, he or she enters a special altered state of consciousness, one property of which is profound hypersuggestibility. Hence, the purpose of the induction and deepening routines: the more deeply the person is hypnotised, the more responsive to suggestion he or she will be. Accordingly, the induction and deepening procedures presented so far ought to be appropriate for a treatment approach that relies heavily on suggestions of change.

Ideas about the correctness or otherwise of the above assertion were addressed in our discussion of theories of hypnosis. More important for present purposes is the issue whether there is any evidence that the hypnotic induction procedures do indeed render the person significantly more responsive to suggestion.

To address this question it is important that the reader understands the following. Even though this working model has very little currency in modern cognitive psychology, it is entirely possible to undertake successful therapy on the assumption that a hypnotic induction renders a person hypersuggestible, say, on the basis that during hypnosis suggestions and posthypnotic suggestions are somehow 'implanted in the person's unconscious mind'. However, we ask the reader to follow our analysis and consider a different paradigm, one that is more consistent with the evidence, albeit mainly from laboratory rather than clinical investigations.

Following a hypnotic induction, there is indeed an increase in measured responsiveness to suggestion. As we have noted in Chapter 3, however, this increase is modest, at least in the context of the psychological laboratory (Kirsch & Braffman 1999).

Now, suppose instead of administering the standard induction and deepening methods, we give subjects a series of instructions. We tell them that we are shortly going to ask them to bring to mind certain ideas and situations and it is most important that they concentrate, using the full powers of their imagination, to create the images, the feelings and the experiences, as vividly as possible. We proceed in this vein for some time and then administer a standard susceptibility scale. Which procedure yields the larger increase in susceptibility scores, these 'task-motivational instructions', as they are called, or the traditional procedures? Actually, they both have more or less the same effect (Barber & Calverley 1962, 1963a, 1963b).

Now, do something more drastic. Replace the standard relaxation induction procedure with its complete opposite! Instead of telling the subjects they are feeling more relaxed, tell them they are feeling more energetic. Say that instead of narrowing their attention on their inner experiences, they are becoming more aware of everything that is happening around them, as though their mind is 'expanding'. In place of a comfortable chair or couch, provide them with an exercise bicycle and have them pedal constantly as you administer your 'alert induction' as it is called. Under such conditions, what happens to their susceptibility scores? They increase overall by the same margin as when a traditional relaxation induction procedure is used (Bányai & Hilgard 1976).

Let us be yet more radical. We dispense altogether with a verbal 'induction' procedure and wheel into the room a gas cylinder containing 'a drug that has a powerful effect on suggestibility'. The subjects inhale the gas, which is actually air, the mask having been 'imbued with a medicinal odour for verisimilitude'. Then they are given suggestions for analgesia. Once more the increase in responsiveness to suggestions is the same after the procedure as it is after a standard hypnotic induction (Baker & Kirsch 1993).

Well, why not, just give the subjects a 'dummy' hypnosis pill? It has already been done! The finding was that for eight different suggestions the same increase in responsiveness was found as for the traditional procedures (Glass & Barber 1961).

DEFINITION OF THE INDUCTION PROCESS IN THE SECOND APPROACH

We emphasise here that these studies have been undertaken in an academic context in which the demands and expectations are different from those in a clinical context. However, we ask you to pause and consider what all of this is telling us about the hypnotic induction in relation to responsiveness to suggestion. Clearly the message is this: the standard induction and deepening process enhances responsiveness to suggestion, not by placing the person in an altered state of consciousness characterised by hypersuggestibility, but by enhancing the motivation, expectancy and commitment of the subjects to deploy their repertoire of cognitive skills to respond to the suggestions that are to follow.

Therefore, another definition of hypnotic induction and deepening is as follows:

A series of instructions and suggestions intended to enhance the subject's responsiveness to the suggestions to follow.

This definition is most relevant to applications of hypnosis that rely heavily on suggestions and images intended to directly alter the habitual behaviours, thoughts, feelings and somatic symptoms of the patient or client. These include the cognitive-behavioural treatment of anxiety disorders such as generalised anxiety disorder and phobia, problems of confidence, performance anxiety, habit problems, including smoking and obesity, and certain other psychological disorders described in later chapters, in which behavioural difficulties are a central feature. Pain and psychosomatic disorders present problems that are covered by both approaches to the hypnotic induction.

In such treatments, the practitioner may adhere to the simple paradigm of 'trance induction' followed by the recitation of direct hypnotic and posthypnotic suggestions. In theory, at least, two important determinants of outcome will be the explicit definition of the medium of treatment as 'hypnotic' and the hypnotic susceptibility of the patient or client. In practice, there will be non-hypnotic determinants that will attenuate the relative contribution of hypnotic susceptibility, which may thus have little influence on outcome. However, susceptibility may still play a significant role for those problems described as 'involuntary' by Wadden & Anderton (1982) as discussed in Chapter 3.

Clearly, rather than adhere to the simple trance model of hypersuggestibility, practitioners should be advised to 'pull out all the stops' and incorporate into their treatment as many techniques and ploys as possible for maximising the impact of their communications and suggestions in the preparation, induction and deepening stages.

The foregoing discussion puts a question mark against the relevance, to the induction and its ultimate purpose, of suggestions of absorption and physical and mental relaxation. However, as we shall see in due course, there are very good reasons for retaining these in many applications of hypnosis.

PRELIMINARIES TO THE SECOND APPROACH

The structure of the hypnotic session for this approach to hypnosis is essentially the same as in the first approach. Likewise, the preparation of the patient, with regard to introducing hypnosis, describing what it is, allaying misconceptions, and so on, will be more or less the same. From then on, however, the two approaches diverge, the emphasis in the first being on absorption, the emphasis in the second approach being on suggestion and suggestibility.

At the beginning of the last chapter, we emphasised the importance of instilling a positive attitude to hypnosis and this may require, in some patients, the dispelling of misgivings and misconceptions. The significance of this is that Spanos and his co-workers (Spanos 1991) have demonstrated that, within limits, the more positive the person's attitude to hypnosis, the more responsive that person will be to hypnotic suggestions.

Another variable that enhances response to suggestion is the person's expectation that he or she is indeed a responsive subject (Kirsch 1991, Spanos 1991). Consequently, it will be useful for patients to be confident that they *are* responsive, however slight this may be. We can capitalise on this in the following manner.

Prior to the induction it is useful, when adopting this approach, to introduce patients to some suggestions that, with the incorporation of certain ploys, most of them will respond to in some way. One guiding principle (which is actually employed in the construction of most susceptibility scales) is the 'foot-in-the-door' effect. That is, one starts off with the easiest suggestions and gradually introduces more demanding ones. A useful way of doing this would be to administer a susceptibility scale such as the Creative Imagination Scale. One problem, however, is that the therapist does not have the required degree of control over the proceedings should the patient prove unresponsive.

A useful starter is a simple ideomotor suggestion. Postural sway may be used but many therapists will have misgivings about the nature of the physical interaction that this entails between them and the patient. Hence we recommend the arm lowering suggestion as described in Chapter 2. Before you begin this, instruct the patient along these lines:

You have probably noticed that when you imagine something, you have some of the experiences that you would have in the real situation. For example, if you imagine something that you are really looking forward to, you feel some of the excitement. Or you might imagine something that you find really amusing and you find yourself smiling or even laughing about it. You might bring to mind an occasion when you were out in bitterly cold weather and you may feel as though you want to shiver. And, like everyone else, you are probably quite good at making yourself feel anxious by imagining something that really worries you. You can use your imagination so well to change the way you are thinking and feeling – sometimes for the good, sometimes for the bad. Right now I want you to imagine this .... .

Administer the arm-lowering suggestion described in Chapter 2. (You are free to choose what you consider an appropriate image for a heavy object.) Now, what happens if the chosen arm fails to move? There is an obvious risk that the patient's confidence and expectations about the effectiveness of hypnosis will be compromised by this lack of response. Here, a tactic stemming from the work of Spanos and his colleagues may be used to good effect. Recall from Chapter 4 that these researchers consider that people do not respond to suggestions when they adopt too passive an attitude. Instead of 'waiting for the response to happen', they should be 'making the response happen'. It is therefore legitimate to instruct the patient to deliberately move the arm, but to try to move it in such a way that it appears to be being pressed down by a heavy weight. We suggest the following instructions:

It's OK to start to move your arm down, but see how much you can do this so that your arm seems to be moving all on its own, pressed down by a heavy book. You will have to concentrate quite hard to do this, but just slowly move your arm down so that it feels like it is being pressed down hard ... that's fine ... keep concentrating ... good.

At the end of this, tell the patient to 'let go of the image and allow your arm and hand to feel perfectly normal again'.

Most people show some response to this suggestion, and again it is important to emphasise to patients how an idea or image can affect the way they feel and behave. In the case of patients with whom you have used the Spanos technique, they will nearly always report at least some success in having the feeling that, at times, the arm seemed to move on its own.

A useful suggestion to follow this with is the 'fruit' imagery described in Chapter 2. Remember to cover all modalities. The patient is to open the eyes at the end and then you can ask about the experiences. It is very important to be positive about *any* response the patient reports (the visual image of the fruit, the feel of the texture of the fruit in the hand, the smell, the taste, and so on). It is very good if the patient reports salivation, as this exemplifies an autonomic response that is clearly triggered by suggestion. Draw the patient's attention to how the ideas and images can affect the way he or she is behaving, thinking and feeling. Most people will report some experience from this exercise. If this is not so in the case of your patient, then this need not be a serious problem. It is useful and true to say to your patient that most people do not respond to *all* suggestions.

You may now proceed to do the 'arms coming together' suggestion described in Chapter 2. Once again, if the patient shows no response, introduce the 'Spanos method', asking the patient to deliberately move the arms together, but create the feeling that they are being drawn together automatically. (It is always a good idea, when giving such an instruction, to say something like, 'You will need to concentrate very carefully for this'. Otherwise the risk is that patients may have the impression that the 'test has failed' and that you are now asking them to do something akin to pretending or cheating.)

If you sense that you have a very suggestible subject, you could do more suggestions, although you do not want to make the process too drawn out. You may administer, for example, a suggestion for hand cooling or glove anaesthesia. You are at liberty to choose imagery that you feel suits the particular patient. One ploy is to ask the subject to raise the hand by flexing the elbow. This may promote a slight cooling effect owing to a change in circulation, which may be amplified by your suggestions. You may test the person's response by gently pinching the backs of both hands for comparison. (We suggest you seek the patient's permission for this.) This may not be necessary, as subjects often report some degree of cooling or numbness without the test. In Chapter 26, we shall discuss ways of potentiating this suggestion in patients who are not responsive to standard imagery.

Another suggestion one may use (in patients who have up to this point been very responsive) is the finger lock challenge. This can be a very convincing demonstration of the effectiveness of suggestion and hence a useful way of building on the patient's expectations for a good response to the treatment to follow. It comes with the risk of a very obvious demonstration of failure should the patient separate the hands with ease. This risk can be mitigated in the following way.

After asking the patient to squeeze the interlocking fingers together as tightly as possible, suggest an appropriate image. The one we recommend is that of the roots of a tree that have become so entangled that they are absolutely impossible to separate. You may now say, 'Now, holding that image and that idea firmly in mind, try to separate the hands'. There is one more trick to incorporate into this technique, but first note this. You have asked your patient to do something which the patient would normally have no difficulty whatsoever in doing, namely separating the two hands. However, the patient has to do this while holding onto an image that would make separation impossible. If the patient is fully committed to doing this, then separating the hands would be inconsistent.

Some subjects will still separate the hands (although this is less likely to happen if your patient has thus far responded well to these suggestions). We therefore advocate (as we do for challenge suggestions in general) that you use an *indirect* suggestion for the attempted hand separation. (Indirect suggestions are discussed in Ch. 10.) In this case, a suitable indirect suggestion may be as follows:

Now, holding that idea and image firmly in mind, you may not be too surprised to find ... how *difficult* it can be ... when you try to pull your hands apart.

The purpose of the pauses here is to create a little suspense on the patient's part and this may enhance the impact of the communication. So, we allow for the possibility that the patient may indeed separate the hands, but, nevertheless (as is very likely under the circumstances), it requires more than the expected effort.

As with the previous suggestions, reinforce any aspect of the patient's response by indicating how an idea or image can automatically affect experience and behaviour.

There are other suggestions you may use in the preparation phase. Chevreul's pendulum is fairly failsafe and many patients are intrigued by it. Some practitioners also show a keenness for arm rigidity; our earlier comments on postural sway apply here. The ones we have mentioned are usually sufficient.

We have spent considerable time discussing this phase of hypnosis in treatment, but, in reality, once you have become practised, it only takes a few minutes and is only usually part of a first session of hypnosis. Always keep in mind the purpose, namely to build up the confidence and expectation of patients in their responsiveness to the hypnotherapeutic procedures to come. You are also gaining a measure of the patient's inherent level of hypnotic susceptibility. Should you discern at this stage that the patient is not very responsive, press on. There is still much to be done and the relationship between susceptibility and outcome is normally not sufficiently robust as to allow you to determine with due confidence whether or not treatment will succeed on the basis of these suggestibility tests alone.

Very occasionally, you will have a patient who gives you the strong impression of overplaying the lack of responsiveness to your suggestions by repeatedly emphasising an inability to respond. This should alert you to the possibility that there are some major problems that perhaps even your patient is not able to acknowledge fully and that make it difficult for this patient to accept treatment. Therapy can tolerate some disparity in the degree of optimism of patient and therapist, but too great a difference does not bode well.

Having thus prepared the patient, you are ready to move on to what may be more formally identified as the hypnotic induction. Say something like:

Now, you've been doing very well and you are ready to experience a hypnotic induction. This is really more suggestions that help you use your imagination so you can feel really relaxed. Remember you are always in control and you stay in touch with my voice. Just allow your eyes to close now.

It is a good idea to spend a minute or so allowing the patient to become used to sitting in the chair listening to you with the eyes closed, so you may use the 'sensory-focusing' procedure described in the last chapter for the first approach to induction. There are several induction methods to choose from; although they still encourage the experience of absorption, they place a much greater emphasis on suggestion and suggestibility than the first approach.

INDUCTION AND DEEPENING METHODS OF THE SECOND APPROACH

Eye-fixation methods

Tell the patient that in a few moments you will ask him to open his eyes again and to raise them up as high as they will go so that he is staring at a point on the ceiling (or the tip of your pencil, in which case you will be standing to the side of the patient, but still able to see his face). Say that as the patient is fixating the point, *inevitably* his eyes will gradually become more and more tired, his eyelids will become heavier and heavier, and gradually his eyes will want to close. When his eyes close, he will feel a sense of relief and relaxation in his eyes that will spread down his face and throughout the whole of his body.

Ask the patient to do this now: 'Open your eyes, and raise them up', etc. Repeat suggestions such as, 'Allow your eyelids to gradually become tired and heavy … heavier and heavier … '. Also suggest that as this is happening, so the rest of his body is feeling comfortable and relaxed.

It is important to observe the rate of blinking. If the person is responsive to this suggestion, then the rate of blinking will increase. Some patients' blinking is characterised by slow, heavy-lidded closing and opening movements, similar to when one is 'nodding off'. Others have more rapid, fluttering movements. Draw the patient's attention to these movements thus:

Notice how your eyes have started to blink more now; how they are feeling heavier and heavier. And as this is happening, you are feeling more and more relaxed.

Time these key words with each blink of the eyes.
When it appears as though the eyes are near to closing, say:

Your eyes are feeling so heavy that they will soon be wanting to close. When your eyes do close, you feel a sense of relief and relaxation that spreads down your face and all the way down your body.

When the eyes close say:

That's fine! Now feel that sense of relief and relaxation spread down from your eyes to your face and down through your body.

Once the eyes close, some patients experience an involuntary flickering of the eyelids. This is a temporary phenomenon but can be a little distracting for the patient, so it is helpful, if this happens, to say:

Notice now how your eyes naturally flicker once they have closed. You will find that as you are relaxing more and more, your eyes will relax completely.

Some patients show only a very gradual, if any, increase in blinking rate, such that, if you were to continue 'to the bitter end', it would take an inordinate length of time for the eyes to close. Indeed, one sometimes reads of cases in which, for example, 'After 20 minutes the patient's eyes closed'. Is there really any point in this? The aim of the exercise is to exploit the patient's responsiveness to the suggestion of eye-heaviness, not to cause the eyes to close because of natural fatigue and discomfort. For this reason, it is sensible to avoid suggestions such as, 'Your eyes will start to prick and burn'.

If, after a minute or so, the patient is not proving responsive, say:

In a little while, your eyes will be ready to close and when they do so you will feel a sense of relief and relaxation all the way down from your eyes, down your face and your body. Before you do that I shall ask you to...

Then administer the suggestions for the eye-roll procedure described in Chapter 6.

A variation of the eye-fixation method is to instruct patients, as they are staring at the fixation spot, to mentally count back in ones, twos, threes, or whatever (depending on their proficiency in arithmetic) from 300. One rationale for this is that it leaves patients with less attentional capacity to reflect on what they are doing. Thus they are more likely to go along with the ideas and suggestions and be more responsive to them.

Eye-fixation with arm lowering

This is an alternative to the simple eye-fixation method. Take the patient's hand, raise it above her head and release it with the instruction 'Keep looking at your hand'. Suggestions are then given that as the patient is staring at her hand, her arm will grow tired and heavy. As this is happening, her eyes too will grow tired and heavy and as her arm gradually falls towards her lap so her eyes will grow heavier and heavier and eventually close when the hand reaches her lap.

Eyes open – eyes closed

This method is recommended as a follow-up to a *successful* eye-fixation induction.

Tell the patient that in a moment you will count from 1 to 10:

As I count from I to I0, at each count you open your eyes and immediately I shall say 'Relax' and your eyes will close again. With each count, the eyes will feel heavier and you will feel more deeply relaxed until, at the count of I0, your eyes will be so very heavy and you will be very relaxed indeed.

Start the first count and intersperse with such suggestions as 'very heavy' and 'very deeply relaxed'. Pace the instructions for opening and closing of the eyes with inhalation and expiration respectively.

A variation of this is to say 'One, two, three … relax'. The patient is to open the eyes at 'one' and to close them at 'relax'. Repeat this until the patient's eyes are almost too heavy to open.

Eye catalepsy

You can follow up a *successful* eye-fixation induction (or eyes open–eyes closed technique) with the suggestion of eye catalepsy. There are variations in the form of the suggestion. Here is one of them that is relatively permissive and indirect (see Ch. 10).

You may have had the experience that your eyes have felt so heavy that it is too much effort to open them. You can allow yourself to have this experience now.

The patient may take this as a cue to try to open the eyes; if not, you can continue with:

In a few moments, I shall count to 3 and at the count of 3, you can be surprised that it can feel like it's too much effort to open your eyes. I − 2 − 3.

Arm-levitation technique

This can be a very convincing technique and there are a variety of ploys for maximising the likelihood of a positive response. The patient is seated comfortably with both hands resting on the lap (or on the arms of the chair if this is more comfortable) with eyes closed. Then ask the patient to make a tight fist with the preferred hand and to press down harder and harder on the leg or chair arm. Then ask the patient to release the fist:

Feel your hand becoming relaxed, loose and cooler again. Your hand may also naturally feel a little lighter, as though it is wanting to move upwards. Notice that as you think about this feeling, you make it happen even more. Just imagine your hand becoming lighter and lighter.

Repeat these suggestions of lightness until you observe any movements, in which case you draw the patient's attention to them by saying, 'Notice how your fingers are starting to move now'.

At some point (though this may prove unnecessary), you can say:

Imagine that in front of you there is a big red balloon filled with helium, with a piece of string hanging down which is wrapped round your wrist. Feel the balloon tugging at your wrist and lifting the arm up.

Keep repeating these suggestions and others (e.g. 'lighter and lighter ... higher and higher ... up and up').

When the arm is moving, it is usually jerky rather than smooth, and you can link the movement with suggestions of increasing relaxation in the usual way.

This is sometimes quite a protracted procedure and if, after a minute or so, the patient's arm shows only a minimum of movement, say, 'I'm allowed to help your arm a little with this one'. Then very gently (allowing the patient to do as much of this unaided) raise the arm by placing your fingers under the patient's or taking a loose hold of the wrist, and, gently lifting, making the suggestions of lightness.

Another ploy for an unresponsive patient is to use the 'Spanos method' as discussed earlier. Say:

Now, in a few moments, I want you to concentrate on your hand and arm and see if you can move your arm in such a way that it seems to you to be moving all on its own. You need to concentrate hard on this. When you're ready, very slowly start to move your arm as though it seems to be moving all on its own.

It should not be of great concern if the arm only moves very slightly, whatever method is used. With a reasonably good response, you may suggest arm catalepsy (see below). Otherwise, after 2 or 3 minutes of this procedure, suggest that the arm is becoming heavy again:

As your arm is feeling heavy again, and as it is gradually falling to your lap, you are becoming more and more relaxed. When your arm reaches your lap, you will be very relaxed indeed.

When concluding this procedure, suggest that all the normal feelings such as heaviness, warmth, and so on have returned to the hand and arm.

Arm catalepsy

If the patient shows a reasonably good response to arm levitation, you may consider suggesting arm catalepsy. When the arm has risen as far as it appears to be going, gently place it in the flexed position with the forearm vertical. As always, for a 'challenge' suggestion, we advocate a permissive and indirect approach, such as:

People often find that when they are doing this, it is very difficult for them to put their arm down.

This may be all that the patient needs to test the suggestion, or you may gently say, 'You might like to try this for yourself'.

Either the patient's arm remains immobile or it does come down, though often with some difficulty. Because of the wording of the question, it is not too much of a problem should the arm come down with little difficulty. Should it remain in the flexed position, proceed as above for concluding the arm-levitation routine.

Eye fixation with arm levitation

You can start the arm levitation with the eyes open, in which case it will be an induction, rather than a deepening routine. One variant is to ask the patient to fixate the hand. Suggest the arm is rising towards the face. As the arm is rising, you suggest that the eyes are becoming heavy and are wanting to close. Suggest that when the hand touches the face, the eyes will close. Also link whatever is happening to suggestions of relaxation. You may also suggest that when the hand touches the face, it will immediately become heavy again and drop down onto the patient's lap; at that moment suggest that the patient will feel very relaxed indeed.

The above routine is probably best reserved for a patient who has shown a good response to your preliminary suggestions.

ADDITIONAL POINTS

Your voice tone when using this approach can, at appropriate times, be more brisk and assertive compared to the calm, soothing tone appropriate for the first approach.

Just as in the previous set of induction and deepening procedures, it is often useful to end up with an imagery technique, such as the ones in the last chapter. Your alerting method will be the same as that described. Prior to alerting emphasis to the patient how well he has done and how on the next and subsequent occasions he will respond more strongly and effectively to the suggestions that are going to help him to overcome the presenting problem.

After alerting, discuss with the patient his experiences as recommended in the last chapter. Also, as previously recommended, ask for a time estimation.

As with the previous approach, there is no need to go through all of these preliminaries and procedures in subsequent sessions of therapy.

FINAL REMARKS ON THE TWO APPROACHES

The two approaches to hypnosis, notably with regard to the choice of induction and deepening methods, are only different to the extent that in the first there is more emphasis on helping the patient experience this state of inner absorption that we have labelled 'trance' and in the second approach there is more emphasis on maximising the patient's responsiveness to suggestion and building up positive expectations of change. Readers will understand that the former approach addresses more the needs of patients who, for example, are troubled by difficult thoughts and emotions that they cannot understand. To such patients, techniques such as arm levitation or eye catalepsy make very little sense. On the other hand, patients keen to change well-ingrained destructive habits need the confidence and expectation that the medium of hypnotic suggestion is going to empower them to achieve such changes. Hence, the second approach is the more appropriate. Of course the difference is only one of emphasis. Induction and deepening routines from both approaches may be combined according to the therapist's judgement.

REFERENCES

Baker S L, Kirsch I 1993 Hypnotic and placebo analgesia: Order effects and the placebo label. Contemporary Hypnosis 10: 117–126
Bányai E I, Hilgard E R 1976 A comparison of active-alert hypnotic induction with traditional relaxation induction. Journal of Abnormal Psychology 85: 218–224
Barber T X, Calverley D S 1962 'Hypnotic' behaviour as a function of task motivation. Journal of Psychology 54: 363–389
Barber T X, Calverley D S 1963a The relative effectiveness of task motivating instructions and trance induction procedure in the production of 'hypnotic like' behavior. Journal of Nervous and Mental Disease 137: 107–116
Barber T X, Calverley D S 1963b Toward a theory of hypnotic behavior: Effects on suggestibility of task motivating instructions and attitudes toward hypnosis. Journal of Abnormal and Social Psychology 67: 557–565
Glass L B, Barber T X 1961 A note on hypnotic behavior, the definition of the situation, and the placebo-effect. Journal of Nervous and Mental Disease 132: 539–541
Kirsch I 1991 The social learning theory of hypnosis. In: Lynn S J, Rhue J W (eds) Theories of hypnosis: Current models and perspectives. Guilford Press, New York, ch 14, p 439
Kirsch I, Braffman W 1999 Correlates of hypnotisability: The first empirical study. Contemporary Hypnosis 16: 224–230
Spanos N 1991 A sociocognitive approach to hypnosis. In: Lynn S J, Rhue J W (eds) Theories of hypnosis: Current models and perspectives. Guilford Press, New York, ch 11, p 324
Wadden T A, Anderton C H 1982 The clinical use of hypnosis. Psychological Bulletin 91: 215–243

8

Further ethical matters and precautions during the preparation phase of hypnosis

INTRODUCTION

Ethical matters and issues of risk and safety are raised at apposite points in this book and we have already touched upon these in Chapter 5. Although at times they concern eventualities that are quite rare in clinical practice, remember that sometimes it only takes one unfortunate and avoidable event in a lifetime's work to have a lasting effect on one's reputation and personal fulfilment in one's chosen profession.

USING THE TERM 'HYPNOSIS'

A question that not uncommonly arises for some practitioners is whether one should always use the term 'hypnosis' with the patient to describe what one is doing. One complicating factor is that hypnotic procedures are very similar to other methods used in psychological therapy. Examples are various relaxation and self-regulation techniques such as progressive muscular relaxation, meditation and autogenic training, covert systematic desensitisation, and guided affective imagery. Indeed, two practitioners may employ virtually the same procedures, one using the designation 'hypnosis', the other denying that hypnosis is being used and calling the procedure 'relaxation', 'meditation', or whatever. There are, in fact, no clear dividing lines between any of these methods and hypnosis for the practitioner who uses both.

Having learned formal procedures of hypnosis, some practitioners may find that on occasions the methods can be introduced in an informal way at certain very apposite moments during treatment. For example, a dentist who is about to start working on a patient, or a physician on the point of conducting a difficult physical examination, may suddenly notice that the patient is unduly anxious. Suppose that the practitioner suggests that the patient might feel more relaxed if she closes her eyes, breathes comfortably and just goes off in the imagination 'to some place where you would rather be now, where you can feel safe … calm … comfortable … where nothing need bother you … etc.' Is the practitioner 'doing hypnosis' and should the practitioner explicitly tell the patient that this is so?

If the answer to both of these questions is 'Yes', then the practitioner must go through the whole business of describing what hypnosis is and is not, reassuring the patient, dispelling misconceptions, and so on. Not only may the practitioner not have the time to do this, but the psychological moment when the relaxation suggestions may be most effective has thus been lost.

On the other hand, what happens if the practitioner goes ahead without introducing the method as 'hypnosis' and afterwards the patient says, 'Excuse me, but were you using hypnosis on me then?' Some people do not like the idea of their 'being hypnotised'; perhaps they have had a bad experience with hypnosis, or they have, as very occasionally happens, an objection on religious grounds. How is the practitioner to reply? Also, in some countries there may be legal repercussions about using hypnosis with patients.

There is no satisfactory answer to this but our recommendation is that where procedures are used that only involve suggestions of physical and mental relaxation, relaxed breathing and pleasant imagery (characteristic of the first approach to hypnosis), practitioners are justified in using the term 'relaxation' if they so wish. When the procedures entail suggestions of more unusual ideomotor responses such as eye heaviness and arm levitation, perceptual changes such as numbness and hallucinatory phenomena, catalepsy of the eyes, arm, etc., age regression, and posthypnotic suggestion, then practitioners should make it clear that hypnosis is being used.

THE USE OF A CHAPERONE

There is a question about whether there are occasions where it is advisable to have a third person, or chaperone, present. This arises because of the belief that when using hypnosis there is a slight risk of a false accusation of improper conduct, which, so far as we know, is always made against male practitioners. This risk is difficult to quantify, as it is well established that doctors, other health service personnel, and psychotherapists have sometimes behaved improperly and have even indecently assaulted their patients and clients. There may, however, be occasions when a patient deliberately makes a false accusation against a practitioner. Also, in theory at least, it is possible that a client may fantasise an indecent assault and confuse fantasy with reality.

Most psychotherapists would probably find it unacceptable to have a chaperone present, even when hypnosis is being undertaken. The mere presence of a third person implies that neither the therapist nor the client is to be trusted and clearly one cannot undertake psychotherapy on that basis.

Also, a client may feel inhibited by the presence of a third person (particularly if that person is a friend). We have, however, heard of instances where a client has insisted on bringing a chaperone and some therapists do feel able to work with this.

Another solution would be to videotape the session, but this would have to be with the knowledge and agreement of the client. Audiotaping the session is a partial solution. In both of these cases, however, there is still the implication of less than 100% trust between therapist and client.

Our impression is that most of the time, most therapists are opposed to the idea of having a chaperone present as a requirement when they are using hypnosis. Some feel that it is advisable, however, for a male therapist to have a chaperone present if the therapy concerns sexual abuse. A key factor appears to be the fact that when using hypnosis, the client's eyes are closed and he or she may be asked to recall incidents from childhood; it is possible that the boundaries between what is actually happening and what the client is imagining become blurred, for example, if the client experiences a vivid 'flashback experience' or abreaction.

It is considered advisable that when a doctor is using hypnosis to facilitate a physical examination, then a chaperone should be present. This may be a requirement anyway, even if hypnosis is not being used. In Britain, also, it is a rule that dentists are always accompanied by a third person, whether hypnosis is used or not. Hartland (1974) describes the case of an obstetrician who was accused by a patient of indecent assault during an intimate examination that was facilitated by the use of hypnosis. The case went to court and the obstetrician was found not guilty. Presumably we have here an actual instance of a false accusation.

If a practitioner suspects that at the conclusion of a session a patient or client may falsely make an accusation of improper conduct, then the practitioner should speak to a professional colleague as soon as possible and describe what happened, and also make a written account of the same.

The matter of the use of a chaperone with children is discussed in Chapter 14.

REFERENCE

Hartland J 1974 An alleged case of criminal assault upon a married woman under hypnosis. American Journal of Clinical Hypnosis 16: 188–198

9

Self-hypnosis

INTRODUCTION

Whichever of the two approaches to hypnosis is adopted, in many of the therapeutic applications it is considered advantageous for patients, in their own time, to rehearse on a regular basis the induction and deepening procedures used in therapy. Not only does this have the effect of reinforcing some of the therapeutic work undertaken in the clinic, but it also encourages a sense of independence and empowerment on the patient's part. The patient is not simply a passive recipient of the treatment dispensed by the all-knowing therapist.

In its simplest and most common form, self-hypnosis is a meditation procedure based on the induction, deepening and alerting routine that has been found to be most suitable for the patient. When a session of hypnosis is confined to these three phases, it is often termed 'neutral hypnosis', no therapy or suggestions specific to the patient's problems being undertaken. Nevertheless, the regular, self-directed practice of 'neutral hypnosis', as with other forms of relaxation and self-regulation, such as meditation, autogenic training and biofeedback, itself has therapeutic benefits. That is, around 15 to 20 minutes of 'time out' spent in this way have been shown to reduce the adverse effects of daily stress (Benson 1975).

WHICH PROCEDURES?

Some practitioners encourage their patients to engage in self-hypnosis after the first session of heterohypnosis. However, it makes sense to delay self-hypnosis until you are sure that the induction and deepening procedures that you have selected are the most suitable for your patient and that he or she is sufficiently accustomed to experiencing hypnosis.

It also makes sense to avoid, for the purposes of teaching self-hypnosis, inductions that utilise overt ideomotor actions. The disadvantage of these methods is that your patient may wish to use a brief self-hypnosis procedure in a public situation such as in the dentist's waiting room or on a bus. A person using an arm-levitation procedure in those situations would become an object of curiosity amongst those present! (Spiegel & Spiegel (1987) teach a standard self-hypnosis routine using an eye-roll induction and an arm levitation that is disguised as a brushing action of the hand against the side of the head.)

Common procedures to use are characterised by those recommended in Chapter 6 for treatment approaches based on the 'trance' concept of hypnosis, and imagery techniques are a natural choice.

A typical standard routine may begin with the Spiegel eye-roll, and eye-closure on a prolonged outward breath. If nothing else, this formalises for the patient the beginning of self-hypnosis. This may be followed by a relaxed breathing technique (coupled with a cue word or symbolic image on the outward breath) and then a progressive relaxation procedure, which should not be too lengthy. Finally, the 'special place' image is a good choice. It is recommended that patients alert themselves by the counting method (from 1 to 5 or the reverse, depending on preference) followed by a few deep breaths and stretching.

TEACHING SELF-HYPNOSIS

The simplest way to teach self-hypnosis is to take the patient through the chosen induction and deepening routine and then make the following suggestions:

Whenever you wish to use hypnosis (or *relaxation*) for yourself, when it is convenient and safe to do so, all you need do is find a comfortable place where you can sit or lie down, close your eyes and consciously relax your body.

At this point, you remind the patient of the routine you have chosen, making liberal use of suggestions that the patient will relax easily, quickly and deeply, and be fully in control.

Then give the following instructions:

You may remain in this relaxed state as long as you wish, but whenever you want to alert yourself again and open your eyes, just count down to yourself from 5 to 1, preparing to open your eyes at the count of 1, and when you open your eyes, you will feel alert, fully oriented, and ready to carry on with the rest of the day, feeling refreshed and recharged.

Also, if at any time you need to open your eyes and take immediate action – say, someone calls you or there is a knock on the door or the telephone rings – you will open your eyes immediately, be fully alert and ready to take the appropriate action.

When teaching self-hypnosis, also give some general positive suggestions such as:

Each time you use your self-hypnosis, you will find yourself becoming more relaxed and calm in everyday situations – not *just* when you're sitting down relaxing but also when you're up and about, even in those situations in which you feel tense and apprehensive. You will find you are able to *control* those feelings . . . . You control *them; they* don't control *you.*

After you have alerted the patient, he or she may then practise the self-hypnosis routine in your presence, with plenty of ongoing positive feedback from you ('Good ... that's fine ... very relaxed ... etc.').

THE PROBLEM OF 'FINDING THE RIGHT TIME'

A good time to do self-hypnosis may be in anticipation of those times or events in the day when one knows one becomes unduly tense. As a rule, it is best not to use self-hypnosis when one is sleepy, as the aim is usually waking relaxation (unless the patient finds that 'having a nap' is the best way of unwinding). Rossi (1982) suggests that there are natural periods in the day, coinciding with the 'rest' phase of the biological 'basic rest–activity cycle', when it is most appropriate to do one's self-hypnosis. Many people, for example, may find the period after the midday meal coincides with one of these phases. Indeed, there is some evidence that hypnotic responsiveness may vary with this cycle (Aldrich & Bernstein 1987).

All this may be hypothetical, as it has to be acknowledged that as a general rule people find it difficult to commit themselves to regular sessions of self-hypnosis, and some research on relaxation tapes suggests that patients may overstate the number of sessions they practise, perhaps to please their therapist (Hoelscher & Lichstein 1984, Hoelscher et al 1986). Some patients may have difficulty finding a time when they are on their own and not likely to be interrupted. Some may leave their self-hypnosis until bedtime; this is not a good idea unless the problem is insomnia. Many feel guilty about 'doing nothing'. Some patients are disappointed with the experience of self-hypnosis and say that they 'do not go as deep' on their own as with their therapist.

The same problems have been reported in the meditation literature and some authorities have recommended a series of 'mini-meditations' throughout the day rather than just one full-length session each day (Carrington 1993). It may be easier and still very useful, therefore, for patients to do their self-hypnosis along these lines.

For example, using the standard self-hypnosis routine outlined earlier, you may suggest that the patient can use all three stages or select just one or two of them depending on the situation. A quick eye-roll and eye-closure and a few moments relaxing the breathing (perhaps with an appropriate affirmation or self-suggestion) need only take a couple of minutes and may be a good way of calming down, forestalling a more acute stressful reaction, and 'getting back in control'. With a few more minutes at the patient's disposal, the progressive relaxation method may be added, or the 'special place' technique.

PURPOSES OF SELF-HYPNOSIS

The following are common reasons for teaching your patient self-hypnosis. They will be taken up again in the chapters on specific applications of hypnosis.

1. A daily period of simple relaxation (15–20 minutes) has been shown to significantly reduce stress indices (Benson 1975).
2. Self-hypnosis can be used when a person becomes aware that stress levels are increasing and there is a need to 'regain control'. It has been demonstrated to be useful in this way (and in 1) with problems such as asthma, migraine, irritable bowel syndrome and panic disorder. It may be used to wind down in preparation for sleep by patients with sleep-onset insomnia.
3. Self-hypnosis can be used as a way of rehearsing affirmations – for example, the goals and reasons for abstaining from smoking or for eating sensibly (such as 'tobacco is a poison' or 'I will eat only what my body requires'), or imagining the results of successful abstention or sensible eating (wearing favourite clothes again, having the money to spend on a desired purchase, etc.). This assists in maintaining motivation and preventing relapse.
4. It can be used to practise anxiety management, anger management and other self-control procedures, and to rehearse in imagination coping with future difficult situations.
5. It may be useful in helping patients cope with the pain and discomfort of certain illnesses.
6. It is useful as a preparation for learning, as being mentally and physically relaxed and focused facilitates learning.
7. It may help the person become more attuned to inner experiences – emotions, memories, fantasies, and so on.

THE USE OF TAPED INSTRUCTIONS

Sometimes it is useful to put the procedures on tape for the patient, particularly if they are complicated, along with additional instructions such as rehearsal of coping strategies. Indeed, patients sometimes request this. Although patients do value listening to the instructions, they may come to rely on the tape and not learn much from it. Also the instructions may need to be modified as the therapy progresses. Some authorities do not regard taped hypnosis as true self-hypnosis.

If you do provide your patients with a tape, always emphasise that it is to enable them to learn the procedures for themselves so they can use them in everyday life *without* the tape.

REFERENCES

Aldrich K J, Bernstein D A 1987 The effect of time of day on hypnotisability. International Journal of Clinical and Experimental Hypnosis 35: 141–145

Benson H 1975 The relaxation response. William Morrow, New York

Carrington P 1993 Modern forms of meditation. In: Lehrer P M, Woolfolk R L (eds) Principles and practice of stress management, 2nd edn. Guilford Press, London, ch 5, p 139

Hoelscher T L, Lichstein K L 1984 Objective versus subjective assessment of relaxation compliance among anxious individuals. Behaviour Research and Therapy 22: 187–193

Hoelscher T L, Rosenthal T L, Lichstein K L 1986 Home relaxation practice in hypertension treatment: Objective assessment and compliance induction. Journal of Consulting and Clinical Psychology 54: 217–221

Rossi E R 1982 Hypnosis and ultradian cycles: A new state(s) theory of hypnosis? American Journal of Clinical Hypnosis 25: 31–32

Spiegel H S, Spiegel D 1987 Trance and treatment. Basic Books, New York

10

Variations in style: permissive, indirect and alert approaches

INTRODUCTION

Having explained the traditional direct methods, we now introduce readers to three ways of varying the style and content of hypnotic suggestions. With practical experience, readers will be able to incorporate these ideas into their work according to their own personal style and approach.

AUTHORITARIAN VERSUS PERMISSIVE SUGGESTIONS

In the past, hypnotic induction procedures and suggestions were given in a very direct and authoritarian manner. This was probably based on the premise that somehow the hypnotist is directly in control of the subject's mental faculties, and that the hypnotist's prestige and 'personal magnetism' are essential to effective hypnosis (compare with Svengali in Georges du Maurier's 1894 novel, *Trilby*).

A dramatic example of an authoritarian suggestion is the command 'Go to sleep!' delivered forcefully by the hypnotist while staring into the subject's eyes. More typical examples nowadays are: 'You are feeling deeply relaxed'; 'Your arm will float up in the air'; 'Your hand is feeling cold and numb'; and 'You cannot open your eyes'.

It is now recognised that the idea that effective hypnosis depends on the power and prestige of the hypnotist is erroneous, and in treatment generally, and psychotherapy in particular, the trend is for a more equitable relationship between practitioner and patient or client. Moreover, there is an (accurate) insistence now that hypnosis is something subjects do for themselves, rather than something the hypnotist does *to* the subject. Consequently, there is a preference for more 'permissively worded' suggestions. Examples (corresponding to the authoritarian suggestions given in the previous paragraph) are: 'Allow yourself to relax at your own pace';

'Your arm may become so light that it lifts off your lap'; 'As you imagine the ice-cold water, you may notice that your hand starts to feel a little cold and numb'; and 'You can allow your eyes to become so heavy that they won't want to open for a while'.

Apart from the reasons cited earlier, one obvious advantage of permissive suggestions is that, should the patient not respond, the authority and credibility of the hypnotist are not as seriously compromised as could be the case with authoritarian suggestions. However, the available evidence from controlled experiments does not allow us to claim that one approach is more effective overall than the other (Spinhoven et al 1988).

Most practitioners appear to favour permissive suggestions but we may speculate that there are circumstances when the authoritarian approach is more appropriate. The personal preference of the hypnotist is not an irrelevant consideration: patients may detect when their therapist feels uncomfortable with the method being used and this could damage their confidence in the treatment. Some patients will prefer a practitioner 'of the old school'; for example, they may maintain the traditional position of deference towards their doctor, and want and expect the doctor to tell them exactly what they are to do. Some situations may call for a very direct, 'no nonsense' approach, for instance an acute emergency or a dental treatment where the patient literally wants the doctor or dentist to 'take over'. In such a case, the patient may be very receptive to firm authoritarian suggestions rather than what might appear to be 'beating about the bush' on the part of the practitioner.

DIRECT VERSUS INDIRECT SUGGESTIONS

Indirect methods have been popularised in recent years by the followers of the American psychiatrist and psychologist Milton Erickson (1901–1980). In Chapter 17, we present a summary of the Ericksonian approach to psychotherapy. At the level of the present discussion, we shall confine ourselves to the business of administering hypnotic suggestions.

The rationale of the indirect approach to suggestion

Using the indirect approach, the hypnotist does not directly state what response is required – for example, by saying, 'Your hand will feel light and rise in the air'. Instead, the hypnotist presents the idea of the response in an implicit or covert manner. The effect of this is often that the response that is the sole focus of the suggestion in its direct form becomes, in the indirect form, secondary to some other focus. For example, instead of saying, 'Your right arm is feeling lighter', one might say, 'I wonder which arm is feeling lighter – the left … or the right?' Or one could say, 'Will your arm start to feel lighter now … or later?' With the subject's focus of attention displaced from the immediate idea of the experience or response – the arm's becoming lighter and moving all by itself – the opportunity arises for him or her to create the intended effect in an unconscious manner, using previous learning experiences. Contrast this with the very explicit way in which the direct method instructs the subject – 'Imagine a helium-filled balloon that is pulling at your wrist'.

This approach is often described as 'naturalistic' because it is assumed that hypnotic phenomena are continuous with everyday experiences. Indeed, the matter of the arm's lifting without apparent conscious effort is an everyday occurrence, likewise not noticing a pain, seeing something that is not there, not seeing something that is right in front of one, recalling a past event so vividly that it seems real, failing to recall something one has only just been told or even done, and so on.

In summary, it is assumed that by giving the suggestions in a covert way, we are tapping into the subject's existing repertoire of previous experiences and learning to achieve the intended response, whereas a direct suggestion limits the subject to immediately available, or 'conscious' resources. Conscious resources, though necessary and useful, are more limited than unconscious resources.

Also, from a slightly different standpoint, we may say that many indirect suggestions put more responsibility on the subjects to create for themselves the experiences that we are helping them to access. For example, in an ego-strengthening routine, we may give the direct suggestion, in a suitable convincing manner, 'You have reached the top of the mountain and are experiencing a wonderful sense of achievement and exhilaration'. This is fine, but you don't necessarily have to work so hard to help patients feel this; it is better that you help patients to create the experience for themselves. One way is to use an indirect form: 'Now you are reaching the top of the mountain, I wonder what words will come into your mind to describe the good feelings that you are about to experience'.

The concept of trance in the indirect approach

The Ericksonian approach to 'trance' is also a 'naturalistic' one. The hypnotic trance is continuous with everyday trance occurrences – times when we are deeply involved in some experience. This is similar to the concept of 'trance' that we described in Chapter 2. However, although in Ericksonian terms trance and suggestion are everyday experiences, hypnosis is still conceived of as an altered state of consciousness in a stronger sense than that adopted by the present authors.

Apart from the more obvious examples of naturally occurring trances, such as day-dreaming and being engrossed in some thrilling music, we may cite periods of surprise, shock, anticipation, suspense, confusion, inspiration, and insight, when our customary way of looking and thinking about things has the opportunity to make a sudden shift. Thus, Ericksonians speak of the potential of hypnosis to assist clients in 'suspending their habitual frame of reference', notably with regard to their presenting problem. Indeed, it appears that much of Erickson's psychotherapeutic work – hypnotic and non-hypnotic – can be viewed as his endeavouring to assist the client in this respect, often by his adopting quite innovative, not to say wily, strategies (see Ch. 17).

The scope of this book puts a limit on how much presentation we can give to Ericksonian hypnosis and indirect approaches generally. Our advice to newcomers to clinical hypnosis is to master the direct methods first, then investigate the use of indirect methods by introducing them into their routine hypnotic work. For the moment, we shall familiarise readers (or those readers who are new to this approach) with some ways of presenting suggestions in the indirect form. Our presentation is thus necessarily limited and selective and may be idiosyncratic in parts.

Styles of indirect suggestion

In most of these, the key suggestion is hidden or implied within a more complex statement. There is considerable overlap in many of the examples given to illustrate different styles.

Permissiveness

Some permissive styles of suggestion are also indirect, such as: 'Allow your arm to become as heavy as it wants to'.

Embedded suggestions

We have already encountered this technique in earlier chapters. The suggestion is contained within a statement and the key words are spoken in a subtly different tone from the rest of the communication. For example: 'You may have noticed that when ... *you are feeling relaxed ... your limbs feel heavy and warm'*. The suggestions, given in italics, are spoken in a softer tone and are separated by very slight pauses. Another recommendation is that suggestions of relaxation and calmness are given as the client is breathing out.

Creating (the illusion of) choice or permission

This form of suggestion is sometimes referred to as a 'bind' or, where the response alternatives are deemed to be unconscious, a 'double bind' (see Erickson et al 1976 and Erickson & Rossi 1979 for a more thorough exposition). The therapist offers the subject a choice of responding, but all possibilities imply the intended response. For example:

Your eyes may start to close now or not for a little while.
  Do you want to relax in this chair or that one? (Answered 'consciously'.)
  Will your left hand or your right hand lift first, or will they lift together?
(Answered 'unconsciously'.)

Indirect implications using the negative

In a similar way to the above, the suggestion is given that something will
not happen at a particular moment, with the implication that it *will* happen
at some other time. For example, in an arm-levitation induction, instead of
directly suggesting that the subject's eyes will be fully closed when the
hand touches the face, one might say:

Your eyes won't be fully closed *before* your hand touches your face.
(Implying that they *will* close fully when the hand touches the face.)

  Similarly:

You won't be deeply relaxed before you are thinking of a place you'd like to be
right now.
  Your hand will not come to rest back on your lap before you have had
enough time to do some useful work on your problem.

Paradoxes

Paradoxical suggestions are similar to the above in that they often use the
negative; they appear to suggest to the subject the opposite response to that
required, but the latter is implied in the wording. For example:

Parts of you may not be as relaxed as other parts.
  Don't go into your trance just yet.
  Make sure that you don't relax too quickly.
  Your eyes may not become heavy enough for them to close completely on
their own.
  Try to stop your hands being drawn together too quickly.

Open-ended suggestions

Rather than describe for the subject a particular experience, the therapist
simply asks the subject to observe what experiences are present at the
time. For example, in the case of the suggestion of glove anaesthesia or arm
levitation, rather than say, 'Your hand is feeling cold and numb (or light)',

the therapist may say:

Notice the different kinds of sensations in your hands.

Here, the (reasonable) implication is that the subject is experiencing different sensations in the hands. The therapist might then go on to say:

You may observe that one type of sensation is more noticeable ... or less noticeable ... than another.

At some point, the therapist may ask what the subject is experiencing and then utilise that sensation to introduce the idea of the desired response. For example, if the subject reports a heavy feeling and the desired response is numbness, suggestions of the heavy feeling changing into a cold, numb feeling may be offered.

Offering a range of alternatives or dichotomies (or covering all possibilities)

This is similar to the above. It is a 'fail-safe' type of suggestion and may be appropriate for less responsive subjects. For example:

Your hands may feel warm ... or heavy ... or comfortable ... or just relaxed.
Your hand may become so light that it will float off your lap ... or it may be so heavy and relaxed that it remains there.

Reference to the subject's experiences from everyday life

Consistent with the earlier mentioned notion that the perceptual and experiential changes that are targeted by suggestions are all encountered naturally, one can introduce a suggestion by first referring to a relevant life experience. One can preface this kind of suggestion with the phrase: 'You have probably had the experience of ...' For example:

... carrying something so heavy that your arm floats up when you let go. (Arm levitation)
... not noticing you have a pain because you are so absorbed in something that is so interesting. (Pain relief)
... when *your eyes feel so heavy and tired* that *they just don't want to open.* (Eye catalepsy)
... coming into the warmth of your home on a cold, frosty day and *your hands feel warm and glowing.* (Hand warming)
... when someone tells you something and you just put it right out of your mind. (Amnesia)

Reference to other people's experiences of hypnosis

For example:

It's surprising how many people find it so hard to move their arm from that position. (Arm catalepsy)
　　Some people, when they relax, feel very heavy, but some have a light, floating feeling. Some people feel warm, and others might have a cool sensation somewhere. Just notice how you experience your relaxation.

As with many of these suggestions, it is important to pause at the appropriate moments to allow the subject's own response to the suggestion to develop.

Creating suspense or uncertainty about what will happen and when

With many indirect styles, the subject is placed in the position of waiting for a response to happen. On this basis, one may argue that the suggestions themselves have 'trance-inducing' properties in the weak sense of the term, and that the response is determined more at an unconscious level than when a direct suggestion is made. For example:

You may not notice a light feeling in your hand before you are aware of a tingling sensation.

Explicit use of suspense or uncertainty may be made by prefacing the suggestion with the following kinds of phrases:

I wonder (if, when, what ...) ... (e.g. ... when you will start to have a numb feeling in your hand).
　　I don't know ... (e.g. ... if your arm will feel so light it will move from your lap).
　　I don't know if you know ... (e.g. ... what that pleasant memory might be).
　　You may not know ... (e.g. ... how deeply you are going to relax today).
　　I wonder how surprised you'll be when ... (e.g. ... your arm starts to move).

Questions

Indirection and suspense may simply be conveyed and elicited by framing the suggestion in the form of a question. For example:

Which sensations do you notice first?
　　Does one of your hands feel a little heavier than the other?
　　Do your eyes want to close now or later?

Confusion

We earlier stated that one may think of confusion as a naturally occurring trance experience. When we are confused, we focus on wherever the confusion lies and try to grasp at anything that seems to make sense. Erickson (Erickson et al 1976) exploited this by deliberately communicating to the subject in a confusing manner, thus encouraging the subject to attend more closely and be more receptive to any statement that made sense. Thus, after confusing the subject, one can slip in the key suggestion in the direct form. For example, a suggestion for age regression may begin:

As you are relaxing ... maybe now ... maybe not quite now ... you can be thinking about today ... and about how today is yesterday when it is tomorrow ... and when today *is* tomorrow. ... But today was tomorrow yesterday ... and this week was next week last week ... and if this year is next year, then *you are now back to last year* ... .

The confusion method is regarded as useful for patients who tend to analyse the hypnotist's suggestions rather than 'go with the flow', and therefore prove resistant to more conventional methods.

The conversational approach

Many of the above techniques can be expanded into an actual induction that, when written down, resembles more an ordinary conversation about hypnosis. This can be useful as a preparation for hypnosis in which the trance experience is emphasised (first approach). The therapist describes to the patient what hypnosis is like, reminds the patient of relevant trance experiences in everyday life (e.g. reading a book or listening to music), describes other people's experience of hypnosis, and so on. All the time, the therapist is using embedded suggestions as above, gradually slowing the pace of the delivery and softening the voice tone, and subtly leading and following the subject's natural inclination to relax and adopt a more attentive and receptive mental set. Some suspense and confusion may be strategically introduced. For example:

I don't know, and I don't know whether you know, or whether you are beginning to wonder, and I am wondering to, just how ... *you are going to experience hypnosis* ... .

Finally, the therapist might introduce into the conversation the 'special place' technique described in Chapter 6. This can be done along the following lines, with suitable pauses:

One of the best ways to experience hypnosis is to *take yourself in your imagination to somewhere where you know you feel safe and relaxed.* A very special place where you can go to in your imagination whenever you want to. It may be a place you've only been to once, maybe on a holiday. Or a place you go to regularly. It can be outdoors, or indoors. You might be on your own or with others. You might be doing something active, or just sitting or lying around. It doesn't have to be a *real* place. It can be just a fantasy, or a combination of both.

Then one can give the indirect suggestion:

Either now or in a little while you may find it easier to *bring such a scene to mind* by allowing your *eyes to close.*

The 'Yes' set

This is not an indirect method but, like the confusion and conversational technique, it illustrates the idea of the trance as a naturally occurring state of receptiveness to suggestion. In its simplest form, the therapist asks the patient a series of rhetorical questions to which the patient is certain to respond by saying 'Yes'. For example:

Therapist	You have come to me today with your problem.
Patient	Yes.
Therapist	And it's been a really difficult time for you.
Patient	Yes.
Therapist	And you want me to help you overcome this problem.
Patient	Yes please.
Therapist	And you agree that it would be really great if you could ... *stop worrying about these things. ...*
Patient	Oh yes!
Therapist	And ... *just learn how to relax* (softening the tone).
Patient	Yes indeed.
Therapist	And do you want to ... *relax right now?*
Patient	Mmm.
Therapist	With *your eyes gently closing ... .*

Therapeutic metaphors and stories

The use of metaphors and stories is another key aspect of the Ericksonian approach to therapeutic communication. In Chapter 13, we provide a brief introduction to this and discuss its application with children in Chapter 14.

Verdict on indirect suggestion

We have already discussed the supposed theoretical advantages of the indirect approach. One practical advantage that is fairly apparent is that, as with permissively worded suggestions but probably even more so, indirect suggestions offer the subject a wider scope for responding, the business of 'passing' or 'failing' being much less clear-cut. We have seen in Chapter 7 that this is especially useful for 'challenge' suggestions.

Nevertheless, and in spite of some rather sensational claims, systematic research on indirect suggestion has not indicated that it is of much consequence to the effectiveness of hypnosis (e.g. Groth-Marnet & Mitchell 1998, Lynn et al 1988). It was originally hypothesised that those subjects who score low on scales using direct suggestions will respond better to indirect suggestions, on the rather vague assumption that 'they bypass the critical faculties' and, for this reason, may be particular effective for resistant subjects. Research on the above has yielded mixed results (Fricton & Roth 1985, Hart 1994, Van Gorp et al 1985).

A reasonable criticism of this research is that, of necessity, such studies have used standard scripts for administering the direct and indirect suggestions. With indirect suggestion, the timing of the subject's response is often uncertain, and appropriate use has to be made of pauses in the delivery. Also, with indirect suggestions in particular, it is important to match them with the apparent readiness of the subject to respond. Ericksonians are strong advocates of the close observation of the client's non-verbal behaviour, particularly with reference to the 'signs of trance' or state of attentiveness and receptiveness to suggestion.

Let us explore this matter a little further. Suppose one begins a session of hypnosis with the indirect suggestion 'Do you want to relax with your eyes open or closed?' Is this really likely to be any more effective than simply telling the person to relax? To answer this, let us take a similar, everyday example. Suppose that you say to a child, 'Go to bed now!' Not uncommonly, the child will resist this instruction, so you might try an indirect approach. You say, for instance, 'Are you going to take Teddy or Snoopy to bed with you now?' Well, unfortunately, children are not so easily fooled!

What you must first do is help the child become more *receptive* to the idea of going to bed. Perhaps you could tell a little story about how Teddy and Snoopy once went for a walk and they became lost. It grew very dark and they became very frightened. Eventually somebody told them the right way home and when they arrived they were very tired and ready for bed. You tell the child this story in such a way as to gain his or her full attention (or, if you like, the child goes into a 'naturalistic trance') and at the end of the story you are ready to introduce your indirect suggestion 'And are you going to take Snoopy or Teddy to bed with you now?' Is not the child now more ready to respond positively?

Now, let us go back to the earlier example. Before you give the choice of relaxing with eyes open or closed, first you use the conversational method to hold the subject's attention, by talking about how *pleasant* an experience hypnosis is, how much the subject will *enjoy* the sense of being *very*

relaxed ..., and so on. When you can see that the person is in a state of positive anticipation ('trance'), *then* is the moment to give your indirect suggestion: 'Now, would you like to relax with your eyes open or closed?'

For this reason, presenting indirect suggestions in a rigid and standardised form, as in the experiments cited, may result in a considerable loss of
impact. Another reason why this may happen is as follows. If you study the
above examples of different styles of indirect suggestion, it seems that
many of them are designed to create a sense of expectancy or suspense that
something is going to happen (but it is not certain exactly what). So we have
again what might be called a 'naturalistic trance' experience. We might
even speak of 'mini-trances' that occur in everyday communication. For
example, when we have something important to tell someone, in order to
prepare the person to be receptive and to maximise the impact of the statement we say: 'Guess what?'; 'You're not going to believe this'; 'Have you
heard the latest?'; 'You might be surprised to know ...', and so on.

So, this may be one basis for predicting that indirect suggestions such as
'I wonder which hand will start to feel lighter first?' might be more effective
than a direct suggestion, such as 'Your right hand is feeling lighter'. But
again the question of timing is important and the subject also needs time to
observe the outcome of the suggestion. Again, suggestions that are presented in a standardised manner cannot take this into account.

ALERT METHODS

Traditional methods of hypnotic induction emphasise relaxation, tiredness,
heaviness, restriction of attention, and even drowsiness and sleepiness.
Alert methods of induction, on the other hand, use suggestions of wakefulness and mental alertness, expanded awareness, increased energy, and
greater clarity of mind. The imagery used is also compatible with such
experiences, as ascending a staircase (rather than descending), climbing a
mountain, flying and running.

Advocates of alert methods point out that there are many practices that
are regarded as trance-inducing that entail great energy and activity on the
person's part (e.g. tribal dances and certain meditative procedures, exemplified by the whirling dervishes). Some laboratory work on this theme was
reported by Ludwig & Lyle (1964).

For present purposes, alert methods may be administered while the subject or subjects sit relaxing in a chair in the same way as traditional hypnosis. We may label this the 'passive–alert' method. By contrast, the subject
may be engaged in some form of continuous activity such as pedalling an
exercise bicycle during the induction (Bányai & Hilgard 1976). We may call
this the 'active–alert' method.

The alert methods do tend to result in more alert subjects (Fellows &
Richardson 1993). These researchers also found that passive–alert hypnosis

had the understandable disadvantage of making some subjects feel very restless. As was noted in Chapter 7, there is little overall difference in the effects of the two types of inductions (alert versus relaxed) on measured susceptibility. However, there is evidence of enhanced responsiveness to suggested posthypnotic amnesia with the alert methods, and reduced responsiveness to challenge suggestions (Bányai & Hilgard 1976, Vingoe 1968, 1973).

Few clinicians have chosen to use alert methods. Don Gibbons in the USA (Gibbons 1979) has been a great advocate, as has Frank Vingoe in Britain, who published some laboratory work (Vingoe 1968, 1973) as well as some clinical work with his colleagues, using alert methods to improve reading efficiency (Donk et al 1970).

Probably the most prominent advocates now of active–alert methods are Eva Bányai and her colleagues in Budapest. They have used them for a wide range of clinical problems (Bányai et al 1993). Of interest is their work on depressed patients, whose problem is one of underarousal, and for whom the reported mood-enhancing experience of the active–alert methods may be more appropriate than relaxation. Another obvious application is with sportspeople.

From time to time in this book, we shall refer to the possible use of alert methods for various problems and disorders. Perhaps they are underused because of an overadherence by clinicians to more traditional methods.

REFERENCES

Bányai E I, Hilgard E R 1976 A comparison of active-alert hypnotic induction with traditional relaxation induction. Journal of Abnormal Psychology 85: 218–224
Bányai E I, Zseni A, Forenc T 1993 Active-alert hypnosis in psychotherapy. In: Rhue J W, Lynn S J, Kirsch I (eds) Handbook of clinical hypnosis. American Psychological Association, Washington DC, ch 13, p 271
Donk L J, Vingoe F J, Hall R A et al 1970 The comparison of three suggestion techniques for increasing reading efficiency utilizing a counter-balanced research paradigm. International Journal of Clinical and Experimental Hypnosis 18: 126–133
Erickson M H, Rossi E L 1979 Hypnotherapy: An exploratory casebook. Irvington, New York
Erickson M H, Rossi E L, Rossi S I 1976 Hypnotic realities: The induction of clinical hypnosis and forms of indirect suggestion. Irvington, New York
Fellows B J, Richardson J 1993 Relaxed and alert hypnosis: An experimental comparison. Contemporary Hypnosis 10: 49–54
Fricton J R, Roth P 1985 The effects of direct and indirect suggestion for analgesia in high and low susceptible subjects. American Journal of Clinical Hypnosis 27: 226–231
Gibbons D E 1979 Applied hypnosis and hyperempiria. Plenum Press, New York
Groth-Marnet G, Mitchell K 1998 Responsiveness to direct versus indirect hypnotic procedures. International Journal of Clinical and Experimental Hypnosis 46: 324–333
Hart B B 1994 Hypnotizability and type of suggestion in the hypnotic treatment of generalised anxiety. Contemporary Hypnosis 11: 55–65
Ludwig A M, Lyle W H 1964 Tension induction and the hyperalert trance. Journal of Abnormal and Social Psychology 69: 70–76
Lynn S J, Weekes J R, Matyi C L et al 1988 Direct versus indirect suggestions, archaic involvement, and hypnotic experience. Journal of Abnormal Psychology 97: 296–301

Spinhoven P, Baak D, van Dyck R et al 1988 The effectiveness of an authoritative versus permissive style of hypnotic communication. International Journal of Clinical and Experimental Hypnosis 36: 182–191

Van Gorp W G, Meyer R, Dunbar K 1985 The efficacy of direct versus indirect hypnotic induction on reduction of experimental pain. International Journal of Clinical and Experimental Hypnosis 33: 319–328

Vingoe F J 1968 The development of a group alert-trance scale. International Journal of Clinical and Experimental Hypnosis 16: 120–132

Vingoe F J 1973 Comparison of the Harvard Group Scale of Hypnotic Susceptibility, Form A and the Group Alert Trance Scale in a university population. International Journal of Clinical and Experimental Hypnosis 21: 169–179

11

Suggestion, posthypnotic suggestion and ego-strengthening in therapy

INTRODUCTION

Much of the practice of hypnosis entails the giving of suggestions and posthypnotic suggestions that are intended, directly or indirectly, to promote the desired changes. Inherent in this process is the assumption that the induction of hypnosis potentiates the suggestions given, that is, increases the likelihood of a response or tends to elicit a more profound response.

We have outlined two theoretical bases, or working models, that may underlie the above contention. One model assumes that the induction of hypnosis guides the subjects into a state of mind that is conducive to enhanced responsiveness to suggestion. This model may be based on a 'strong' or 'weak' interpretation of the hypnotic trance, as discussed in earlier chapters. Another model posits that by defining the context as 'hypnosis', most notably by conducting an hypnotic induction ceremony, we enhance the subjects' commitment and expectation that they are going to respond to the suggestions to follow.

These two working models are not mutually incompatible and the procedures that they generate are very similar. However, we recommend that, when engaged in therapy, you do not simply rely on the idea that because you have hypnotised your patient, whatever you say, in whatever way you say it, is automatically going to be acted upon by the patient. Far from it. Instead, think about how you can maximise the impact of your suggestions in ways that are not exclusive to hypnosis – the building-up of positive expectancies, the use of voice tone, the customising of suggestions and imagery to the patient's own life experiences, and so on (see also our discussion of therapeutic suggestions in Ch. 7).

THERAPEUTIC SUGGESTIONS DURING HYPNOSIS

It is usually most appropriate to give your suggestions in a calm and convincing, but not overdramatic, way and to repeat them using variations on the words you use (e.g. 'Your body is becoming very heavy... heavy and comfortable... feel the heaviness in the whole of your body'). Emphasise key words with an appropriate change of stress.

You might improve on the effectiveness of the suggestions by linking the desired outcome with some other activity or experience. The form of the suggestion then becomes:

As X is happening, you will do/think/feel Y.

Here 'X' is termed a cue or anchor for the desired response. For example, you may say:

As I count from I to I0, let your hand become cold and numb.

You may further improve on the effectiveness of your suggestion by using a cue or anchor that is apposite to the intended outcome. This is usually an image, as in the example of a bucket of ice and water for eliciting glove anaesthesia or a bridge leading back into the mists of time in the case of age regression.

We should say here that, for non-clinical purposes, the evidence from the laboratory has not indicated that appropriate imagery is of central importance to hypnotic responding (Kirsch 1991). However, our impression is that in clinical practice it may be helpful to use images chosen by the subject.

POSTHYPNOTIC SUGGESTION IN THERAPY

Posthypnotic suggestions in therapy often take the form of instructions that you might give the patient or client in the normal way (e.g. 'Every time you reach for a cigarette just think of what it's doing to your lungs!'). Once again, underlying the use of posthypnotic suggestion is the assumption that the hypnotic induction renders the patient more likely to respond, or to respond more strongly. As before, we can choose between different models (e.g. strong trance, weak trance or expectancy) on which to base our use of posthypnotic suggestion. However, we consider that there is a strong case for advocating that more attention be paid to the research literature before deciding what rationale one is to adopt for the use of this technique. In our experience, the 'strong trance' model can easily depict posthypnotic suggestion as having the properties of a magic spell (and the hypnotic trance, a 'state of bewitchment').

Research findings on posthypnotic suggestion

As one would expect, the probability that subjects will respond to a posthypnotic suggestion is positively correlated with their measured hypnotic susceptibility, and susceptible subjects do experience a certain compulsion to respond (Barnier & McConkey 1998). Some theories of hypnosis (e.g. that of Woody & Bowers 1994) may explain this in terms of the subject's loss of executive control over the stipulated response, so that it is executed in automatic fashion. However, this kind of explanation may be of less cogency in the context of treatment, in which the posthypnotic response may first occur hours or even days after the session of therapy. Moreover, studies (e.g. Barnier & McConkey 1998) indicate also that responding to posthypnotic suggestion involves the active participation of the subject, who must be motivated and prepared and feel expected to respond. Also, in laboratory studies, subjects do not always respond when they are not under the surveillance of the experimenter (Spanos et al 1987).

A rather neat demonstration of factors influencing posthypnotic suggestion was reported by Fisher (1954). He gave a posthypnotic suggestion to 13 subjects, seen individually, of medium or high hypnotisability. The suggestion was that they would scratch their right ear whenever he or any of his assistants said the word 'psychology'. All subjects responded positively after alerting. After some time, without explicitly cancelling the suggestion, the experimenter subtly altered the tone and content of the interactions with the subject to convey the impression that the experiment was now completed. This went on for between 5 and 10 minutes, during which period only two of the subjects continued to give the posthypnotic response in a consistent manner. Nine of the subjects stopped responding altogether. Finally, the experimenter subtly altered the conversation again, intimating that the experiment was actually still in progress. Now, 11 of the subjects (including the nine non-responders in the previous phase) gave the posthypnotic response.

These kinds of experiments are sometimes cited as 'debunking hypnosis'. This is not the case. However, they reveal that hypnosis involves the fascinating rich and subtle interplay of a range of cognitive and social psychological processes. Much of this understanding is lost, however, when we simply ascribe what we superficially observe to some hypothetical 'trance' state, about which scientists currently know very little but at some indeterminate time in the future will all be explained.

Guidelines on the use of posthypnotic suggestion in therapy

How can we use the above knowledge in therapy?

A posthypnotic suggestion is *not* a magic spell (or in negative terms, a curse!). It quickly decays in strength unless consolidated by the naturally occurring processes of conditioning and cognitive restructuring. It is usually easily over-ridden by conscious control or existing competing habits. The suggestion has to be aimed at responses that are appropriate to the context, valued by or acceptable to the subject or patient, and demonstrably within the subject's repertoire or potentialities.

Posthypnotic suggestions have the following form:

From now on, when/whenever/each time/each and every time X (*stimulus*), you will Y (*response*).

Box 11.1 gives some good examples of posthypnotic suggestions. The following are some guidelines for using posthypnotic suggestion in therapy:

1. We recommend that X and Y should be discrete and identifiable stimuli or responses. For example, in the case of examination anxiety, instead of just saying: 'From now on, whenever you sit an exam you will feel confident', say something like:

As soon as you put your pen on your answer paper, you will bring this memory (of being confident) to mind and all the good feelings that go with it.

(Prior to this suggestion you will have encouraged your client to recall and rehearse in imagination a memory in which your client felt especially confident.)

2. In framing the above kinds of suggestions, always endeavour to identify as precisely as possible X (the salient trigger) and Y (the appropriate response). For example, if you are a dentist working with a dentally phobic patient, identify the stimulus that starts off the panic, say the switching on of the dentist's drill. In other cases of anxiety, sometimes the triggers for the beginning of an anxiety attack are internal stimuli such as 'butterflies' in the stomach or the thought 'I'm going to pass out'. Likewise determine what is the most appropriate response to the trigger. To accomplish this, you will need to carefully take the patient through the sequence of events – internal and external – that precede the problematic feeling or behaviour.

3. Use your tone of voice, demeanour, and so on to be convincing.

4. Repeat the suggestion several times.

5. Especially when you have adopted the second approach to hypnosis (Ch. 7), use the following ploy. If the patient has responded well to previous suggestions, say arm levitation and eye heaviness, you may say, 'Just as your arm became light when I suggested this, and just as your eyes became heavy when I suggested this, so ... ' (and then give the posthypnotic suggestion).

6. Sometimes it may be useful, in the earlier formula for a posthypnotic suggestion, to interpose between the 'X' and the 'Y' a mediating image or action by the patient that is designed to 'cue in' the desired response. The

Box 11.1 Examples of posthypnotic suggestions in therapy	
Examples	Applications
From now, each and every time you feel these anxious sensations in your stomach, you will immediately take in a deep breath, and as you breathe out your whole body will relax.	Anxiety management
As soon as you start to notice your heart beating, the thought of that relaxing scene will come to mind.	Anxiety management
Each and every time you feel the urge to expose yourself, the image of that terrible scene will come to mind.	Exhibitionism
If, at any time, your hand moves to scratch your skin, even when you are asleep, you will immediately withdraw your hand again and experience a sense of relief and relaxation (Waxman 1989).	Eczema
As you reach to pull your hair, you will immediately become aware of what you are doing and allow yourself the choice of pulling your hair or leaving your hair alone (Barabasz 1987).	Compulsive hair pulling
Every time you have those negative thoughts (specified) in that situation, you will immediately replace them by these new realistic thoughts (specified).	Cognitive therapy
Whenever you start to get anxious about going to the toilet, you will immediately say to yourself 'Stop! Relax! I am in control! I do not have to go to the toilet right now' (Walker 1988).	Irritable bowel or incontinence phobia
Between now and when I see you again, you will have a dream at night that will help you understand your problem.	Psychodynamic therapy
The moment your pen touches the paper, you will experience this same feeling of relaxation and you will concentrate fully on your examination.	Exam nerves
While you are brushing your teeth in the morning, you will remember to use your inhaler (Gainer, unpublished work, 1999).	Compliance with asthma treatment

first two examples in Box 11.1 illustrate this, the outward breath and the relaxing image each serving as a cue to relaxed feelings. Sometimes the cue or anchor has no intrinsic relationship with the response or experience. One of the most common examples of this is the use of a simple gesture that has been explicitly linked to the desired experience. For example, your intention may be to help the patient feel calm in a situation that she finds very difficult to cope with. You ask the patient to imagine a situation in which she normally feels confident. Ask the patient to signal to you when these feelings have been brought to mind, then say:

Now, while you are experiencing these confident feelings, press your thumb and forefinger of your preferred hand together. As you are doing that, connect the feelings in your thumb and finger with those good feelings.

Good! Now, whenever … X … , you will bring your thumb and forefinger together and immediately these feelings of confidence will come flooding back and you will cope with the situation just as you want to.

It is a good idea for the patient to rehearse this several times.

In Chapter 12, we shall present the use of the clenched fist in an anchoring method for coping with difficult feelings such as excessive anxiety or anger. An anchor may also be an image or a word spoken to oneself. In the third example given in Box 11.1, one could use a word that the person associates with the 'terrible scene'. In fact, this was done in a case reported by Wright & Humphreys (1984). The cue word was 'police' which was associated with the patient's arrest for indecent exposure, a terrible experience for the patient and one that was used as an image in a covert sensitisation procedure (see Ch. 20).

7. The posthypnotic suggestion may be incorporated as a self-suggestion in the patient's self-hypnosis routine.

Posthypnotic suggestion as an adjunctive technique

We do not recommend that you rely solely on posthypnotic suggestion to promote the kinds of changes your patient is striving for. For example, in Chapter 12 we describe how you can use memories of difficult experiences and the technique of future rehearsal to assist the desired changes and new methods of coping and we shall demonstrate how posthypnotic suggestion can be used to facilitate such procedures.

EGO-STRENGTHENING

Ego-strengthening in clinical hypnosis appears to have been popularised by John Hartland (1966) and is a way of helping people to enhance their self-confidence and self-worth. It is similar to the approach of Emile Coué, namely that of repeating positive suggestions to oneself (e.g. 'Every day in every way I am getting better and better'), the idea being that somehow these suggestions take hold in the person's subconscious mind and exert an automatic influence on feelings, thoughts and behaviour.

Applications of ego-strengthening

Ego-strengthening and general positive suggestions of well-being may be incorporated into most applications of hypnosis. We warn below of the inappropriateness of relying on them as the main therapeutic technique. It is better to use them to reinforce any progress that patients are making and to help them build a feeling of self-confidence and self-reliance, trusting themselves that they have the strength and resources to handle the inevitable strains and pressures of life.

The following is the original ego-strengthening routine of Hartland, taken from the earliest edition of this book (Hartland 1966). Hartland used the term 'sleep' as a metaphor for hypnosis, but this practice has declined since his original writings.

Hartland's ego-strengthening routine

You have now become *so* deeply relaxed ... *so* deeply asleep ... that your mind has become *so* sensitive ... *so* ... receptive to what I say ... that *everything* that I put into your mind ... will sink *so* deeply into the unconscious part of your mind ... and will cause so deep and lasting an impression there ... that *nothing* will eradicate it.

Consequently ... these things that I put into your unconscious mind ... will begin to exercise a greater and greater influence over the way you think ... over the way you feel ... over the way you behave.

And ... because these things *will* remain ... firmly imbedded in the unconscious part of your mind ... after you have left here ... when you are no longer with me ... they will continue to exercise that same great influence ... over your *thoughts* ... your *feelings* ... and your *actions* ... *just* as strongly ... *just* as surely ... *just* as powerfully ... when you are back home ... or at work ... as when you are with me in this room.

You are now so *very deeply asleep* ... that *everything* that I tell you that is going to happen to you ... *for your own good* ... *will* happen ... *exactly* as I tell you.

And *every feeling* ... that I tell you that you will experience ... you *will* experience ... *exactly* as I tell you.

And these same things *will continue to happen* to you ... *every day* ... and you *will continue to experience* these same feelings ... *every day* ... *just* as strongly ... *just* as surely ... *just* as powerfully ... when you are back home ... or at work ... as when you are with me in this room.

During this deep sleep ... *you* are going to feel physically *stronger* and *fitter* in every way. You will feel *more* alert ... *more* wide awake ... *more* energetic. You will become *much* less easily tired ... *much* less easily fatigued ... *much* less easily discouraged ... *much* less easily depressed. *Every day* ... you will become so *deeply interested* in whatever you are doing ... in whatever is going on around you ... that your mind will become *completely distracted away from yourself.*

You will no longer *think nearly so much about yourself* ... you will no longer *dwell nearly so much upon yourself and your difficulties* ... and you will become *much less conscious of yourself* ... *much less pre-occupied with yourself* ... and with your own *feelings.*

Every day ... your nerves will become *stronger and steadier* ... your mind *calmer and clearer* ... *more composed* ... *more placid* ... *more tranquil.* You will become *much less easily worried* ... *much less easily agitated* ... *much less easily fearful and apprehensive* ... *much less easily upset.*

You will be able to *think more clearly* ... you will be able to *concentrate more easily.* You will be able to *give up your whole undivided attention to whatever you are doing ... to the complete exclusion of everything else.* Consequently ... *your memory will rapidly improve* ... and you will be able to *see things in their true perspective* ... *without magnifying your difficulties* ... *without ever allowing them to get out of proportion.*

Every day ... you will become *emotionally much calmer* ... *much more settled* ... *much less easily disturbed.*

Every day ... you will become ... and *you* will remain ... *more and more completely relaxed* ... and *less tense each day* ... *both mentally and physically* ... even when you are no longer with me.

And *as you become* ... and *as you remain* ... *more relaxed* ... *and less tense* each day ... so you will develop *much more confidence in yourself* ... more confidence in your ability to *do* ... not only what you *have* ... to do each day but more confidence in your ability to do whatever you *ought* to be able to do ... *without fear of failure* ... *without fear of consequences* ... *without unnecessary anxiety* ... *without uneasiness.*

Because of this ... *every day* ... you will feel *more and more independent* ... *more able to 'stick up for yourself'* ... *to stand upon your own feet* ... *to hold your own* ... no matter how difficult or trying things may be.

Every day ... you will feel a *greater feeling of personal well-being* ... a *greater feeling of personal safety* ... *and security* ... than you have felt for a long, long time.

And because all these things *will* begin to happen ... *exactly* as I tell you they will happen ... *more and more rapidly* ... *powerfully* ... *and completely* ... with every treatment I give you ... you will feel *much happier* ... *much more contented* ... *much more optimistic* in every way.

You will consequently become much more able to *rely upon* ... *to depend upon* ... *yourself* ... *your own efforts* ... *your own judgement* ... *your own opinions.* You will feel much less need ... to have to *rely upon* ... or to *depend upon* ... *other people.*

This ego-strengthening routine has proved very popular and in our experience many therapists, particularly medical and dental practitioners, swear by it. It is, however, true to say that it is not to everyone's taste. It is rather lengthy and some people find it too authoritarian in tone; this conflicts with the more egalitarian, client-centred approach of modern therapies. Another criticism is that it does not make use of an important resource that all people possess, namely their imagination. Also, the suggestions do not indicate *how* the person is to achieve these desirable feelings. *How* is the person going to come to feel confident, for example?

Unless there are good feelings present to begin with, the whole thing may backfire. For example, you cannot simply use this procedure to lift the mood of a depressed person. One of us (Heap 1984) has described the case of a depressed patient whose relatives funded a 12-session course of treatment with a Harley Street hypnotherapist (on the questionable assumption that 'that's as good as you can get'). The entire fee had to be paid in the first session. The therapy consisted solely of sessions of ego-strengthening. Despite being assured by the hypnotherapist that his treatment had a 95% success rate, by the 11th session the patient had to inform the therapist that he was in fact feeling worse. The hypnotherapist then suggested he ask his relatives to fund a further course of 12 sessions. Soon afterwards, the patient was admitted to hospital, having made a serious attempt on his life.

This unfortunate story illustrates another point. For ego-strengthening suggestions to stand any chance of success, there must be a good therapeutic relationship.

Indeed Heap (1991) has questioned whether suggestions such as 'You are feeling more confident', 'Your nerves are getting stronger' and 'You are beginning to stand up for yourself' can really be responded to in the automatic manner of the response to a hypnotic suggestion (compare with 'Your arm is getting lighter' or 'Your hands are feeling warmer'). These suggestions do not specify *discrete* thoughts, behaviour, feelings and imagery that we said earlier should characterise posthypnotic suggestion in therapy. It seems more likely that whether a patient responds positively to these general kinds of suggestions would depend greatly on the patient's faith in the therapist, and whether these good feelings are already being experienced, rather than on the patient's hypnotic susceptibility.

Heap's ego-strengthening routine

The following is a routine used by one of the present authors (MH) that is somewhat shorter than Hartland's and which may be a useful way of rounding off a session of hypnosis when progress seems to be under way.

As you are relaxing and letting go, you may at some time be thinking of how many things you have learnt to do and *how* you learnt to do those things – everyday things like reading and writing, walking and talking. (*Others as appropriate.*) You have learnt to do all these things automatically, so you don't even have to try to do them.

Now as you're relaxing, and each time you relax like this, either with me or on your own, you can be learning just from the experience, how to relax and be calm in everyday situations; not *just* when you're sitting or lying down, but also when you're up and about and active .... How to feel in control so when you do start to experience any anxious thoughts and feelings, *you* can control *them, they* won't control *you.*

You are learning all this from the experience of relaxing, in the same way that you have learnt so many things just by experiencing them. And as you are learning that you can control these anxious thoughts and feelings, so you will find it easier and easier to put aside these thoughts and feelings when they do arise, just like when someone's trying to bother you and distract you and you ignore them and carry on with what you're doing – they soon go away, and you don't even notice when they have gone.

So each and every time you are aware of any unnecessary thoughts or feelings of anxiety or self-doubt, you can think to yourself '*I* can control *them*. They won't control *me!*' and you can immediately switch your attention away from yourself and towards whatever you're doing and whatever is happening around you.

And it might surprise you when you realise some time later that those anxious thoughts and feelings have gone away.

So in this way you can start to feel more confident in your ability to handle any tense or anxious thoughts and feelings and any doubts about yourself. So, you will feel more confident to face up to things and enter situations which previously you may have avoided … feeling more calm, more in control and more ready to take on the things that you wish to do … *do* the things you *want* to do … *say* the things you *want* to say … in your own way. You can be learning all this *now* as you are relaxing … just from the experience of relaxing.

So just continue to relax for a little longer and imagine all these suggestions finding a place deep down in your mind where they can work automatically and effectively whenever you need them in your everyday life.

As the patient is improving, the tenses may be suitably altered; for example, 'You are now noticing that you are starting to feel more confident'.

Ego-strengthening routines using symbolic and metaphorical imagery

The following are two examples from Stanton (1990) of routines that have the advantage of making use of imagery. As with any imagery method, it is a good idea to check with the patient that the kind of images you are about to use appeal to him or her and that there are no adverse memories or feelings associated with them. The first metaphor is associated with Hitchcock (1981).

Patients are asked to visualise a cloud hovering nearby. When they have signalled that they have created that image, the therapist then instructs them to put into the cloud all the reasons for their lack of assertiveness. (The instructions may be adapted to a patient's particular problems.) It is suggested that these reasons are like computer programmes that maintain their unwanted behaviour and can be erased. The therapist further suggests that as they are drifting along in this relaxed way, if any further reasons come to mind, they are to put them in the cloud also, so that it becomes darker and darker. Eventually it will become 'inky black' and they are to signal when this happens. They are then to study the cloud and they will see a source of light behind it that is at first dim but becomes increasingly bright. When they have signalled that this has happened, the therapist explains that the light is in fact the sun, 'the sun of your own desire to be free of everything that has been preventing you from living life to its fullest'. The therapist then counts to 5 and suggests that with each count, patients will become aware of the warmth of the sun, burning away the cloud completely. They are then able to bask in the warmth of the sun, 'feeling the sun's rays penetrating every cell of their bodies, bringing a sense of assertiveness and self-confidence'.

The second ego-strengthening imagery that Stanton uses comes from Gibbons (1979). Gibbons promoted the use of alert methods of hypnosis (see Ch. 10), which he called 'hyperempiria', a term that never caught on. This is one of his examples (Gibbons 1979, p 175–176).

Patients picture themselves standing at the top of a tall, snow-covered mountain, looking down into a valley below. As they are focusing on this image, it soon becomes as vivid and real as if they are really there. Down in the valley below, at the very foot of the mountain, they can see the place that they have been trying to reach. They have come as far as the mountain top, but all along the mountainside, standing between them and their goal, are barriers and obstacles that represent all the things that have been standing between them and the things they want to accomplish.

They are then instructed to bend down and pick up a handful of snow and examine it. They notice how soft and powdery it feels. It is similar to how their own resolve has been at times – 'soft and powdery, when it ought to have been firm and strong'. They then start to pack the snow together in their hands, compressing it into a snowball as they add still more snow, so that it becomes firm, round and hard. As they do so, they feel their own courage and resolution becoming stronger and firmer too, hard and firm as the snowball that they are preparing for its trip down the mountainside.

They then imagine walking over to a very steep incline at the side of the mountain and gently rolling the snowball down the mountain towards the obstacles below. 'Slowly, slowly the snowball begins to roll down the mountainside; and slowly, slowly it begins to grow. It's growing and grow-ing and increasing in size with every foot *(metre)* it travels'. As the snowball rolls down the mountain, 'it grows to the size of a boulder, and then it becomes an avalanche, sweeping everything before it as it continues on all the way to the bottom'.

Now patients can see that their way ahead is clear and the obstacles have all been swept away. They then begin their own descent down the mountainside, 'where your courage has gone before to clear a path for you.' And so they stride down the mountainside, their confidence and resolve continuing to grow just like the snowball. 'They are going to continue growing and getting stronger by themselves, just as the snowball did. And soon your confidence and resolve will become so strong that they, too, will sweep away every obstacle in their path, and you will easily be able to attain whatever goals in life you have set for yourself, just as easily as you now see yourself walking down the mountainside'.

The therapist then gives posthypnotic suggestions that in the coming days and weeks 'the processes we have begun on the mountainside will continue of themselves'. The patients' resolve will continue to grow and strengthen with each new day until they are able to accomplish everything they have set out to do.

You may wish to adapt the above routines to suit your own personal style. In fact, there is absolutely no reason why you should not make up ones with which you feel most comfortable. There is a great deal to be said for improvising your own routines, tailored to the needs and interests of the particular patient you are seeing.

Summary of guidelines on ego-strengthening

1. Ensure that you have established good rapport between you and your patient and that your patient has trust and confidence in you and the therapy you are offering.

2. Ensure that some good feelings are already there to be amplified. For instance, the suggestions may be used to 'round off' a good session of therapy when some progress has been evident. Don't just rely on them alone for therapy, especially with depressed patients.

3. Sound convincing! Don't just speak in a droning monotone.

4. Be realistic! For example, you can suggest that the patient will be able to cope with the frustration of any setbacks that are part of the process of recovery.

5. Use the technique described earlier for enhancing the impact of posthypnotic suggestions; namely, tell patients that just as they have already responded to suggestions (specified), so they will (for example) find that their confidence is growing with each day.

6. Customise the suggestions to the needs of the individual patient. (For example, it is no use, and indeed may harm rapport, saying to patients that they are going to become more assertive with people, if they have never considered this to be a problem.)

7. Use memories of real experiences that the patient can recall when confident feelings were present – for instance, when the patient experienced a great sense of achievement. (Earlier in this chapter and in Ch. 12, we describe the technique of 'anchoring' feelings, and this may be useful here.)

8. Make use of symbolic or metaphorical imagery as in the examples from Stanton (1990). It is also a good idea to elicit from patients their own personal metaphors or images which symbolise their poor self-regard, and to modify them accordingly. An illustration of this is as follows. A client, Oya, (seen by MH) who was training for a certain profession, suffered from bouts of depressed mood, self-doubt and lack of confidence. She had aspirations to succeed in her chosen career but saw her ideal as a set of goalposts in the far distance. Her therapist asked her how she could modify

this image so that it was more constructive and useful for her, yet still realistic. We shall not disclose to you what she came up with but allow you to do the exercise for yourself. The client found it useful to remind herself of her reconstructed image every time her self-doubts started to trouble her. One lesson of this is that an image can have much more impact (negative and positive) on how one is feeling than the equivalent idea expressed in words.

9. Explore the use of alert methods, described in Chapter 10, particularly for use in self-hypnosis.

REFERENCES

Barabasz M 1987 Trichotillomania: A new treatment. International Journal of Clinical and Experimental Hypnosis 35: 146–154
Barnier A J, McConkey K M 1998 Posthypnotic responding: Knowing when to stop helps keep it going. International Journal of Clinical and Experimental Hypnosis 46: 204–219
Fisher S 1954 The role of expectancy in the performance of posthypnotic behaviour. Journal of Abnormal Psychology 49: 503–507
Gibbons D 1979 Applied hypnosis and hyperempiria. Plenum Press, New York
Hartland J 1966 Medical and dental hypnosis and its clinical applications. Baillière Tindall, London
Heap M 1984 Four victims. British Journal of Experimental and Clinical Hypnosis 2: 60–62
Heap M 1991 Role and use of hypnosis in psychotherapy. In: Heap M, Dryden W (eds) Hypnotherapy: A handbook. Open University Press, Milton Keynes, ch 2, p 15
Hitchcock H W 1981 A 'shotgun' attack on extreme shyness. Medical Hypnoanalysis 7: 165–168
Kirsch I 1991 The social learning theory of hypnosis. In: Lynn S J, Rhue J W (eds) Theories of hypnosis: Current models and perspectives. Guilford Press, New York, ch 14, p 439
Spanos N P, Menary E, Brett P J et al 1987 Failure of hypnotic responding to occur outside the experimental setting. Journal of Abnormal Psychology 96: 52–57
Stanton H 1990 Using ego-enhancement to increase assertiveness. British Journal of Experimental and Clinical Hypnosis 7: 133–137
Walker L G 1988 Hypnosis in the treatment of irritable bowel syndrome. In: Heap M (ed) Hypnosis: Current clinical, experimental and forensic practices. Croom Helm, London, ch 16, p 167
Waxman D 1989 Hartland's medical and dental hypnosis, 3rd edn. Baillière Tindall, London
Woody E Z, Bowers K S 1994 A frontal assault on dissociative control. In: Lynn S J, Rhue J W (eds) Dissociation: Clinical and theoretical perspectives. Guilford Press, New York, ch 3, p 52
Wright A D, Humphreys A 1984 The use of hypnosis to enhance covert sensitization: Two case studies. British Journal of Experimental and Clinical Hypnosis 1: 3–10

12

Behavioural techniques for self-control

INTRODUCTION

In this chapter, we describe some common behavioural methods for the control of tension and anxiety that illustrate the use of the basic hypnotic procedures that we have already described. In addition, we introduce the technique of rehearsal in imagination. That is, patients are asked to imagine successfully using the self-control procedures to cope with those situations that they find difficult. This is also done using situations from the past that they recall as being particularly difficult to cope with, and using situations that they expect to encounter in the near future. These are examples of *covert* behaviour therapy and we shall present more covert methods in Chapter 20.

PARADOXICAL INJUNCTION

The reader will encounter this expression (or 'paradoxical intention') a number of times in this book. It refers to the instruction to the patient to intensify a symptom or deliberately engage in some problematic behaviour or troublesome thoughts (hence the alternative label 'symptom prescription').

Ask patients to close their eyes and to notice how they feel physically and what their body is telling them. After some time, ask them to imagine a scale from 0 to 10 which measures how tense or relaxed they are. A 0 means completely relaxed, 10 means as tense as possible, 4 or 5 is somewhere in between. When they have given the rating ask them where in the body they notice the tension. Ask them to focus on this part for a while and see if they can make the tension more noticeable, that is raise the tension by just one point simply by imagining this happening. Or perhaps they can imagine how they would feel if the tension did increase by one point.

They are not to increase the tension by deliberately clenching any muscles or holding their breath, but they are allowed to think of a situation in which they often feel tense. (Please note: if the rating is already high, say 7 or more, proceed without the instruction to raise the tension further.)

Allow patients some time to try this and then say:

Let me know when you have succeeded or when you think you've spent enough time on this. Sometimes it works, sometimes it doesn't.

After a response, say, 'Now let's see if we can bring the tension down by at least one point' and proceed with a breathing technique.

BREATHING TECHNIQUES

We have already described the use of breathing techniques as methods of induction and deepening, whereby suggestions of relaxation are coupled with exhalation and inhalation. Instruction in these further techniques does not normally require an induction, but the sensory-focusing procedure described in Chapter 6 is a good method of preparation. There are many variations on this theme and readers can invent their own.

Ask patients to focus on their breathing. To start with, you can suggest the sensations of the air flowing through the nasal pathways – 'The cooler, drier air flowing in, and the warmer, moist air flowing out'. Continue with the first breathing-induction method described in Chapter 6.

The 'coloured vapour' technique

Ask patients to give their tension a colour and to imagine that each time they breathe out they are breathing out their tension in the form of a vapour – 'the colour of your tension'. Suggest that with each breath they are blowing some of their tension away in the form of this vapour, and as it drifts away they are left feeling more calm and relaxed. Maybe the colour remaining is changing – growing fainter or becoming a colour associated with calmness and relaxation. Finally, ask patients to tell you when they have spent enough time on this and what the rating of their tension is now.

The 'blowing bubbles' technique

Another image is that of blowing a steady stream of bubbles. Remind patients how, when they were younger, they probably played at blowing bubbles through a loop. 'If you blow too hard, it breaks the film; if you don't blow hard enough, you get no bubbles at all'. You can then ask them to imagine that they are blowing a steady stream of bubbles with each outward breath and that each bubble is carrying a bit of their tension away. You can also ask patients to 'blow the bubbles' by breathing out through the mouth, and then inhaling through the nose.

The 'hand-on-abdomen' technique

The focus of attention on the breathing process can now be switched to the abdomen by asking patients to place one hand on the abdomen (just above the navel) and focus their attention on that. Remind them again of the pattern of breathing described above and suggest a warm, comfortable feeling passing all the way down the front of the body each time they breathe out. Remark on the fact that as they breathe in, the hand rises very slightly and as they breathe out, the hand falls. This is the reverse of the characteristic style of overbreathing or hyperventilation.

The technique can be further augmented by asking the patient to place the other hand gently on the chest and to imagine the chest muscles relaxing so that the hand hardly moves at all. This two-handed approach to hyperventilation control was developed at Papworth Hospital, Cambridge (see Wilkinson 1988).

A variation of this technique for abdominal pain and nausea will be presented in Chapter 25.

VARIATIONS ON THE CLENCHED FIST TECHNIQUE

The clenched fist technique was described by Stein (1963) and has proved to be very popular since. Basker (1979) reported its successful use in treating people with agoraphobia and Stanton (1997) has presented some case illustrations. It demonstrates the use of anchoring, described in Chapter 11. The anchor used is a clenched fist, but if you prefer you may use another gesture; for example, the patient may press together the thumb and forefinger. These techniques may warrant, during the first session of hypnosis, an induction approach of the second kind described in Chapter 7, as it is important to maximise the impact of your suggestions here.

Negative anchor for tension control

Administer instructions for paradoxical injunction by asking patients to imagine being in a situation in which they know they would feel tense and anxious. Say:

Don't spare any details. Imagine it as vividly as you can. Imagine everything that could go wrong does go wrong.

By imagining this situation, you might experience some of those tense and anxious feelings that you would have if you were really there. Or you can imagine what it would be like to have those feelings ... where in your body you would experience them ... and what kind of anxious thoughts you would be having.

Ask patients to signal when they have done this. Then ask them to slowly make a fist with the non-preferred hand but remind them to breathe comfortably throughout and not tense any other part of the body. As they are doing this, they are to imagine all the tension in the body streaming down into that hand. Say:

Imagine the tension flowing down to that fist, collecting in your hand, leaving the rest of your body relaxed and comfortable. Think that you are now holding all your tension in that hand.

They are then instructed to take in a deep breath, and as they are breathing out, they are to slowly release the fist and imagine all the tension leaving the hand and evaporating in the air around them, leaving the hand and the whole of the body relaxed and comfortable.

One variation is to ask patients to release the hand while counting from 1 to 5 (or 5 to 1). This can be combined with the release of a deep breath. Another variation is to instruct them to release the fist quickly, and symbolically 'throw the tension away'.

The technique is practised several times in the session using the same or different problem situations.

Anchor for positive feelings

Repeat the above, but this time ask patients to think of a situation in which they feel, or have felt, confident and in control. One way of doing this is to ask them if there is any situation they can bring to mind in which they have, or have had, the confidence and resources that would help them cope with the problem situation they rehearsed for the negative anchor. Ask them to bring this situation to mind and say:

By imagining this situation, you can experience some of those confident feelings and inner strengths right now. When you have a feeling of that confidence, or imagine what it would be like if you had that feeling right now, make a fist with your preferred hand and imagine all those good feelings streaming down into that hand. Hold on to those good feelings now so they are there in your hand, ready to hand, for you to use right now.

When patients have clenched the fist, tell them that once they have made that connection they can relax the hand again. You can then repeat the above for several positive situations.

Combining anchors

The techniques of negative and positive anchoring may be used separately, or you may combine them as follows. Having done the above procedures, you can now ask patients to bring to mind the first situation again – the one they find difficult. When they signal they are there, ask them to make the fist with the non-preferred hand as before and then to imagine dispelling the tension by slowly releasing the fist. As they are doing this, ask them to stay in the situation and make a fist with the preferred hand. Say:

And now imagine bringing all those good, confident feelings and strengths right into this new situation, and handling this situation in the way you wish ... confident and in control ... etc.

You may repeat the combining of the anchors one or more times until patients feel that they are now more confident about the difficult situation.

Using the clenched fist procedure for anger control

When using the clenched fist procedure for dispelling anger concerning a specific event in the past, it may be better to introduce the following variation. As the Roman philosopher Seneca pointed out, anger is almost always associated with a sense that the world (particularly the world of people) has treated us unfairly. (We can, of course, be angry at the unfair or cruel treatment of others.) Hence, whereas we tend to perceive fear and anxiety as something to be completely rid of, we are inclined to feel justified in holding on to our anger. Consequently, when asking patients to dispel the anger by releasing the clenched fist, one might give the instruction:

Only let go of as much of that anger as you feel ready and able to do right now. Let the remaining anger stay in your hand.

When patients have done this they are to completely relax the hand, allowing the remaining anger to return to their body. It may be that you will be doing some further work on this anger at a later stage.

COVERT REHEARSAL OF SELF-CONTROL METHODS

Having gone through any of the above procedures, it is very useful to ask patients to imagine using them to cope with various difficult situations they encounter in daily life.

Covert rehearsal of situations from memory

It is very often the case that patients have memories of their not coping that 'stick in the mind' and still upset them when they think of them. We cannot cite any research evidence for this, but our contention is that using these memories to rehearse a self-control method, for example an anxiety management technique, can be particularly effective. Examples of such memories are the occasion of a first panic attack, an activity that had to be completely abandoned, or a situation that patients had to leave, as they felt totally unable to cope. The memory is often one of being 'completely out of control', 'unable to do anything' or 'overwhelmed'. Perhaps, then, the value of 'replaying' such memories, this time successfully using a self-control strategy, is that it implants the message 'I did not have to feel completely out of control (or overwhelmed)' and 'There *was* something I could have done'. The intention, however, is not to somehow re-encode the memory so that it is thenceforth recalled as one in which the patient coped successfully.

In Chapter 19, we shall describe various methods of assisting the patient in the process of bringing to mind important memories, particularly from the remote past. For present purposes, it is usually sufficient simply to ask the patient to 'Go back in time to the memory you described earlier when you … '. It is important also to ask the patient if it is all right to do this. Also, ask the patient to signal when he or she is ready to describe the memory and then say, 'Now just describe what is happening as it happens'.

Encourage the patient to use the present tense (e.g. 'I am standing in the queue at the supermarket … '). Proceed slowly, asking the patient such questions as 'What do you see now?', 'What are the sounds you can hear?' and 'What feelings are you noticing?' If the patient finds it too distressing to bring this memory to mind, then there are ways of helping and these are described in later chapters. This matter was also discussed in Chapter 6.

When the patient starts to describe the feelings of anxiety you can say:

OK. Now this time I want you to imagine remaining in the situation, but *(for example)* now start to clench your left fist as you did earlier … .

Take the patient through the self-control procedure. Throughout this, encourage the patient with appropriate comments such as 'That's fine!', 'Good!' and 'Well done!'

Replay this several times until the patient reports being able to imagine handling the situation in this new way and coping with it satisfactorily. There may be more than one memory that you wish to work with.

Future rehearsal in imagination

Having rehearsed the self-control procedures using memories of previous situations, it is useful to repeat the exercise using an imagined future event.

The ideal is when the patient is faced in the immediate future with a difficult situation, as this will be very much at the forefront of his or her mind.

Ask the patient to imagine going forward in time to the actual event, and repeat the procedure described for rehearsing the self-control technique using remembered events. Persist until the patient reports being able to cope successfully with the situation using the chosen technique. Again in later chapters, we shall describe methods for overcoming difficulties that the patient may encounter with this approach and that need addressing.

The significance of the future rehearsal technique is as follows. Many patients with anxieties and phobias will come to therapy saying, 'I just can't imagine coping at all with (*whatever their problem is*)' and, 'When I imagine myself in that situation, all I see is me going out of control'. They mean this literally. Hence, our contention is that if you can bring such a patient to the point where he or she is genuinely able to say, 'Yes, I can imagine myself coping' and this seems to the patient to be a realistic possibility, then that patient has probably made great strides in overcoming the problem, although in the end, of course, the final proof comes only when the patient faces the real situation.

POSTHYPNOTIC SUGGESTION

The next stage is your posthypnotic suggestions. These will be as follows.

For a breathing technique, a posthypnotic suggestion might be something like:

From now on, each and every time you notice these anxious feelings (*e.g. in your stomach*) you will give them a colour and as you breathe out, with each breath, you will imagine breathing out your anxiety in the form of a coloured vapour, and with each breath you will feel more calm, more confident and more in control.

A similar posthypnotic suggestion can be given for the 'bubbles' technique.

For the negative anchoring technique, you can give the posthypnotic suggestion:

Each and every time you are in a situation in which you are feeling unduly tense and anxious, you can make a fist with this same hand and allow all that tension to flow down into the fist. Then when you release the fist, all the tension will leave your hand and you will feel more calm, more relaxed and more in control.

For the positive anchor:

Each and every time you need those same positive feelings and resources, you can make a fist with this same hand, and immediately you will bring to mind these confident feelings and ways of thinking ready to hand, to bring to bear in that situation and to help you cope with it in the way you want to, feeling calm, confident and in control.

The posthypnotic suggestion for the double-anchoring method can be constructed from the above two.

SELF-HYPNOSIS

As part of the patient's self-hypnosis, it is a good idea for him or her to covertly rehearse the chosen self-control method. We recommend that you suggest to patients that several times a day they take time out from what they are doing, do a brief sensory-focusing or self-relaxation routine, bring to mind the problem situation (and maybe create some anxiety) and then imagine coping with it, using the technique rehearsed in the session.

Sometimes, putting the instructions and suggestions on an audiotape may be helpful so that the patient may listen to the tape, say, every day. You will need to judge how committed your patient is to doing this. More realistic may be an instruction to make occasional use of the tape at the patient's discretion.

EGO-STRENGTHENING

Reinforce the self-control procedure you have chosen with ego-strengthening. Prior to this, ask your patient to go in imagination to his or her 'special' or 'safe' place. Give some general ego-strengthening suggestions such as those of Hartland or Heap given in Chapter 11. Finally, give a posthypnotic suggestion such as:

Each and every time you practise these procedures, either with me or on your own, they will work for you more quickly, more automatically and more effectively in your everyday life.

Finally, alert your patient in the usual manner.

REFERENCES

Basker M A 1979 A hypnobehavioural method of treating agoraphobia by the clenched fist method of Calvert Stein. Australian Journal of Clinical Hypnosis 7: 27–34
Stanton H E 1997 Adorning the clenched fist technique. Contemporary Hypnosis 14: 189–194
Stein C 1963 Clenched-fist as a hypnobehavioral procedure. American Journal of Clinical Hypnosis 2: 113–119
Wilkinson J B 1988 Hyperventilation control techniques in combination with self-hypnosis for anxiety management. In: Heap M (ed) Hypnosis: Current clinical, experimental and forensic practices. Croom Helm, London, ch 11, p 115

13

Metaphor and story technique

INTRODUCTION

In our discussions so far of the use of hypnosis in clinical practice, we have laid great emphasis on the theme of effective communication, that is maximising the impact of the suggestions we make to the hypnotic subject and patient. We have studied ways of doing this, both for routine hypnotic suggestions (e.g. 'Your arm is feeling so light it wants to rise in the air'; 'Your hand is feeling cold and numb'; and 'You cannot open your eyes') and for the therapeutic messages we give to patients in the form of, for example, posthypnotic suggestion and ego-strengthening.

In this chapter, we explore ideas concerning therapeutic communications that are related to the indirect style of hypnotic suggestion, presented in Chapter 10, and therefore favoured by the Ericksonian approach.

LITERAL ANECDOTES

One way to present therapeutic suggestions and messages indirectly is to talk about the experience and the solutions of other patients. (In Ch. 10 we described a similar ploy for simple indirect suggestions.) This is probably something that many therapists do anyway. Such disclosures should not, of course, breach confidentiality. One may also offer anecdotes concerning oneself and one's colleagues. For example, Erickson (Erickson & Rossi 1979) told a man with tinnitus the story about how he once spent the night in a factory and learned naturally, as the workers there had already done, to block out the din of the machinery.

Therapists will have differing views on how far they wish to take this approach. We know of therapists who actually make up fictitious accounts (or embroider accounts of actual cases), so when they say, 'There was once a patient who ...' they are not telling the truth. We imagine that some readers may have misgivings about going so far.

This is an actual example of an anecdote that one of us (MH) occasionally uses.

A patient (let's call him Bill) whom I was seeing came to his appointment one day with a big smile on his face. He had been severely depressed and was now doing very well indeed, but he just could not stop dwelling on bad thoughts. Well, when I saw him he said, 'I've just hit on a very good way of getting rid of these bad thoughts. When I was in the Navy, we had an expression "Not wanted on voyage" when we tipped any rubbish overboard. So now, as soon as I start to think these bad thoughts, I immediately say to myself, "Not wanted on voyage" and imagine tipping them overboard. And it really works!'

There are a number of therapeutic messages here for the depressed patient. One simple message is that other people suffer from severe depression too. Another is that they get better. Also, other depressed patients are plagued with bad thoughts as well. Eventually, a way can be found of stopping this habit. One way is to think of a slogan and an image that one can use to cut short a chain of negative thoughts.

It is important that the patient on the receiving end of this anecdote is able to make use of the information. For example, Bill had reached a point in his recovery when he was able to employ his technique successfully. The patient to whom you are relating this story must also be at that stage. Perhaps 1 or 2 months prior to Bill's appointment, his technique would have had no effect. Also, the intention of the communication is not that the patient should adopt Bill's particular method. Most people have not had his naval experience to draw on. However, the anecdote may encourage patients to search for their own symbolic imagery for dispensing with unwanted thoughts. The story may also serve as a prelude to a more direct therapeutic intervention to assist the patient with some form of thought-stopping procedure.

Two questions arise from this discussion. The first is why it should be that putting the messages in the form of an illustrative story should be any more effective than advice offered more directly. Second, there is the question of where the role of hypnosis lies in this method. We shall defer answering these questions until we have described an extension of this approach, namely communicating by metaphor.

METAPHORICAL ANECDOTES AND STORIES

This technique involves relating anecdotes and stories to the patient (or asking the patient to imagine various scenes) that are metaphorically related to his or her presenting problems and their possible solution.

The anecdote may be very brief or protracted. A ploy that some favour is to embed the anecdote in a longer story. For example, one could start by talking about a friend and then say that this friend had another friend, who told him a story about another person ... etc. The effect may be to cause the listener to focus more closely on the story and thus have less chance to adopt an analytical attitude to it.

Later on in this chapter, we give some metaphorical anecdotes that we have picked up in our own work. Here is one example:

A circus arrives in town and everybody is busy pitching the tents, practising their acts, attending to the animals, and so on. A passer-by stops to watch what is going on when suddenly she notices that outside a tent is an enormous adult elephant with a piece of rope fastened round one of its legs and tied to a wooden stake, stuck firmly in the ground. The woman immediately asks to see the owner of the circus and points out that the elephant can easily escape. All it has to do is to give a tug on the stake and it can walk away free. The owner of the circus explains to the woman that there is no such danger. The elephant has been tied to the stake ever since it was a small baby. Once it struggled and struggled to escape but was not strong enough and it has long since stopped. Now it doesn't realise that it has grown up and has all the strength and power to free itself.

Let us for the time being note that those who use this kind of approach consider that the patient must be in a receptive mode for the communication to be effective (as with hypnotic suggestions generally). One way to do this is to use formal hypnosis, although this is not a necessary condition; for example, one can adopt a more 'conversational' style that holds the person's attention, as described in Chapter 10. Note also that the therapist makes no attempt to explain the message of the story to the patient.

Rationale

As to why communicating at the metaphorical level may be effective in therapy, some take the view that, like the indirect suggestions, the patient's conscious mind addresses the literal meaning of the communication, whereas the metaphorical meaning is accepted by the unconscious mind. We do not take this working model of the human mind literally and would prefer other explanations. It seems that putting the message in the form of a story may encourage patients to be more actively engaged in constructing a personal meaning than when they are given the message in its most explicit form. As a rule of therapy, it is far better when patients actively construct for themselves new ways of understanding and tackling their problems than when these are provided by the therapist. The approach also stimulates the imagination; pictures are formed in the patient's mind and, as a general rule, 'A picture is worth a thousand words'.

That is, much information is compressed into a small amount of cognitive space.

The effectiveness of communication by allegory and symbol is evident in the fact that our language itself is replete with figurative expressions, catch-phrases, similes, proverbs, and so on. For instance, for greater effect, we may say, instead of 'Jack is very enthusiastic', 'Jack is as keen as mustard'; instead of 'Mary is unperturbed by it all', 'Mary is as cool as a cucumber'; and instead of 'Steve is very witty', 'Steve is as sharp as a knife'. Similarly, whilst it is certainly true that both sides contribute to any relationship, we might prefer to say, 'It takes two to tango'. When somebody is becoming too bossy, we say, 'He's getting too big for his boots'. When a wife seems to be dominating her husband, we say, 'She's the one who wears the trousers'. We describe somebody who always spoils our enjoyment of things as 'a wet blanket'. And how many times do we warn somebody not to 'throw the baby out with the bathwater'?

We often find it more telling to quote a proverb than to give a full explanation of a point we wish to convey. For example, when somebody is behaving in a hypocritical manner, we say, 'People who live in glasshouses shouldn't throw stones'. Indeed, often all we need to do is to give the opening words of the proverb – 'A rolling stone!', 'A stitch in time!', 'Too many cooks!', and so on. Again much meaning is encoded in a few words.

In every culture, there is also a large store of stories, fables and legends that convey important truths with great drama and impact, more effectively than an abstract statement of the lessons contained in each one. Every new story, novel, play and film contains a collection of themes that, however modern the setting, date from antiquity. What, for example, is the story of Adam and Eve? A literal account of the beginnings of human life? Or a wonderful story, as rich now in the poignant truths that it conveys about human existence, as it was when it was first told? Likewise, we have the parables of Jesus, mirrored by similar stories in the scriptures of other great religions.

Our shared stories, fables and legends are also codified in such a way that they may easily be conveyed and brought to mind in shorthand fashion. Thus we may merely mention, say, the hero or villain of a well-known story to convey a telling point. 'Remember Icarus!' might be a warning to someone who is the current favourite of an unpredictable boss. Likewise, we may say, 'At the moment he has the Midas touch', 'I feel like King Canute', 'This is simply the Emperor's new clothes', and 'It was another case of the tortoise and the hare'. Similarly, we frequently add vividness to our descriptions of people or situations when we allude to characters from stories and dramas, such as when we refer to someone as 'a Don Juan', 'a Scrooge', 'a bit like Jekyll and Hyde', and 'a Walter Mitty character'. Similarly we may declare, 'I'm in a Catch 22' or 'She wants her pound of flesh!'

All this suggests, if nothing else, that there must be some advantage in communicating through the imagination in symbolic and metaphorical forms, drawing from the accumulated pool of wisdom that is contained within the stories, fables and legends that we all seem to know and are able to share.

Examples of metaphors and stories

Accordingly, we believe that there is a rational basis for the strategic inclusion of metaphors and stories in therapy, both during hypnosis and out of it. The story must convey empathy and understanding and the hope of a satisfactory outcome. You cannot be sure that your patient will be able to take on board your story and use it to address the targeted problem. However, if such is not the case, then no damage has been done, such as any disappointment or loss of credibility had you expressed your message in a more direct fashion.

The examples we give below concern general themes, common to many patients (e.g., depression, lack of self confidence, anxiety about the future, fears of condemnation and rejection, and fear of failure).

The journey

The metaphor of a journey is an appropriate one for many patients. They usually know their destination (i.e. what they wish to achieve) but in order to reach it, they may have to confront problems and situations about which they have anxieties and lack confidence. For example, clients, who have been out of work for some time because of problems with depression or severe anxiety, will be faced in the course of their improvement with the prospect of starting work again. Perhaps they are concerned about how they will cope on their first day back at work or, if they have lost their job, they are faced with the prospect of looking for work, going for an interview, being with people they do not know, and so on. Another example of this is that some people who are overweight find that whenever they manage to successfully lose weight, there comes a point when, for some reason, they start to become anxious. One reason may be that they may be losing the protection that they perceive their being overweight offers them in some way. In the case of people with phobias, whatever treatment they are having, at some stage they have to confront the situations they are afraid of, and this may, at first, precipitate a great deal of anxiety.

If any of these fears seem to be present, one could acknowledge them by telling the patient a story on the theme of a journey in which the traveller knows the destination and is keen to arrive there, but there are places on the journey which he has to pass through which provoke anxieties and misgivings. There are also places on the journey that are unfamiliar and the traveller is not sure how to cope. Also, as the journey progresses, places come up over the horizon for which he may be unprepared. Sometimes things come to a halt and the traveller makes no progress for a while and even has to retrace his steps. Sometimes the traveller takes a wrong turning and it takes some time before he is back on the right road, so that perhaps he needs to ask for help to get moving again, or to be pointed in the right direction. However, with persistence, the traveller reaches the destination feeling stronger and wiser for having made that journey.

The map

A similar theme is the idea of trying to find one's way around an unfamiliar place using a map. We all have a map of our personal world and, just like an ordinary map, it informs us of what choices we have available to us, the various ways of getting from A to B, where we can and where we cannot go, and so on. Parts of the map may be missing, in which case attempting to visit the places involved will be fraught with difficulty and anxiety ('fear of the unknown'). A map may be faulty and it may be out of date. This is a difficulty that is particularly apposite to problems that many patients have; that is, they, and indeed to some degree all of us, tend not to revise and update their personal maps of the world as a result of their experiences. For example, a person who is very unassertive and deferent may be said to be using a map that, when that person was, say, a young child and living with very authoritarian parents, or attending a very strict school, was very appropriate. But now the person has left all that behind, has grown into an adult and people have different expectations of her and will respond to her in a different way than when she was a child. However, if the person still uses the old map as a guide, then the anxieties that existed as a child will persist, and the choices about how to react in any situation will be limited. The person may avoid situations because of a fear of rejection or disapproval, in which case we can say that she has not allowed herself the opportunity to test out the validity of the map and to amend it accordingly.

All of this is of course good cognitive therapy (see Ch. 21) and it can be a useful way of introducing the patient to the ideas behind cognitive therapy in preference to a rather dry and abstract exposition.

One can present the ideas to the patient in the form given, or one can construct a story which contains all of these themes, say, one about a person who visits a city with a map and becomes completely lost and very confused. This person goes into a shop and discovers that there are in fact new maps and the map she is using is completely out of date. And so the story unfolds and proceeds to a satisfactory conclusion. If the patient seems to have grasped the various analogies in the story, one can then say to her, 'How old is *your* map?'

The man, the boy and the donkey

The next story was told to one of us (MH) by a patient. The patient originated from one of the countries in the Middle East. The story is perhaps appropriate for someone who is overly concerned about what other people think and say about him or her.

A man and his young son set off on a journey from their own village with a donkey. As the three of them are walking along, they come to the first village on their journey. Some of the villagers notice them and in loud voices cry, 'Look at that man and his son, walking along with their donkey. Their donkey is healthy and strong, so why doesn't the father get on the donkey and save his energy?' On hearing this, the father climbs onto the donkey and the three of them set off for the next village. On arriving there, some of the villagers notice them and in loud voices cry, 'Look at that! The father is riding on the donkey while his poor little son has to walk in the heat of the sun. The father is big and strong, so why doesn't he get down and let his son ride on the donkey?' On hearing this, the father climbs off the donkey and the son gets on. On arriving at the next village, some of the villagers see them coming and in loud voices cry, 'Look at that! The son is on the donkey while his father has to walk! Surely the donkey is strong enough to carry both of them?' On hearing this, the father climbs up onto the donkey with his son and they are carried on their way. At the next village, some of the people see them coming and in loud voices cry, 'Look at that! The poor donkey is having to carry both the father and his son! That is very cruel and selfish!' Eventually the father and son arrive at their destination, and the entire village turns out to watch them coming, everyone pointing and laughing at them. For now the man and his son are staggering along carrying the donkey between them!

Wintertime

Metaphors and stories that are apposite for people who are suffering from depression may concern themes that resonate with the bleakness and sense of helplessness that the person experiences, but convey hope that things will be better and the good times will return. Such themes may be represented by wintertime, when everything dies, when there is no colour, when the mornings are dark, and daylight lasts only a short time. However, gradually spring emerges, the days lengthen, the sun reappears, the trees and flowers start to bud and will soon be in bloom, and so on. Sometimes the weather takes a turn for the worst again and winter seems to come back, but it is always temporary.

The portrait of Oliver Cromwell

This is a story that may be helpful for somebody with problems of self-consciousness and lack of self-confidence. The moral of the story seems to be that self-confidence has more to do with accepting our faults and weaknesses than holding on to an unrealistically ideal image of ourselves.

One of the greatest of all Englishmen was Oliver Cromwell who lived about 350 years ago. In those days, kings and queens were very vain and when they had their portraits painted, woe betide the artist if he did not produce a picture that depicted the sitter in the most magnificent light! Oliver Cromwell had no time for kings and queens and he fought with and defeated the king at that time, Charles I, and had his head cut off. Oliver was an ugly man and his face was covered with warts and boils. However, when *he* was having his portrait painted, he said to the artist, 'Mr Lelly, I desire you would use all your skill to paint my picture truly like me, and not flatter me at all; but remark all these roughnesses, pimples, warts and everything as you see me, otherwise I will never pay a farthing for it'.

(The Oxford Book of Quotations, 2nd edn.
Oxford University Press, New York, 1953, p 167)

Thanks to Oliver, even today we still say to one another, 'Accept me with my warts and all'.

For historical reasons, this anecdote may not appeal to confirmed monarchists or to Irish people, whom Cromwell treated with great cruelty.

Taking the plunge

One variation of this approach is to use the symbolic imagery and analogies that the patients themselves spontaneously use. This was illustrated in Chapter 11 in the case of ego-strengthening imagery. Also, to illustrate apposite themes one may use memories from the person's own life. One can, for example, remind patients of the first time they dived into a swimming pool (if indeed this did occur). They may have stood on the edge and looked into the water and may have experienced a sense of fear and yet, looking around, could see other children jumping and diving in the water, enjoying themselves with nothing bad happening to anybody. Yet, although the reasonable side of the person could confirm this, the fear still persisted. In the end it was only by 'taking the plunge' that they were able to convince themselves that their fears were unfounded.

METAPHORS FOR BEREAVEMENT

The following are two metaphorical stories that one of us (Aravind, unpublished manuscript, 2000) has constructed as part of his counselling approach to patients with intractable grief as well as those with terminal illness. The first of the stories addresses the question, invariably asked by the bereaved person, 'Why did it happen when it did?'

May I tell you a story that my grandmother used to tell me when I was a child? I did not understand it much at that age, but now for me it answers lots of questions that we ask about death, why it is out of anyone's control, and why it doesn't seem to have a reason. It has comforted many people and helped them to understand the timing of the death of their loved ones. It goes like this.

Once, in a certain village, there lived a man who was privileged to travel to Heaven and to Hell whenever he wished. When he returned from his trips, the villagers would gather around him to hear about their loved ones who had gone either to Heaven or Hell and how they were doing. He was very good at passing messages and regards between them. At one such gathering, he told them that he had learnt how death happens to all of us. It is all written up in a book, the precise time we start our life and the precise moment when we have to leave this world for Heaven or Hell as the case may be.

The chief of the village then wanted to know how this is done with such precision. The man replied that two angels are sent to us at exactly the designated time and we have to follow them. Nobody can refuse their instructions. If the angels fail to inform the person at the precise moment, then that person will become immortal, but this has never happened; there has never, ever been a mistake.

The chief then asked the man if, during the next trip, he would look up in the book what would be 'his time'. The man came back and informed the chief the precise time of his death, which happened to be only a few weeks away! The man had checked this three times and there was no mistake. The chief was surprised because he had no reason to die when he was so young and when he had money, authority and everything that made him happy. So he decided to cheat the angels by building a 10-inch thick steel room with an airtight door that could only be opened from inside. Just to be absolutely sure, he went in the room *2 days earlier* than 'his time', with all the food and drink that he needed to survive for 4 days, sealing the door from the inside.

Safe inside his steel room, the chief ate his breakfast, dinner and supper and day one went by, likewise day two, and he was still alive. To be absolutely sure, he spent the third day in the steel room. On the fourth day, 2 days after his time to die, he prepared to come out. He was greatly excited, as he was still alive, and jubilant about cheating the angels. But as he opened the door, the angels were waiting there, telling him that it was his time to leave this world at that precise moment.

The chief then declared that the angels had missed their rightful chance and so he did not have to follow their orders. To his utter dismay, however, all those present shook their heads and told him that there was no mistake on the part of the angels. Then the penny dropped: while he was sitting in the dark in his steel room, he had lost track of time and it so happened that he opened the door at the precise moment that was destined for him.

Patients seem to have no difficulty in accepting the moral of this story, namely that death is something that is unavoidable and the precise time is a matter of chance only. Therefore, there is no place for the question 'Why?' and especially 'Why him (or her)?' This seems to take away half of the 'wall of grief' and is more acceptable than the usual clichés such as 'It is God's will', 'She has gone to heaven', 'God has taken her away' or 'He gave his life for others' (making him a hero). This and the next story are also very useful in helping cancer patients set aside their preoccupation about dying very soon.

The second major issue in the loss of a beloved one is the feeling the bereaved person has about being 'left alone'. The deceased may have done things that the bereaved never did in their life, and after the death, the latter assume that they have a duty to do all those things, at the same time being unable to do so without the presence of the deceased. This is an illusion that stems from extreme hurt, but the bereaved person genuinely becomes caught up in it and it causes great distress.

To explain that everyone leads a more-or-less independent life and the person has never been solely reliant on the deceased, another metaphor is introduced. It also prepares the deceased for the process of saying goodbye at the end of the therapy session. The 'metaphor of life' is as follows:

When we start our life in the womb, our mother provides the place, the nourishment and the love for us, the embryo, to do all the growing ourselves. It is like being put in a boat in which we grow until we make our big launch into the wide world. So we sail our boat by ourselves for 9 months and then, when we are born, we start to sail our boat (our life) in the wide world. The world is like a vast sea and we all sail together side-by-side at the same speed, 24 hours a day, no more and no less. Some move away and some come and take those empty places. When we catch a fish, we share it with others close by and when we catch lots we give some away. We shout at one other and we laugh together. We give advice and we do many things for each other, while each person carries on sailing his or her own boat himself or herself. ... Always. ... No one can sail anyone else's boat and nobody ever did. We all sail our own boat, always, and are still sailing.

Now, we all have our final port, predestined and fixed. When we reach that port we have to leave our boat and say goodbye to everybody. No one can go any further and we cannot leave our boat an inch before that port either. We have to take the boat to the destined port even if part or most of our boat is damaged or lost. Even when there is only one plank of wood left, still we have to make that journey, right up to the port before we can leave this world, and then we have no choice but to leave our boat at that point.

For some people, their port is only a few hours' journey away; for others, it is a few months, years or tens of years away. When we reach that port, we know it: we have reached the end of our journey. But, at the same time, we never know where our port is until it is just in front of us. Therefore it is worthless and futile to calculate or forecast where it could be. Such a preoccupation also makes you lose valuable time when you could, say, be catching more fish, as there are people out there needing them. Or you miss all the sunshine that is there.

This story can be a way of motivating those who are grieving and who feel that there is nothing that they want to do for the rest of their life without their loved one by their side. It also helps to cushion the impact of grief when it is anticipated. Likewise, it is very useful in dissuading patients, when they are told that they have cancer or similar illnesses, from losing all hope and becoming resigned to spending the remainder of their life in 'death-watch'. It helps to motivate them to think that they *are* living, albeit with a serious problem, and not dying, *yet*, and to look forward and think what they can do to improve the quality of their life and that of their family.

The therapy continues by acknowledging that when tragedies happen the person has to struggle with many unanswered questions, yet at the same time needs to move on as 'your boat has to sail on with all the rest'. The person is therefore given plenty of time to talk and to give vent to any negative feelings, with the therapist now and then guiding and leading. Then the therapist begins to help the patient to answer all of those questions, which are always tied up with the negative feelings. Eventually the therapist re-introduces the metaphor of the boat (of the deceased person) that has arrived at its port. 'X (the deceased's name) is looking at you and saying to you that he (or she) has reached the port and it is time to leave his (or her) boat. But X cannot do that without saying a proper goodbye to you and he (or she) cannot hang on any longer.' The therapist then guides the patient through a 'saying goodbye' ceremony that is invariably accompanied by great emotion. Finally, the therapist can say:

You are sailing your boat as you have always done … all by yourself. And you don't need the *physical* presence of X to manage from now on. But you know in your heart that the wisdom that X gave to you will always be there, out in front, for you. Now it is time for you to sail your boat, looking forward all the time and catching all the fish and enjoying the sunshine on the way and not missing any of this.

This allows the patient to start new relationships and new ventures in life without guilt as:

Life is built with one brick upon another and then upon another … and so, also, love. And as long as we can keep all those bricks, our life will remain stable and successful.

FINAL COMMENTS

Using these methods is very much a matter of experience and judgement. Some writers (e.g. Langton & Langton 1983) have developed entire therapeutic programmes around the telling of stories. We do not recommend this, except possibly in the case of children, who are naturally very receptive to ideas conveyed in story form. There are books available which offer the reader entire scripts for particular problems. Again, we do not recommend working in this way. Instead, at the most, we suggest that you use this method as an adjunct to therapy, probably more the 'icing on the cake' rather than the cake itself.

We cannot quote any good research evidence for the effectiveness of the techniques. It is important that this work is done if the techniques are to be used to any great extent; it is undesirable to allow one's therapeutic practices to wander too far from the available evidence for their efficacy. In the present case, the evidence has some catching up to do.

REFERENCES

Erickson M H, Rossi E L 1979 Hypnotherapy: An exploratory casebook. Irvington, New York
Langton S, Langton C 1983 The answer within: A clinical framework of Ericksonian hypnotherapy. Brunner/Mazel, New York

14

Basic procedures with children

GENERAL CONSIDERATIONS

Hypnotic susceptibility in children

A number of studies have shown that hypnotic susceptibility peaks between 9 and 13 (Olness & Kohen 1996). Children who are, at an early age, encouraged by their parents to engage in fantasy-related activities, such as telling fairy tales and magical stories or creating make-believe plays, have higher than average hypnotic susceptibility (LeBaron et al 1988).

Myers (1983) administered the Creative Imagination Scale to 1302 children and adolescents and found higher scores in females than males from the ages of 8 to 17 (see also Ch. 3). However, London & Cooper (1969) using the Children's Hypnotic Susceptibility Scale (London 1963) and Morgan & Hilgard (1978/79) using the Stanford Hypnotic Clinical Scale for Children found no sex difference (see also Barber & Calverley 1963).

Children's experience and behaviour during hypnosis

Eye-closure

Except for more mature children and for adolescents, the methods of induction and deepening that we have described in Chapters 6 and 7 are often unsuitable for children, and increasingly so the younger the child. For example, young children will not be inclined to maintain eye-closure and often keep opening their eyes to look around. Hence, it is not a good idea to insist on continuous eye-closure. Indeed, 5- to 8-year-olds may simply be told to close their eyes as and when they please.

Relaxation

The same considerations apply to suggestions of relaxation. Children under 5 rarely physically relax to a state of immobility. Children aged between 5 and 8 may physically relax but may still move about a great deal. Eight to 12-year-olds may relax more easily and deeply, but it is better not to rely entirely on direct suggestions to 'relax', rather to allow them to actively participate in a guided imagery routine that is itself intrinsically relaxing.

Absorption and trance

A key aim is to engage the child's attention and encourage the child to become absorbed in the real or imagined events in the way we have described in earlier chapters. However, particularly in younger children, their inquisitiveness and curiosity on the one hand, and their vivid imagination on the other, result in their constantly being 'in and out of trance'. This need be no great obstruction to the therapeutic process, and once therapists have accustomed themselves to this, children can be the most rewarding subjects for hypnosis.

PREPARATION AND PRELIMINARIES

In Chapter 32, we shall discuss in more detail the preparation of the child for therapy and certain professional issues. Here we shall focus mainly on preparation for hypnosis generally. Working effectively with children (whether or not one is using hypnosis) requires experience, patience, a certain temperament, and so on, and advice on this is beyond the scope of this book. However, we do give some guidance on how to adapt hypnosis to suit children and young people of all ages.

Particularly with young children, there is no advantage in spending a great deal of time explaining what hypnosis is, and in fact with the younger children, the methods will blend naturally into the interaction that one is already having with the child. With the more structured imagery methods, the idea may be conveyed that the child is going to spend some time having a nice daydream that will help him or her sort out the problem that has been identified and, if this is a key aim of the therapy, the expectation may be created that he or she will find this very relaxing. It is only common sense to use simple words that the child understands, but it may still be necessary to explain some words. For example, the child's understanding of the word 'relax' can be assisted by reference to examples from his or her everyday life.

At least in clinical practice, to help with the choice of induction and the kinds of images and fantasies to describe to the child, it is most desirable to ascertain the child's likes and dislikes, favourite television programmes, videos and computer games, hobbies, things they are good at, pets, favourite persons (including hero figures), and so on. If the child is going to be encouraged to use self-hypnosis, then, as with adults, this is a consideration when choosing the induction and deepening methods.

As Gibson & Heap (1991, p 176) advise, it is also a good idea to appeal to the child's 'sense of adventure and curiosity, rebelliousness, and appreciation of challenge and suspense'. For example, if one is using toys and puppets with a very young child, one might begin:

Look at poor Teddy! ... He's been crying. ... Do you know why? ... Shall we find out? ... Shall I ask him? (Therapist 'listens' to Teddy.) ... Oh dear! (Therapist 'listens' again.) ... Oh no! ... Can you guess? ... etc. (drawing out the suspense).

Or with an older child:

I wonder how X (e.g. the child's favourite sportsperson) manages to calm herself down before a match. Shall we find out?

In the above examples, we see the use of expressions such as 'I wonder', 'Do you know ... ?' and 'Shall we find out?' Others may be: 'I bet you don't know ... '; 'Can you imagine how ... ?'; 'I'm very curious to know ... '; 'I bet you can't tell me ... '; and 'I really don't know how ... '. We discussed the rationale of these kinds of ploys in Chapter 10. Also, during the preliminary phase and the induction and deepening methods, the visual and kinaesthetic modalities are preferred and one's choice of words will reflect this.

It is extremely important to inform the child what is to follow after each step or stage. Make sure that you obtain permission to use a particular image that the child is happy with, or give a number of options or allow the child to come up with one of his or her own. Avoid doing anything by surprise unless you say that the child is going to have a pleasant surprise in a moment.

With older children and adolescents, one's approach and style will come to resemble those that one adopts for adult subjects, and standardised methods may be more successfully employed, say for the purposes of research.

INDUCTION AND DEEPENING METHODS WITH CHILDREN

Although one's choice of approach to induction and deepening is limited by the age and maturity of the child, and what kind of interaction the child is able to actively engage in, we wish to emphasise as always that choice of method should be informed by what the purpose of the therapy is and what assumptions are being made about the role of hypnosis in this. The distinction that we have drawn between the approach and methods described in Chapters 6 and 7, namely those that focus on suggestion and suggestibility and those that focus on the trance experience or absorption, can be mirrored in the preparation and choice of induction and deepening routine in children.

Very young children

At a very young age, up to 4 years, physical contact such as moving or stroking the arms, and lots of animation, are the best modalities. One may also use toys, dollies, teddy bears and puppets to play out certain activities and themes that are relevant to the child.

Story techniques

Most young children are able to become involved in listening to a story, and for them storytelling is a natural choice of induction. Clearly, one must tailor the story to the purpose of the intervention. For example, when one is helping anxious children relax one might tell them the story of how their favourite characters met with some adventure and afterwards sat down and calmed themselves, then went off into a nice dreamy sleep, and so on. Indeed, we shall see later that a whole session of therapeutic hypnosis, including the induction, may consist of the telling of a story that mirrors the child's problems and their solution.

Stories should be tailor-made to suit the child, taking account of his or her likes and dislikes, interests and hobbies, etc. It is a good idea to include people who are special to the child, and even pets, in the story. It may be easier to use familiar fairy tales that one adapts for the child or published therapeutic stories.

Miscellaneous guided fantasy techniques

These tend to merge with the story technique and may be used for induction or for deepening purposes. One can use the 'safe' or 'secret' place method or a more structured fantasy such as walking down steps to a beach, as described in Chapter 6, or even favourite hobbies and sports. An adaptation is to incorporate magical themes that may appeal to the child, such as flying to the child's secret place on a magic carpet or zooming off in a space ship to some distant planet. While the child is engaged in this imagery, you can slip in your suggestions of relaxation or whatever is appropriate.

The magic television

Invite children to sit comfortably, close their eyes, and imagine that they are looking at a special or magic television set. (With very young children, it may be suggested that the television is actually in the room; hence, one might say, 'I bet you can't see my special magic television' etc.) Sometimes it is helpful to say that they are sitting comfortably in their own living room and are there with their parents. Prompt them to switch on the television or video to start watching their favourite programme. Nowadays we may suggest instead that they are playing a favourite video or computer game. Encourage them to tell you about the programme (this helps if you are not familiar with it) and add your comments, making sure that they are complimentary.

Because it is a special television, you can invite them to take the place of a favourite character or play an additional part alongside their hero figure. This theme can continue as a deepening method and as a medium for therapy.

Covert modelling

One can include this method (which will be further described in Chapter 20) in any of the above approaches. One of the children's hero figures is chosen and they are encouraged, say, to imagine the hero in a situation where they need to relax or 'switch off'. It may be suggested that this hero has a very special way of doing this. One might say, 'This is a secret method; not many people know about it, so don't tell anyone else'. Children then imagine watching the hero as he or she relaxes or whatever, and then are encouraged to go through the procedure with their hero.

Staring at a coin or finger nail

This is a common induction method with children and adolescents. Draw a 'happy face' on the thumbnail. Perhaps they can give the face a name, let's say 'Charlie'. Or instead, give children a coin or a small object to hold between the thumb and the index fingers. Ask them to extend the whole arm, if necessary with your help, to a straight and rigid position slightly above the shoulder. Once this is achieved, tell them to keep staring at the object or nail.

As you are staring at it, it is going to get heavy ... very heavy ... more heavy ... more and more heavy ... very, very heavy ... Because it has become so heavy, your fingers (arm) may start getting tired. (With the thumbnail procedure, you could suggest, 'Charlie is getting so tired ... so tired', etc.) Very tired ... so tired ... At any moment from now the coin (your arm) will drop because it is really heavy. You won't be able to hold it (to keep the arm up).

Watch for loosening of the grip and the moment the coin or arm is about to fall. For the coin method, when it has dropped say:

That's fine! Wonderful! Don't worry – I'll pick up the coin for you and you can have it back when we have finished.

After the coin has fallen, suggest arm heaviness coupled with suggestions of relaxation, drowsiness or sleepiness, until the arm rests on the lap or on the arm of the chair. In the case of the thumbnail procedure, give the same suggestions when the arm starts to drop. Gently guide it to a comfortable resting place. Eye-closure may happen spontaneously or it may be suggested along with the arm heaviness.

A variation that can be used with older children, adolescents or even adults is not to draw anything on the thumbnail but, as the person is staring at it, to suggest that it turns into a television screen. It will show their favourite place or programme. Suggest that as they are watching their favourite place or programme, the arm will get heavy and soon fall while the screen will remain where it is. While the arm is coming down, give deepening suggestions as usual. Then invite the child to become actively involved with the favourite place or programme and use that for further deepening as well as for introducing therapeutic suggestions or metaphors.

Arm levitation

This induction method was described in Chapter 7 and can be adapted for use with children of most ages provided they are happy with the idea. The accompanying image is that of a balloon tugging at their wrist. With the children's permission, ensure that the nearside arm rests on the arm of the chair or on their lap. With younger children, one can mime tying the balloon to the wrist while the eyes are open, or they can hold on to the string tightly. A variant is to suggest that they can place the hand on top of the balloon, which can then push the hand up.

Proceed with the children's eyes open or closed. (When eye closure is desired you can suggest to them that they can do all this easily if they have their eyes closed.) At some stage, to test their involvement, ask what colour the balloon is. Acknowledge this by repeating the colour aloud. Indicate that the balloon is filled with a special gas called helium and it is pulling on their hand. You can gently press down on the wrist and say the balloon would easily lift the arm if you were not holding it down.

Then say that in a moment you are going to take your hand away. Create some suspense in the aforementioned ways (e.g. 'I wonder if you know what's going to happen next'). Take your hand away and wait for the hand and arm to lift in the air. If there is any delay, you can remind them that the balloon is very big and the pull on the wrist is very strong, then suggest the arm is lifting up and up. As it floats up, continue to acknowledge this and encourage further movement. You may say, 'I wonder how far up it will pull your arm and what a surprise is waiting for you when it does this'. You may also say that the balloon is being blown about by a strong wind and the hand is swaying with this.

When the arm reaches shoulder level, tell them that the pull is so strong that the balloon unties itself from the wrist, or it slips out of their grip, and just floats away to the far top corner of the room, where it sticks to the ceiling. Suggest that, to their amazement, the arm is still floating and swaying because it has become so light. Say, 'Feel that lightness in that floating arm' (thus suggesting some degree of dissociation).

Then suggest that the arm is getting heavy and tired and it will come down slowly to rest where it was before. Suggest that when that happens, they will feel relaxed, dreamy, drowsy ('sleepy' in younger children) and they may want to close their eyes if they are not already closed. You can augment this by guiding the arm, gently holding on to the wrist and taking it as slowly as you want. Continue repeating the above suggestions, adding words like 'more and more dreamy', 'very, very relaxed', etc. ('deeper and deeper' in older children).

The beach ball and bucket

This is another active induction method that may be used in groups as well as individually.

Think of a beach ball. What colour is it? (E.g. 'red and blue'.) Good. A lovely red and blue beach ball. Think of a big bucket with water in it placed next to you. What colour is it? (E.g. 'yellow'.) Good. It's not all that full of water, so when you put your red and blue beach ball in it, the water won't spill onto the floor.

Now you can put the ball in the bucket and watch the ball bobbing on the water. Now, see what happens when you place your hand on top of the ball. (If necessary help by lifting the hand and placing it on the imaginary ball.) There. Now, I wonder if you can push the ball down? Don't worry about spilling any water. I'll mop it up later.

I wonder how much you will enjoy this game? As you are pushing the ball down, the water will push it up. (If appropriate, hold the hand and gently lower it and then lift it up, repeating this to produce the movement that you are suggesting.) Now, I wonder how long you can keep on doing that? You push it down, and the water pushes it up! Down ... Up ... etc.

When the movement has been well established say:

In a moment, I am going to clap my hands and the bucket and ball will move away from you, just like magic, to the far corner of the room. And I wonder if that hand will carry on going up and down on its own just as it's doing now? And will you see the ball still bobbing up and down in the bucket in the corner of the room all by itself?

Note the suggestion of dissociation – 'that hand' instead of 'your hand' – and the suggestion of a visual hallucination. Then give a gentle clap and say (in a surprised way):

> That's right! It's going up and down .... Up and down. And as it's going up and down, you may begin to get floppy, relaxed, drowsy, sleepy and dreamy. (Choose to suit the age of the child.) As your arm is moving up and down, it is getting heavier and heavier ... more heavy ... very, very heavy. As it's getting heavier, you are getting more dreamy ... more drowsy ... more relaxed ... more sleepy. ... That's right .... The hand is coming down. When it comes to rest on your lap or the arm of the chair, I wonder how surprised you'll be when you feel so very deeply and wonderfully relaxed. Maybe you'll be more relaxed than you've ever been ... more than you have ever experienced any time before.

If there is a delay, you may gently bring the arm down and say, 'There. Now it's good to feel so wonderfully relaxed' or 'It's so lovely to feel beautifully sleepy' etc. Further deepening is rarely required.

Other relaxation methods

Progressive relaxation, as described in Chapter 6, can be a good method of induction in more mature children and adolescents, as well as a technique for deepening. Likewise the breathing techniques described in the same chapter.

Verbal triggers

Verbal triggers, such as 'relax', 'now' and 'deep' may be incorporated into the above procedures. They can then be used on their own for deepening purposes by suggesting to the child that from that moment on, every time the trigger words are spoken by you, 'you may want to' or 'you will be able to' or, simply, 'you will' become more deeply relaxed. For example, you may say, '*Now*, I would like you to take a *deep* breath. Every time you take a *deep* breath, you will *relax* more and more deeply'.

SELF-HYPNOSIS

Most of the above methods may be used by the child for the purposes of self-hypnosis, although some of them are not suitable for use in any public place such as the classroom. We noted in Chapter 9 that, contrary to the instructions that we may give to patients, we have to accept that many will not use self-hypnosis on a regular basis, and that perhaps many will find it easier to have more frequent brief periods of self-hypnosis during the day. The same may apply to children who are seen as outpatients. However, some therapists use the method of recording a session of hypnosis and the child listens to this, say, at bedtime. Whatever the case, although the parents will be informed that their child has been instructed to use self-hypnosis or self-relaxation, it is usually not a good idea that they put pressure on the child to keep up regular practice.

POSTHYPNOTIC SUGGESTION

As with adults, these may be used with children, due regard being paid to the advice in Chapter 11. We advocate the use of more indirect forms of posthypnotic suggestion with children, particularly those that create some suspense and the anticipation of surprise. For example:

From now on, I bet you'll really be the boss of that scary feeling when it comes along. You'll take a deep breath and blow it out slowly. And then what will you notice? Will a quarter of it have gone … or half of it … or most of it?

EGO-STRENGTHENING

All that was said concerning ego-strengthening in adults in Chapter 11 applies to children and adolescents also. Ego-strengthening in children, however, can normally be used at the start of treatment. Here is a routine that one of us (KKA) uses.

After describing all of the child's positive qualities, achievements, and so on, say something like:

Your mum and dad … and your grandparents (specified) … and all those people you know … and care about … do care about *you* … always. They do really … genuinely … and sincerely appreciate what you do. Your mum and dad love you … very, very much indeed … and carry on loving you … even when you are not so good. … And do you know … how much your mates are envious of your achievements … in spite of your shortcomings?

One may also use the standard ego-strengthening scripts given in Chapter 11, but children may find these too dry and may prefer storytelling and fantasy techniques. This is where the therapist's knowledge of the child comes into play along with the therapist's ingenuity and creative skills, as he or she devises an ego-strengthening routine for the individual child. Where storytelling or television techniques are used, you can suggest that the child's hero or heroine is commenting on the child's positive qualities (most useful when the child has a bad paternal relationship or has a feeling of not being liked). Shortly, we shall also present some metaphorical fantasy procedures that may be used for ego-strengthening purposes.

Case example

Leroy, an 8-year-old child who was affected by parental divorce and an authoritative stepfather, excelled in mathematics. However, he was ashamed of his small stature. He revealed to his therapist (KKA) that once he was asked by his teacher to stand up and tell the rest of the class how he had scored the highest marks in maths. So the ego-strengthening image was that they were all coming out of school and everyone was *looking up to him*. At that precise moment during hypnosis, he sat upright, holding his chin up. He was instructed to anchor that feeling in both fists. Furthermore, his hobby was making model aeroplanes and he had an in-depth knowledge of various fighter aircrafts. This information was used in an imaginary television quiz in which he was a participant. He knew so much more than the quizmaster that everybody applauded him. This marked a significant turning point in his treatment.

When these images are being given to and described by children, tell them to notice the good feelings that they are now having and emphasise that feeling by repeating such statements. Reinforce all of this by saying that you are sure that everything being said is true and this should make them feel proud of themselves and that they are as good as anybody else if not better.

SELF-CONTROL PROCEDURES

In Chapter 12, we described self-control techniques for adults that use breathing and anchoring procedures. Again these can be adapted for use by children of a suitable level of maturity. With smaller children, the breathing techniques that use the imagery of blowing bubbles can be introduced by playing at blowing real bubbles. Positive and negative anchoring may be effected by use of an object (imagined or real) such as a lucky mascot or talisman (Hartmann & Golden 1990) or a favourite word or phrase.

The following method, similar to the clenched fist technique for releasing tension, is used by one of us (KKA) with children.

Release of negative feelings

Before attempting to teach children this method, it is important to establish what sort of significant negative feelings there are and the extent to which harbouring these feelings may contribute to the children's problems. Following hypnotic induction and deepening, invite children to visualise a situation or experience that will generate these negative feelings. Observing the body language, the therapist encourages them to experience these feelings and to indicate when they are able to do so. Children often succeed at this. Then ask them to place all these feelings in the centre of their chest, take a deep breath and, as they are breathing out, to push it all down through their arms into their open hands. With permission, it may be helpful to 'guide the flow of negative feeling' by running your 'caring' fingers from the shoulder down into the open hands, with the idea that all the negative emotions are being collected in their hands. Enthusiastically encourage them to 'drain' every bit of the negative emotion with every breath they take. To avoid the effects of overbreathing, it is stressed that they should gather all of the negative emotions into their hands by the time they have repeated the above process no more than three times.

Check with them that they have succeeded in draining all the bad feelings into the hands. Then encourage them to compress the feelings into a solid ball and throw them away as they would throw a stone into a pond or hurl it into a deep wood, so that it will have gone for ever and never be seen again. Typically, relief, comfort and great satisfaction can be evident in the children's facial expressions.

Encourage them to practise this two or three times as appropriate with different scenarios. Repeat that this will help them be confident that they have now learned an effective way of ridding themselves of persistent troublesome feelings and of being able to appreciate the freedom to enjoy life. Give further suggestions that it is better to offload negative emotions as and when these emotions happen and they can practise this procedure at any time and at any place.

This is a very useful procedure, and can be used for ego-strengthening purposes. Variations include images of walking along a beach and throwing all the negative feelings into the sea, watching the waves taking them away; dropping them into a deep chasm in the mountains; or sending them up in a space rocket so that the sun can burn them to ashes.

USING STORYTELLING WITH CHILDREN

It is probably the case that therapeutic storytelling is used more with children than with adults, and the reasons for this are not hard to provide. Sometimes with children a whole session of hypnotic therapy may consist of the telling of a story. Formal hypnosis may be used, particularly with older children, but the important thing is that the children are involved in the story and are free to make comments and to offer ideas of their own.

There are a number of very good papers and texts on how to construct therapeutic stories for children and some of these are given in the reference list at the end of this chapter. Some guidelines for constructing a story are as follows.

It is important, of course, that the story mirrors in a metaphorical way the child's problem and its possible resolution. The central character in the story usually represents the child who has some problem or difficulty that is analogous to the child's own. The character may be another child, a grown-up, or even an animal, and some stories have even used plants, trees and inanimate objects for the characters. The content of the story must be appealing to the child, and it is therefore important to establish what are the child's interests. For example, it is not a good idea to construct a story around a voyage across the sea if the child has no interest in this. Elements of the child's life, including family, friends and other significant people, may be paralleled in the story. Therapeutic stories often have magical themes (depending on the child's level of maturity) and usually include a wise person who helps the child. This is of course analogous to the therapist and this wise person may be represented by a hero figure, a benign wizard, a fairy godmother, a wise owl, and so on. It is important that the way this person helps the main character is such as to empower him or her, so that the message is given that the child has the means to overcome the problem. Often the story will have some kind of ordeal or crisis with which the child successfully deals and emerges triumphant. This acknowledges the struggle the child is having with the targeted problem.

A tape recording of the story may be made during the session or at a time convenient to the therapist without the presence of the child. We prefer the former, as the spontaneous input from the child makes it more special. The child may play this whenever he or she wishes (e.g. just before going to bed).

A good example of a therapeutic story is provided by Mills & Crowley (1986, 1988) for a boy with nocturnal enuresis. The boy liked circuses and the central character in the story was a small elephant, Sammy, who had to carry, along with the other elephants, buckets of water as part of their work at the circus. Unfortunately Sammy kept spilling his water, no matter how hard he tried. The 'wise person' in this story is 'Mr Camel' who counsels Sammy and reassures him, by referring to various examples, that he has the means to overcome his problem. A crisis occurs when there is a fire and the elephants have to carry buckets of water to the fire so that it can be put out. Sammy carries his water all the way there and emerges triumphant. The boy's difficulties in overcoming his problem are acknowledged in the story by Sammy's struggle to overcome his problem – it did not just happen overnight by magic.

Metaphorical fantasies

The British educational psychologist Gwyneth Benson (Benson 1984, 1988) has described a number of fantasy methods that may be used to augment therapy with children and adolescents.

Metaphor of the 'subconscious mind' for 'reprogramming habits'

Although we shall later criticise the way in which the idea of 'the unconscious (or subconscious) mind' has been used in the clinical hypnosis literature, we do acknowledge, that as a metaphor, it may provide a useful working model for the therapist and patient to work together on the latter's problems. The following script emphasises the 'secret' nature of 'the subconscious mind' and this may appeal to children and young people, who metaphorically speaking, have secrets about themselves that they wish to be 'kept in a safe, private place'.

Because you're relaxing so well and because you're learning to drift into a really deep trance by relaxing in this way, this is giving you control of your subconscious mind. Your subconscious mind is that very secret, private part of your mind where all your feelings are stored ... all your memories ... everything that's ever happened to you. It's also that part of your mind where your habits are stored ... things that you've learned to do so thoroughly that you do them automatically, without even thinking about it. ... Things like cleaning your teeth and riding a bike. But we all have habits that we've learned just as thoroughly, but that we wish we hadn't learned at all. Habits like getting worried and upset unnecessarily ... habits of getting angry and losing your temper at the wrong moment ... habits of rushing into things without thinking ... or maybe biting your nails or smoking. ... All sorts of things that are difficult to change. But when you're very relaxed like this and you have control over your subconscious mind, this is your opportunity to change habits that you want to change ... to tell yourself to stop doing things you don't like doing ... and to teach yourself the new habits that you want to learn. ... Habits of being calm and relaxed ... habits of just taking things in your stride without getting worried and upset ... habits of thinking before you rush into things.

Now, imagine you have a videotape of all your habits and you can play it through and watch it. I don't know what habits you would like to change, but when you find one you don't like, stop the tape, rewind it and then play it back the way you would like it to be. I'll stop talking while you do that and when you've changed as many habits as you would like to today – and remember you do have to practise new habits well to make them really stick – then give me a signal to let me know, perhaps by lifting a finger or a hand. There's no hurry. Take your time and make a good job of it.

The magic biscuits

The following is an ego-strengthening routine that provides children with a technique that they can use for themselves in their everyday life.

Now we are going to make some rather special biscuits. Imagine you've got a big mixing bowl in front of you. First of all, I want you to put into that bowl all the happy memories you can find. We don't want any bad ones so use a sieve to keep the bad memories out. Nothing is too small to go in so I want you to search out all your happy memories ... all the good times ... all the fun and all the laughs. ... Put them all in the mixing bowl. Signal 'Yes' when you've done that.

And now I want you to put in the names of all the people who are important to you. All those people who care about you and want things to turn out well for you. ... Signal when you've done that.

And now put in every single good thing you know about yourself. If you're like most people of your age, you probably only notice the bad things but you'll be surprised how many good things there are when you start looking. ... The more you look, the more you'll find. Put them all in and make a good mixture ... because all the things that you're putting in that mixture are the things that everybody needs to make them feel strong and safe and happy, to make them feel confident and calm and relaxed and ready to tackle any problems that come along.

Now make yourself some biscuits and then eat as many as you feel like eating today. If you have any left over, put them somewhere safe so that you can nibble one any time you feel a bit low or things get difficult. But you can make yourself more biscuits when you go to bed at night ... when you're relaxed just before you fall asleep ... because every day you'll be finding more and more good things to put in them.

The following two scripts are similar and may be used following, say, the 'magic biscuits' method.

Tidying a garden

When you're feeling strong after eating the biscuits, there's another thing I'd like you to do. I want you to do some gardening. This garden I want you to sort out has got very overgrown and covered in weeds. So get rid of those weeds! Pull the roots up and get rid of them by throwing them on a bonfire. And, as you clear all the weeds away, you'll be amazed how many good healthy plants you find underneath that were just waiting for a chance to grow. Let the sun get to them. ... Water them. ... Move them around if you want to and watch them growing stronger and stronger ... making the garden into a showplace ... a garden you can be really proud of ... looking just the way you want it to look ... somewhere you can be proud to invite other people in to admire.

Tidying a desk

There are other things that you can do to help yourself while you're relaxing and letting yourself drift deeper and deeper ... with every breath you take and every word I say. I want you to imagine now that you've got a desk in front of you ... and this desk has got everything to do with your life in it ... a different drawer for different things in your life. ... Some are locked ... some are open ... some are full and some empty. But it's about time that desk ... your life ... had a really good sort-out. So I want you to go through that desk now ... as much of it as you feel you can do today ... and give it a really good tidy-up. Don't worry if you can't do it all. ... Do just as much as you can without upsetting yourself. Throw away all the old rubbish in there ... any old bad memories that you don't need any more. Get rid of them! Dust the drawers out. Make sure the important things that you want to keep are in a nice safe place ... and have a clean, tidy drawer ready for the things you need for your future. If you find any particular problems in there that need sorting out before you can throw them away, just parcel them up and put them on one side for the time being and we'll deal with those later. I'm going to stop talking now while you tidy that desk up. Take as long as you need to make a really good job of it. ... Sponge off any dirty black stains so that it's all clean and fresh. ... When you've finished let me know by giving me the 'Yes' signal you used before.

This routine may then be followed by the 'parcels' technique for identifying problems to work on, which is described in Chapter 19.

New metaphors for the new millennium

The above heading was coined by the British educational psychologist Geoff Callow (Callow, unpublished work, 2000). Readers themselves may wish to construct their own versions of the above metaphors and may wish to adapt them to the interests and obsessions of contemporary youth. One obvious theme is computers and video games.

Callow has constructed a number of such fantasies on the theme of 'reprogramming', that is 'examining old, inappropriate feelings, thoughts and behaviours and substituting new programmes of more appropriate feelings, thoughts and behaviours'. Following induction by imagining a journey down through a 'hypnotic funnel' that becomes more and more translucent to sight and more opaque to sound (save that of the therapist's voice), the children find themselves in their special place. They are then invited, with the aid of the therapist, to 'run new (software) programmes within themselves'. One metaphor is 'The Island where it never Rains', 'where all unwanted thoughts, feelings and behaviours are thrown' and 'everything withers, dies and biodegrades'. Should anything escape, around the island is a lake full of scavenger fish that 'eat, digest, and excrete anything that spills into the lake from the island'. Moreover, any residual unwanted feelings, thoughts and behaviours ending up on the shores of the lake are devoured by 'antibiotic ants'. New, appropriate feelings, thoughts and behaviours are generated by a 'hypnotic way-finder'. A 'composter' shreds and digests the remains of the old habits and provides new fertile soil where these new, appropriate thoughts, feelings and behaviours may grow. And so on. Finally we revisit 'The Dark Forest of Discarded Dreams' where the 'dark clouds of hopelessness and despair' may be 'rolled back' and 'the sun can shine through'.

REFERENCES

Barber T X, Calverley D S 1963 'Hypnotic-like' suggestibility in children and adults. Journal of Abnormal and Social Psychology 66: 589–597

Benson G 1984 Short-term hypnotherapy with delinquent and acting-out adolescents. British Journal of Experimental and Clinical Hypnosis 1: 19–28

Benson G 1988 Hypnosis with difficult adolescents and children. In: Heap M (ed) Hypnosis: Current clinical, experimental and forensic practices. Croom Helm, London, ch 29, p 314

Gibson H B, Heap M 1991 Hypnosis in therapy. Erlbaum, Chichester

Hartmann W, Golden G A 1990 A 'magic' aid for hypnosis and suggestion in crisis management: A brief communication. International Journal of Clinical and Experimental Hypnosis 38: 157–161

LeBaron S, Zeltzer L K, Fanurik D 1988 Imaginative involvement and hypnotizability in childhood. International Journal of Clinical and Experimental Hypnosis 36: 284–295

London P 1963 Children's Susceptibility Scale. Consulting Psychologists Press, Palo Alto

London P, Cooper L M 1969 Norms of hypnotic susceptibility in children. Developmental Psychology 1: 113–124

Mills J C, Crowley R J 1986 Therapeutic metaphors for children and the child within. Brunner/Mazel, New York

Mills J C, Crowley R J 1988 Sammy the elephant and Mr. Camel. Magination Press (Brunner/Mazel), New York

Morgan A H, Hilgard J R 1978/1979 The Stanford Hypnotic Clinical Scale for Children. American Journal of Clinical Hypnosis 21: 148–169

Myers S A 1983 The Creative Imagination Scale: Group norms for children and adolescents. International Journal of Clinical and Experimental Hypnosis 31: 28–36

Olness K, Kohen D J 1996 Hypnosis and hypnotherapy with children, 3rd edn. Guilford Press, New York

The application of hypnotic procedures in psychological therapy

In previous chapters we have stressed the importance of making explicit the purpose for which any hypnotic procedure is being applied. This theme is developed in Chapter 15, when we consider the various approaches that one might adopt in order to help someone with a psychological problem. Whenever one engages in any treatment, it is always based, implicitly or explicitly, on a set of assumptions about the patient's problem and how one's intervention can assist with this. We call this the 'working model'. In psychotherapy there are a number of major approaches or schools of therapy that are based on divergent assumptions about how and why people come to experience problems, and which inform therapeutic practice accordingly. We present a review of these in Chapters 16 to 21 and describe the adjunctive application of hypnosis in each case. We do not subscribe to any particular school; rather we contend that hypnosis is especially well suited to an eclectic therapeutic approach and we develop our ideas on this in Chapter 22. In Chapter 23 we return again to considerations of risk and safety.

Orientation to the psychotherapies and the concept of a 'working model'

Case example

Suppose that you have a patient or client, Judith, who describes her problem along these lines. She has worked as a dental receptionist for several years and has always enjoyed her job. However, for several months she has noticed that she has felt gradually more anxious at work, particularly when talking to patients and when using the telephone. At such times, she feels hot and sweaty and her breathing rate increases. She becomes more and more aware of these symptoms and feels very self-conscious as she thinks that other people are noticing them too and that they are thinking that she is stupid for being so anxious. When on the telephone, she tends to stammer sometimes and again she thinks the person on the other end of the line must think there is something wrong with her. When not at work she is fine, but she has begun to dread going into work, particularly after a weekend or holiday break. She is worried that she will eventually have to give up her job and she then might not have the confidence to work again. For her this would be a disaster, as next year she and her fiancé are marrying and they are buying a house. She thinks that if she can't work then they will not be able to afford a house and that her fiancé will have second thoughts about marrying her. Before all of this, she did not have such problems although she does recall that she was always self-conscious in class at school and never liked to read aloud or answer a question.

DIFFERENT APPROACHES IN PSYCHOTHERAPY

How can we help Judith? One approach might be to teach her how to control her symptoms of anxiety by some form of anxiety management technique, and how to avoid stammering on the telephone. Perhaps also there have been changes in her working conditions that have created more stress for her and so we could help her be more assertive with her employers in asking them for help. All of this exemplifies what is termed 'behaviour therapy'.

Instead of, or as well as, this, we might take the approach that Judith is making her problems a great deal worse by worrying too much. For example, is it really the case that people are taking that much notice of her anxiety and thinking so badly of her? And how much does it matter what other people think anyway? Isn't she being unrealistic in thinking that she is going to be dismissed when no-one has ever complained about her work? Even if she were to lose her job, is it reasonable for her to think that she might not work again? And would her future husband really reject her because of their not being able to afford a house? Taking all this into consideration, we might be able to help Judith by encouraging her to see that her worries are completely out of proportion. This exemplifies the approach of cognitive therapy.

On the other hand, we could ask whether there is actually more to Judith's problems than either of these approaches is able to reveal. Is it just coincidence that they have loomed up when she and her fiancé have decided to marry? Perhaps Judith, despite her expressions of joy and excitement at the prospects of married life, at some deeper level, has unacknowledged anxieties about being able to leave her parental home, commit herself to a lasting relationship, and undertake the responsibilities of married life. We might ask what has been her experience of married relationships, such as her parents' relationship? Also, it seems that she has always had some problems of self-confidence. Maybe we should help Judith, not by focusing on the immediate problems at work, but by exploring with her the wider concerns in her life and where the source of her anxieties really lies. We may loosely call this the 'psychodynamic approach'.

There are many other ways that we might set about helping Judith. If we adopted a humanistic approach, for example, we would not make any assumptions at all about Judith and her problems. We would consider that what are identified as her difficulties are not simply 'silly problems' to be got rid of and that have nothing to do with 'the real Judith'; rather they are important parts of her self and her life that *belong to her*, and the role of therapy is to help her come to her own understanding of them. Thus we would encourage Judith in the search for her own meaning in what is happening in her life.

There are not necessarily any clear-cut differences in the above approaches and there is actually considerably more similarity in practice than in theory. Some therapists only work with one approach, while others describe themselves as 'eclectic' or 'integrationist' and may work at different levels.

The chapters in this section of the book explore the ways in which hypnotic procedures may be used to augment a course of therapy based on the behavioural, cognitive, psychodynamic or humanistic approach. We use the term 'psychotherapy' in a broad sense to cover all formal psychological therapies. Our account has been prepared with regard to readers who are only vaguely familiar with the distinctions between the various schools of psychotherapy, so we must apologise to more experienced readers if they find our treatment of these matters unduly simplistic. Also, we are presenting this material from the standpoint of how hypnosis may be applied within these approaches, and therefore how we describe them may be selective and somewhat idiosyncratic. For a more detailed presentation, the reader is referred to Bloch (1996).

THE CONCEPT OF THE 'WORKING MODEL'

In this book, we are attempting to develop and clarify certain key themes that ought to underlie our understanding of hypnosis and how it is applied in therapeutic practice. Readers will have noted our eagerness to base our claims about hypnosis and its clinical application on that body of knowledge that is informed by the results of scientific enquiry. We nevertheless acknowledge that in many therapeutic systems, mainstream as well as unorthodox, it is not easy to provide convincing scientific justification for what one is actually doing at any given time with any given patient. This is true both for the assumptions underlying the treatment and the efficacy of that treatment. Thus, there will always be some schism between knowledge and practice, although we should strive to avoid any outright contradiction between the two.

In this chapter, we outline another important theme, namely that of the 'working model'. By this we shall try to bridge the above-mentioned gulf that is inevitable between knowledge and practice. Though analogous to a scientific theory or hypothesis (see below), the working model is more flexible; it is still amenable to scientific enquiry and disproof, but at the same time, due acknowledgement is given to its *usefulness* in informing clinical practice.

Whatever your profession, you will use hypnosis with only some of your patients – maybe the majority, maybe not. With those patients, you may use hypnosis at every session; with others, you will only apply it strategically, as and when required. With some cases, there will be only one session of therapy and this may be mainly taken up by hypnotherapeutic procedures.

Whatever the case, at any given time you will be explicitly or implicitly basing your use of hypnosis on a model of (a) hypnosis and the particular hypnotherapeutic technique you are employing and (b) the particular problem you are working on at the time.

By 'model', we mean a set of assumptions that inform the conduct of your therapeutic interaction with your patient. For example, suppose you are helping a patient who has high levels of anxiety. You teach your patient a self-hypnosis technique for daily practice that includes relaxing suggestions and imagery. Here, your working model may be something like this: your patient experiences excessive anxiety because of a tendency to dwell on worrying thoughts and images. Repeatedly rehearsing in imagination positive thoughts and images will counteract this tendency, and the patient's reported levels of day-to-day anxiety will diminish. Also, negative kinds of thoughts cause higher levels of sympathetic arousal (increased heart rate, blood pressure, sweating, etc.) whereas this is lower when the thoughts and images are positive.

Consider another example. Suppose you are helping a person to overcome an unfortunate tendency to have outbursts of physical violence. During hypnosis you suggest that the patient will have a dream before your next session that will help the patient understand why the problem exists. Here, your assumptions may be that the patient's violent outbursts are related to some emotional difficulties, the nature of which the patient is not entirely consciously aware of. Dreams are expressions of unconscious conflicts. Instructions delivered during hypnosis are accepted by 'the unconscious mind'.

Of course there are many more assumptions made in the above two examples but we have listed the main ones. Incidentally, we call the assumptions about how the patient has come to acquire particular problems the 'formulation'. This will be part of the working model and will be derived from the therapist's assessment of the patient and by reference to existing knowledge about the particular problem in question.

The working model as a scientific theory

What we have identified as a 'working model' is analogous to a scientific theory. A theory is a set of assumptions that generates predictions that can be tested by a strategically designed experiment. One outcome of the experiment will support the theory (although not *prove* it) and another outcome will fail to support or even refute the theory, so that it needs to be modified or abandoned altogether.

In the case of the working model, a subset of the predictions generated by it describes therapeutic applications. The model may therefore be tested by carrying out the particular therapeutic procedures indicated (experiment) and observing the outcome. (This brings us into the domain of 'evidence-based therapy', although the kinds of evaluations that are required in that context go far beyond the observation of individual cases in routine clinical practice.)

There is a very important and far-reaching principle that requires careful consideration when evaluating the validity of theories and models underlying therapeutic practice. While a positive therapeutic outcome supports the model, it does not *prove* it. In fact, therapeutic predictions of a model or a theory turn out to be rather unreliable ways of testing its validity. Let us explore why this is so with reference to a very telling case example.

Testing the working model

In the behavioural treatment of headaches, one procedure that has been used is biofeedback. The assumption of this treatment is that people may control a specific autonomic activity by receiving feedback of the level of that activity and being aware that a change in one direction is desirable and in the other direction is not. Feedback is usually by means of a continuous tone or the position of a needle on a dial. (The assumed process here is operant conditioning and this is explained in Ch. 20.) Thus, problems that are associated with high levels of that activity may be alleviated by biofeedback.

By the process of biofeedback, people may be trained to regulate the activity of muscles that are not normally under direct conscious control. The index monitored is the electrical activity of the muscles and the procedure is known as EMG (electromyographic) biofeedback. Similarly, people may be trained to alter the blood flow to the hands by monitoring finger temperature. The mechanism in this case is vasodilation (hand-warming) or vasoconstriction (hand-cooling). Vasodilation in the extremities may be associated with vasoconstriction more centrally in, for example, the head.

Subjects may also be trained to regulate, within limits, their hand temperature, by hypnotic procedures, specifically by hypnosis and self-hypnosis with suggestions of hand-warming or hand-cooling and suitable imagery. For example, in the case of hand-warming, the images may be of the hands immersed in warm water or resting on a hot water bottle. The assumption here is not that the hands are heated up by imaginary warmth, but that a physiological reaction will occur to the idea of hand-warming, similar to that which would occur if the hands were really experiencing warmth from an external source. This reaction is again vasodilation, a homeostatic response that causes the surface temperature of the hands to rise and therefore lose heat in order to restore the original temperature.

Now let us consider two clinical problems, tension headache and migraine. Let us assume that tension headaches are caused by excessive chronic tightness of the muscles across the forehead and scalp. Let us further assume that migraine headaches are associated with engorgement of blood vessels in the forehead (following an initial vasoconstriction).

From all of these assumptions, we can now make the following predictions. Tension headaches may be reduced in frequency, duration and severity by giving patients sufficient training in EMG biofeedback, specifically to reduce activity in the muscles of the forehead and scalp. Likewise, migraine headaches may be reduced in frequency, duration and severity by giving patients sufficient training either in thermal biofeedback, or in the use of suggestion and imagery, both targeted at hand-warming. These predictions have been tested in numerous studies and while the outcome of treatment may not be 100%, by and large the findings have supported the working models (e.g. Alladin 1988, Andrasik & Blanchard 1987, Blanchard et al 1991, Friedman & Taub 1985, Lisspers & Öst 1990).

However, this does not constitute proof of the models; other models may predict the same outcome, for example one that assumes that these therapeutic methods promote a general relaxation response independent of EMG and hand temperature changes. Accordingly, we should test other predictions generated by the models. For example, the models predict that patients who are able to raise the temperature of their hands the most or reduce the EMG reading the most will benefit the most from the procedure. Another prediction generated by the biofeedback model is that giving patients *false* feedback indicating successful EMG reduction or hand-warming should lead to a less successful outcome than true feedback of success. A third prediction of the biofeedback model is that it should not make any difference to the outcome if patients are given the usual training but are not given information that this will help alleviate their headaches.

Experiments have been conducted on all three predictions with mixed results, and with enough negative findings to lead us to question the self-regulation models outlined above. Some relevant references are Andrasik & Holroyd (1980), Epstein & Abel (1977), Friedman & Taub (1985), Gauthier et al (1985), Holroyd et al (1977, 1980) and Johansson & Öst (1982).

All of this poses a dilemma for therapists who use EMG biofeedback for tension headaches or hand-warming imagery or thermal biofeedback in the treatment of migraine. On the one hand, the evidence shows that significant numbers of patients benefit from these procedures but the working model that predicts this appears to be unsound. Clearly, if we accept these findings, then the conclusion is that the therapeutic procedures work for reasons other than, or in addition to, those predicted by the model. Indeed, some writers have offered more elaborate models that take into account these findings (Cohen et al 1980, Gauthier et al 1981).

However – and this is the important lesson – this is not a sufficient reason simply to abandon the procedures. But why should a treatment be successful while the underlying model is unsound?

Reasons for a successful outcome

First, many medical and psychological problems have a natural tendency to wax and wane over time or to improve on their own without treatment. Hence, it may be that a patient whom you appear to have successfully treated would have improved anyway during the time of treatment.

Second, many problems respond significantly to the 'placebo' effect. People who are suffering (i.e. 'patients', from the Latin 'to suffer') are reassured by the process of diagnosis and treatment and this in itself may have a remedial influence on their illness or problems, likewise their expectation of improvement.

Third, some therapies are effective (more so than mere placebo) for what are termed their 'general' effects rather than the effects specifically assumed by the underlying model. For example, many different forms of psychotherapy and counselling may be effective because of certain common characteristics, notably the opportunity for clients to talk openly about themselves in an accepting and non-judgemental atmosphere. In the case of hypnosis, we shall be presenting in later chapters quite intricate therapeutic techniques that require the use of very specific imagery. However, in the background there is always the possibility that it is merely the effect of general relaxation associated with hypnosis itself that is the therapeutic component of the treatment.

Finally, the specific ingredients of a treatment may be therapeutically active but for reasons other than those predicted by the model. For example, Alladin (1988) has shown, consistent with the original model, that hand-warming suggestions are better than hand-cooling suggestions for migraine relief. The reason for this, however, may have nothing whatsoever to do with any temperature changes in the hand, but merely that we tend to associate hand-warming with comfortable and relaxing situations, whereas the idea that one's hands are cold probably evokes more unpleasant images and memories.

Implications for practice

There are a number of important lessons in all this. First, it is entirely possible for a treatment to be based on a completely invalid model or theory and to be no more effective than placebo and yet to have a strong following and to flourish indefinitely. At the beginning of Chapter 1, we described how, at any time in history and across every culture, there is an extraordinary and virtually unlimited range of treatments for human physical and psychological illnesses and disorders, some of which have survived for centuries, without any proper evidence to support their theoretical foundations and their remedial efficacy beyond placebo. (Indeed some methods such as trepanning and bloodletting were positively harmful.) It is likely that this applies currently in our culture to what is termed 'alternative' or 'complementary' medicine but we should not try to claim that mainstream Western orthodox medicine itself is entirely free of such treatments.

A second possibility is that the model underlying the treatment may be valid, but the treatment itself is ineffective. In many such cases we might say that the treatment is 'process based' (or has a rational basis) but is not 'evidence based'. An example would be a relaxation method that we use as a treatment for chronic hypertension. It may be the case that although a session of this method does indeed result in a lowering of blood pressure, the effects are too short-lived to be of clinical significance for the hypertensive patient. In such a case we would abandon this treatment or look for ways of rendering it more clinically effective.

Third, as we saw earlier, the working model may be invalid but the treatment is effective (and here we mean more effective than just placebo) for reasons not predicted by the model. In such a case, we are justified in continuing with the treatment. Nevertheless, it makes sense to investigate the real reasons for the treatment's success, as refinements may be introduced that may enhance its efficacy.

It is sometimes legitimate when successfully applying a model that is known to be invalid, to regard it as a metaphorical or an 'as if' description of the problem and the remedial process. For example, in a later chapter we shall question the validity of the notion of 'the unconscious mind' but nevertheless suggest that, as a metaphor, it generates therapeutic techniques that may be efficacious. The following is a less contentious example. One technique for alleviating acute pain experienced by children is to show them a 'magic' object such as a toy or pebble and suggest that as they rub it, the pain streams down the arm and into the object. Simple techniques such as these seem to work often enough to apply them with confidence. However, one would not seriously propose that pain is thereby demonstrated to be the result of a blockage of a fluid that can be released by the influence of the imagination!

All of this may seem obvious, but remember this: metaphors are only metaphors. All too often in the business of psychotherapy, what start off as metaphorical constructions turn into literal truths. Thus the servant becomes the master.

Ethical implications

Of course the ideal would be to use treatments that are both of proven efficacy and based on valid models and theories of the human body and mind. It is, as we have seen, possible to be an effective therapist without aspiring to this ideal. However, as therapists, we have an ethical obligation to be honest and open with our patients and clients and those who refer them to us. It behoves us to challenge and question our ideas and practices and to engage in this debate with others. Indeed, we hope that readers will already be questioning, in a constructive way, some of the assertions that we have already made about hypnosis in this book.

Practitioners must also continually avail themselves of the up-to-date research evidence on the validity of their ideas and methods and modify and even abandon them on the basis of the evidence. Moreover, practitioners in an established health-care profession have an obligation to that profession and to their peers to use only those theories, models and practices that are consistent with the rational and scientific knowledge that informs the conduct of that profession. We have already admitted that it is often very unclear as to whether, say, a particular psychotherapeutic procedure can be said to be scientifically based or not. However, it should not be *incompatible* with existing knowledge.

Another point, no less important than any of the others we have discussed, is that whatever working model you are relying on at any time in therapy, if you are accepting it as literal and valid, then invariably you are making some important assertion about the way the mind and body function, and even about human life itself. Again this is an assertion of power and the rule is always that power must be accountable.

Some models are ambitious theoretical structures that make profound claims about the human condition. Psychoanalytic theory epitomises these, and the therapy that is derived from it is equally profound, a prolonged and veritably gothic struggle played out by both participants – analyst and client. More expedient are behavioural and cognitive theories, and the therapeutic procedures that they generate are accordingly more focused and immediate to the client's complaints. Each of these systems generates a hierarchy of working models that may be tested for their validity in terms of both their therapeutic and non-therapeutic predictions. These will be the focus of our attention in the chapters to follow.

REFERENCES

Alladin A 1988 Hypnosis in the treatment of head pain. In: Heap M (ed) Hypnosis: Current clinical, experimental and forensic practices. Croom Helm, London, ch 15, p 159
Andrasik F, Blanchard E B 1987 The biofeedback treatment for headache. In: Hatch J P, Fisher J G, Rugh J D (eds) Biofeedback: Studies in clinical efficacy. Plenum Press, New York, p 281
Andrasik F, Holroyd K A 1980 A test of specific and non-specific effects in the biofeedback treatment of tension headache. Journal of Consulting and Clinical Psychology 48: 575–586
Blanchard E B, Nicholson N L, Radnitz C L et al 1991 The role of home practice in thermal biofeedback. Journal of Consulting and Clinical Psychology 59: 507–512
Bloch S (ed) 1996 Introduction to the psychotherapies. Oxford University Press, Oxford
Cohen M J, McArthur D L, Rickles W H 1980 Comparison of four biofeedback treatments for migraine headache: Physiological and headache variables. Psychosomatic Medicine 42: 463–480
Epstein L H, Abel G G 1977 An analysis of biofeedback training for tension headache patients. Behaviour Therapy 8: 37–47
Friedman H, Taub H A 1985 Extended follow-up study of the effects of brief psychological procedures in migraine treatment. American Journal of Clinical Hypnosis 28: 27–33
Gauthier J, Bois R, Allaire D et al 1981 Evaluation of skin temperature biofeedback training at two different sites for migraine. Journal of Behavioral Medicine 4: 407–419
Gauthier J, Lacroix R, Cote A et al 1985 Biofeedback control of migraine headaches: A comparison of two approaches. Biofeedback and Self Regulation 10: 139–159
Holroyd K A, Andrasik F, Westbrook T 1977 Cognitive control of tension headache. Cognitive Therapy and Research 1: 121–133
Holroyd K A, Andrasik F, Noble J 1980 A comparison of EMG biofeedback and credible pseudotherapy in treating tension headache. Journal of Behavioural Medicine 3: 29–39
Johansson J, Öst L G 1982 Self-control procedures in biofeedback: A review of temperature biofeedback in the treatment of migraine. Biofeedback and Self Regulation 7: 435–442
Lisspers J, Öst L G 1990 Long-term follow-up of migraine treatment: Do the effects remain up to six years? Behaviour Research and Therapy 28: 313–322

16

Introduction to psychodynamic and humanistic approaches

INTRODUCTION

In this chapter, we shall look at a small number of significant figures from the field of psychotherapy whose ideas and practices are important in understanding the thinking behind much of the use of hypnosis within a psychodynamic and humanistic framework. We remind readers of our comments in Chapter 15, namely that we are presenting a highly selective and idiosyncratic review, focusing only on those themes that have a bearing on the aforementioned task. The typical reader we have in mind is the professional who has little knowledge of the various schools of psychotherapy and requires an understanding of the various ways in which hypnosis is applied within each one.

We are using the term 'psychodynamic' here in a more general sense than some readers would prefer, namely to cover the wide range of psychotherapies that are orientated to the emotional experience of the client. The assumption is that many problems that clients bring to psychotherapy may be understood as manifestations of emotional conflicts that they are unable to resolve and may not even be able to fully acknowledge. Humanistic approaches are not so dissimilar from psychodynamic approaches when it comes down to practice, and the two tend to merge.

PSYCHOANALYSIS

The founder of psychoanalysis, Sigmund Freud (1856–1939), as we mentioned in Chapter 1, began by using hypnosis and in fact made some useful contributions, but he abandoned it in favour of other methods, notably free association, dream analysis and interpretations based on transference.

Methods of psychoanalysis

Free association is the technique whereby the client is asked during the therapy session to say whatever comes to mind. It is important that the therapist does nothing that might discourage this, such as to infer that what the client is saying is unacceptable in some way. This process is viewed as encouraging the emergence of unconscious material and thus promoting the cathartic release of blocked emotions and a greater understanding on the client's part of the reasons for particular problems. To facilitate this process on behalf of the client, the analyst from time to time may interpret what the former says in terms of psychoanalytic theory. The analyst may likewise interpret any dreams that the client reports. Dreams are presumed to be the expression, in symbolic form, of unconscious material that may be relevant to the analysis.

Transference refers to the process whereby the patient comes to project onto the therapist desires, feelings, fantasies, and so on that have an important bearing on the patient's problems and psychological development generally. For example, the patient may fall in love with the therapist, feel rejected by the therapist, feel angry and hostile towards the therapist, want to know all about the therapist, feel jealous, may dream about the therapist, and so on, in ways that relate to the patient's relationships with significant others from early life, notably those involving parents. It is as though the patient's underlying neuroses are recreated in the therapy session. Hence, by working through the transference issues, the patient is able to resolve particular problems.

Although transference is traditionally associated with psychoanalytic therapies, transference issues may arise in any therapeutic context and they can be utilised productively.

Theoretical concepts

Freud developed a tripartite theory of the human mind in terms of the ego, the id and the superego. In the simplest of terms, the ego is the executive conscious part of the mind that is concerned with negotiating everyday life in an adaptive way. It is logical and reality-centred. The id is associated with the unconscious mind; it is concerned with the selfish fulfilment of basic drives such as sex and aggression. The superego is equivalent to the conscience or an internalised strict parental figure.

In order to protect the ego from overwhelming anxiety and guilt, various defence strategies are deployed whereby the offending thoughts, urges, fantasies and memories are kept out of consciousness. The main defence mechanism is repression. However, repression does not guarantee good psychological adjustment, particularly when excessive psychic energy is required to maintain the defence.

As well as the unconscious, Freud also identified the 'preconscious'; pre-conscious material is controlled by ego functions and is anything that is potentially available for conscious expression but is not in consciousness at a particular time.

Summary of important themes for clinical hypnosis

Important theoretical themes for the present discussion are the idea of representing the mind as different functional parts that communicate with each other; the notion of an unconscious mind (associated with the id); defence mechanisms, notably repression, that afford (incomplete) protection to the person from the conscious experience of overwhelming anxiety and guilt; and the idea that therapy progresses by encouraging the conscious expression of unconscious material and the resolution of such. Important practical themes here are that the therapist is essentially passive and there is a reliance on the development of the patient–therapist relationship over and above anything the therapist may actually do.

Practitioners of hypnosis who base their therapy on the psychoanalytic approach (and here we are not generally referring to properly trained psychoanalysts, but would include a significant number of lay therapists) adopt the simple idea of a conscious–unconscious mind split, and the idea of bringing into consciousness repressed material, notably traumatic memories, from the unconscious. What we may call the resolution phase of therapy may be the release of the 'pent-up' emotions associated with the memory elicited (abreaction) and the insight gained in identifying the cause of the problem.

NON-DIRECTIVE OR CLIENT-CENTRED THERAPY

Another influential person to consider is Carl Rogers (1902–1987). He developed non-directive, client-centred or 'Rogerian' psychotherapy (Rogers 1951, 1961). This is a humanistic therapy, based more on a philosophy than an elaborate theoretical structure. However, there is a set of general assumptions. First, we are all innately good and effective. We become ineffective and disturbed only as a result of faulty learning. Also we are free to make decisions for ourselves and are responsible for them. However, freedom is a double-edged sword; the realisation that one has freedom implies that we are responsible for ourselves and the world that we personally create. The focus of therapy is on the client's view and interpretation of his or her world, rather than the therapist's.

We may contrast this approach with psychoanalysis and (in a later chapter) behaviour therapy and cognitive therapy, each of which has a theory by which the therapist interprets what is wrong with the client and what are the remedies. In this respect, these other therapies may be said to adopt a medical model. This does not mean that they are based on an organic interpretation of the client's problems but that they provide a theory of the underlying pathology independent of any understanding that the client may have of his or her particular difficulties.

In contrast, client-centred therapy provides the setting whereby clients can take responsibility for their problems and decisions. This is arrived at again through the relationship and not so much with anything that the therapist actively does. The therapist provides a relationship of trust, warmth, empathy and unconditional positive regard that encourages clients to talk about themselves and their feelings. Therapy is a process of authenticating the client; that is, therapists demonstrate by their communications that they have heard what clients have to say and are in empathy with them.

In particular, therapists reflect back to clients the emotional content of their communications. For example, the client may say, 'My parents give my sister all their attention; I don't get anything'. A cognitive therapist (see later chapter) might – if this is a real problem – ask the client to review the evidence for this and encourage the client to challenge this way of thinking. A client-centred therapist would show the client that he or she has heard and understood the meaning of the communication and is in empathy. The therapist might say, 'It sounds like you are really sad about this'.

Thus the *process* is the key factor. By demonstrating that the client is being given unconditional acceptance, the client feels more relaxed and comfortable with communicating information about which she feels anxious, guilty and ashamed. For example, the client might go on to say, 'Sometimes I really hate my sister'. This may be the first time that the client has been able to express and even acknowledge this thought and to experience the feeling that goes with it. Again the therapist remains nonjudgemental even if the client goes on to say, 'And sometimes I feel like killing her!'

By the therapist's adopting an understanding and non-judgemental attitude, the client may be able to acknowledge troublesome emotions and conflicts, dispel feelings of overwhelming anxiety and guilt about them, and resolve them in her own way. By this process, the client's sense of guilt, anxiety and inadequacy diminishes and her self-regard improves. So we have again the idea of the revealing of unconscious material. A two-stage, reciprocal or cyclical process appears to underpin the therapy, namely the communication to the therapist of conscious activity by the client, which facilitates the expression in the client's consciousness of material below the level of consciousness, which is communicated to the therapist, and so on. Rogers, however, did not formulate an elaborate theory of 'the unconscious mind' in the same way as did Freud.

Also, we see again the importance of the relationship over and above content, or any *techniques* that the therapist may employ. In fact, it is fair to say that the client-centred therapist resists the use of any active ploys and procedures that involve the therapist in taking responsibility for the client's problems on the client's behalf.

GESTALT THERAPY

Fredrich Perls (1893–1970) was the founder of gestalt therapy (Fagan & Shepherd 1970, Perls et al 1973). This belongs to the humanist/existentialist school of psychotherapy, but for present purposes we highlight one obvious difference between this and the Rogerian approach. In gestalt therapy, the therapist is very much more active and instructs the client in a range of techniques. Why this is so may be not entirely to do with any advance in knowledge over Rogerian therapy as this quotation from a book on gestalt therapy may reveal (Fagan 1970, p 96).

To justify his hire, the therapist must be able to assist the patient to move in the direction that he wishes, that is to accelerate and provoke change in a positive direction. We are rapidly leaving the time when the therapist, in the absence of more specific knowledge, relies on 'something' in the relationship that will result in 'something' happening. We are approaching the time when the therapist can specify procedures that promote rapid change in a way that the patient can experience directly and others can observe clearly.

This sounds very much like an appeal for therapists to use 'techniques'. But what is a technique in psychotherapy? Here is our definition:

A technique is a prescribed way of responding by the therapist or, under the direction of the therapist, by the patient, deliberately aimed at accelerating the desired behavioural, cognitive, emotional or physiological changes.

It is important to remember that techniques are tools to be used selectively by therapists to assist their endeavours. Unfortunately, therapeutic techniques have now become a commodity, to be sold in books and on workshops and training courses, in a manner little different from the products on sale at a supermarket, offering much ('Cure psychological problems in under 15 minutes with this latest powerful technique'), endorsed by celebrity therapists, yet often unsupported by any real evidence for their effectiveness.

In fairness, it should be said that gestalt therapy uses techniques in a very client-centred fashion. Like gestalt psychology, it is concerned with 'the whole', that is, the person's whole personality or being, including the parts that the person denies or disowns. The aim of therapy is for clients to discover, explore and experience their 'wholeness', resulting in integration of all parts. Once we 'become ourselves' totally, then we can realise our potential for growth.

The focus of the therapy is on the 'here and now'. Like Rogerian therapy, clients are encouraged to take responsibility for their experiences, thoughts and behaviour. This is done by various exercises and techniques that focus on the here and now experience. For example, the therapist may observe that while talking, the client is clenching the hands. In a sensitive manner, the therapist can draw the client's attention to this, and, perhaps ask the question 'What does it feel like your hands want to do?' Perhaps the hands are expressing feelings of anger that the client is not consciously acknowledging. The therapist can then encourage the client to allow the hands to give further expression to this anger, and to discover more about what it is about.

Another technique is to discourage the client from 'gossiping'. This is something that lots of clients and patients do. That is, rather than, for example, confronting someone with the fact that they feel angry with him or her, clients will come along to the session and inform the therapist of this. It is important that clients take full responsibility for the fact that they are angry. Of course, the solution may not be for the client to express the anger to the person concerned; the consequences for this, in reality, may be most unfortunate (e.g. if the other person is the client's boss and has the power to dismiss the client) or the person concerned may no longer figure in the client's life. One technique is therefore, the 'empty chair'. The therapist asks the client to imagine that the person with whom, for example, he is angry, is sitting in the chair opposite. 'Now,' the therapist may continue, 'tell X what you really feel about her.' Another use of the empty chair technique is for the client to imagine that another 'part' of himself is sitting in the chair. For example, in the case of a patient with bulimia, the therapist might suggest that the 'part that wants to binge' is sitting in the chair opposite. The client is then encouraged to have a dialogue with the 'other part' and this may mean that he gets up and sits in the other chair in order to give expression to that 'part'.

Gestalt therapists also employ a similar technique when analysing dreams. This technique is based on the assumption that each element of the dream represents a part of the dreamer. This is of course probably an impossible hypothesis to demonstrate convincingly by empirical means; nevertheless, it can be a useful working assumption. Thus, when relating the dream, the client can be encouraged to be each part of the dream and experience what it is like.

We can thus use the concept of 'parts' in therapy in an informal and expedient manner, such as when we talk to the patient about 'the part of you that hurts now', 'the part of you that is angry', 'the part of you that wants to be thin', 'the part of you that wants to stuff yourself with food', 'the part of you that wants to leave your partner', and so on. The client experiences problems when parts of the self are dissociated, denied or disowned in some way. Thus therapy is about helping clients communicate within themselves – that is, between the different parts of themselves.

Case example

An example of this 'disowning of a part' is Amy, a patient (seen by MH) who attended a session of therapy looking very troubled and as the session progressed, it became apparent that something was on her mind that she was having difficulty in disclosing. This woman was in a very unsatisfactory marriage and had been badly treated by her husband, who had been unfaithful to her many times, but she had always stood by him. Eventually she took in a deep breath and said, 'Doctor, I have something to tell you'. She then said, 'I've been with another man'. She continued, 'I feel so guilty and ashamed. I feel dirty'. However, when describing how she felt when she was with this man, she said, 'I felt like a woman again; I felt wanted'. We can see how one can conceive of this lady's problems in terms of parts. There was a feminine part of her with unfulfilled needs. She had denied this part of herself for so long and now this part of her was 'dirty' and made her feel guilty.

TRANSACTIONAL ANALYSIS AND EGO-STATE THERAPY

Another influential psychotherapist has been Eric Berne (1910–1970). He wrote a popular book called *Games People Play* (Berne 1967) which actually became the title of a hit song in the 1960s. The contribution that Berne made that is relevant here is his idea of ego states. He developed a tripartite model of personality and human interaction, called transactional analysis based on three states, the parent, the adult and the child (compare with Freud's superego, ego and id). The parent is the internalised parent figure; the child is the part of us that we bring from our childhood into our adult world; and the adult is the 'grown-up' part that has to deal with the realities of life in an effective way. An interaction between two people can be defined in terms of which states are communicating. For example, a married couple may be having an argument in which they behave as two children. Or one partner may be very sad and frightened, just like a child, and the other partner plays the role of the comforting parent. All possible interactions are valid and useful, but in any close relationship there has to be flexibility to ensure that all needs are met. For example, a relationship in which one spouse always plays the parent role to the other partner's child is very restrictive and unfulfilling.

We can also conceive of communications within oneself in identical terms. Sometimes we feel very upset and need our 'parent part' to comfort us. However, instead of an understanding and nurturing parent part, we might have an intolerant, nagging, parent; thus we attack and belittle ourselves when, for example, we fail to achieve what we set out to do.

This notion of 'ego states' is used in clinical hypnosis in a much wider sense and relates to the ideas of other writers such as Paul Federn (1952), a colleague of Freud. Ego states are construed as parts of a person's personality each associated with a common pattern of responses and experiences. They can be thought of as having a certain functional autonomy, surrounded by barriers that have varying degrees of permeability. Ego states are a feature of normal development, as manifested by the very obvious tendency for different aspects of a person's personality to be dominant at different times and in different situations (viz. the tyrannical boss who becomes the meek husband when he arrives home).

Good psychological adjustment is evident when ego states are regularly manifested in ways that are adaptive to the situation and when there is a harmonious relationship amongst them, rather like a happy family. However, ego states may develop as a defensive response to trauma or internalised parental conflicts. They may be poorly integrated and dissociated from the 'core personality' so that one can speak of a person's personality as being in various degrees of fragmentation. The ultimate expression of this is multiple personality disorder.

Importance for clinical hypnosis

The leading exponents of ego-state therapy are two American psychologists, John and Helen Watkins. They construe the aim of therapy as to resolve conflicts between ego states and to re-integrate them into the 'family of the self' (Watkins 1993). The ego-state therapy that they have developed incorporates hypnosis, but is much too elaborate to be presented here and the reader is referred to more detailed expositions in Watkins & Watkins (1997) and to the April 1993 issue of the American Journal of Clinical Hypnosis (vol 35(4)), which contains a number of papers on ego-state therapy by experienced clinicians. We shall in a later chapter present a way of using the concept of ego states for the resolution of difficult memories.

Ego-state therapy and the more informal use of 'parts' in therapy lend themselves well to the augmentative use of hypnosis. Indeed, Hilgard's neo-dissociation model (Ch. 4), with its concepts of permeable amnesic barriers, the executive ego, and the hierarchical arrangement of cognitive control systems, provides a natural theoretical framework for ego-state therapy.

The reader will now perceive that we have moved from talking simply in terms of a conscious–unconscious mind split and conscious–unconscious communication, to a somewhat more elaborate model or metaphor in terms of 'parts' of the self. Rather than repression, we are now using the idea of dissociation, a more flexible concept (some would say too flexible), and one that is not restricted to abnormal phenomena. Nevertheless, we still have the idea that therapy facilitates the conscious representation and integration of cognition and affect.

Once again, we contend that the idea of 'ego states' or 'parts of the person' only provides a 'working model' on which to base our therapeutic practice. As such it has its limitations and it is not always appropriate. It is a metaphorical way of understanding the problems that clients bring to us but there are occasions when it is entirely inappropriate to think in these terms. The model can be taken far too far. An unfortunate manifestation of this is the epidemic of 'multiple personality disorder' or, as it is now known, dissociative identity disorder, in some countries such as the USA. At least one reason for this has been too zealous an application of the idea of parts or ego states into which clients have been indoctrinated.

REFERENCES

Berne E 1967 Games people play: The psychology of human relationships. Penguin, Harmondsworth

Fagan J 1970 The tasks of the therapist. In: Fagan J, Shepherd I L (eds) Gestalt therapy now: Theory, techniques, applications. Harper Colophon, New York, ch 7, p 88

Fagan J, Shepherd I L (eds) 1970 Gestalt therapy now: Theory, techniques, applications. Harper Colophon, New York

Federn P 1952 Ego psychology and the psychoses. Basic Books, New York

Perls F S, Hefferline R, Goodman P 1973 Gestalt therapy: Excitement and growth in the human personality. Penguin, Harmondsworth

Rogers C R 1951 Client-centred therapy. Constable, London

Rogers C R 1961 On becoming a person: A therapist's view of psychotherapy. Constable, London

Watkins H H 1993 Ego-state therapy: An overview. American Journal of Clinical Hypnosis 35: 232–240

Watkins J G, Watkins H H 1997 Ego states: Theory and therapy. W W Norton, New York

17

Ericksonian approaches to psychotherapy

INTRODUCTION

In Chapter 10, we looked at styles of hypnosis, notably the indirect method, and in Chapter 13, we covered the use of metaphor and story technique. Both of these approaches have been promoted by the followers of the American psychiatrist and psychologist, Milton Erickson (1901–1980). For many years, Erickson was a leading figure in the field of hypnosis, both as a clinician and as an investigator of hypnotic phenomena, especially the more unusual manifestations. However, he is also remembered as an innovative psychotherapist of unusual insightfulness. In his later years in Phoenix, Arizona, he became something of a guru figure for young therapists who were keen to learn from him and train others in his approaches. That he was such an inspirational figure may be partly due to the physical disabilities that he had to surmount in his lifetime, including two bouts of polio, the first of which occurred in childhood and nearly killed him. In his final years, he was confined to a wheelchair.

Erickson's approach to psychotherapy does not fit neatly into any of the major schools that we are describing in the present section of this book. His approach to therapy is often described as 'strategic'. Our impression is that strategic therapy is usually more often undertaken with couples and families than with individuals. He appears to have been something of a radical in his time, if we remember that the orthodoxy then was classical psychoanalysis, with its strict rules on how analysts conducted themselves and organised the therapy sessions. For example, Erickson had no problems about seeing his clients at his own home (where they would see his wife, children and family pets). Or he might go to their own homes or even meet them somewhere in town. He had no rule about how long a session of therapy might last; it could be a few minutes or a few hours. Although this is common enough now, he was unusual at that time in that he would sometimes see clients with their spouses or families at some or all sessions, and even spouses in the client's absence. He would tell the client stories about himself and his life experiences, something that a psychoanalyst and many psychotherapists would never contemplate doing. He was often very authoritarian and directive.

He sometimes commanded his clients to undertake some task or even 'ordeal', such as a journey or a new hobby. Sometimes the purpose for this would not be apparent to the client. For example, he once instructed a young man with a bedwetting problem to stay several nights in a hotel in a neighbouring city and, amongst other things, deliberately worry about how embarrassed he would feel when the maid discovered his wet bed (Haley 1973, p 86–88).

Erickson was also occasionally deliberately offensive. For example, a man in his 50s who was disabled by a stroke, a very proud Prussian German, was brought by his wife to see Erickson. He appeared to be extremely angry by his predicament. Instead of offering him sympathy, Erickson proceeded to insult him and all his countrymen, telling him that they were 'horrible animals … not fit to live' and 'better used for fertiliser' (Haley 1973, p 310–313). Needless to say, all turned out for the good in the end!

He also made use of symptom prescription. There are many examples of this ploy in his work; for instance, he might instruct a client with a weight problem to go away and *gain* a specific amount of weight.

Behind all of this seemingly disparate and incoherent way of working, it appears that Erickson was guided by certain principles and beliefs about human nature and how people become stuck in their lives.

UNCONSCIOUS RESOURCES

One of the fundamentals of the Ericksonian approach is that clients have the resources at their disposal to solve their personal problems. In all likelihood, by the time they have come to therapy they will have tried all conscious ways to overcome their problem. Hence, the means whereby they may come to resolve it are not immediately obvious to them. In other words, the possible solutions may be said to be 'unconscious'. Thus, we have an 'unconscious mind' that contrasts with the Freudian conception; namely that it has the potential to be resourceful and creative and it acts in the best interest of the person. Some Ericksonian writers extend the domain of the unconscious mind to cover all mental and physical processes that are not consciously directed; these include the regulation of vital activities such as respiration, blood flow and digestion.

So, the therapist does not provide clients with the answers, but helps clients to discover them for themselves. Clearly, then, the means of solving a particular problem will not necessarily be the same for two different clients. Therefore Ericksonian psychotherapy can be construed as being very client-centred, although, as we have seen, the therapist is often very active and may be very direct in planning the most appropriate therapeutic strategy.

UTILISATION

Any attribute, habit or skill however seemingly problematic, has the potential to be deployed as a positive resource in the person's life. This is not too controversial if we think, for example, of a characteristic such as aggression, which may cause someone (and others too) a great many problems, yet can prove a great asset if re-channelled, say, into some sporting activity. This approach to a problem is called 'utilisation'.

Strictly speaking, utilisation means to put to good use something that is not intrinsically designed for the purpose in question. In the clinical context, this means using for therapeutic benefit whatever is available from the client or the immediate situation, even what may be regarded as 'problems', such as resistance. In terms of what we discussed in the last chapter about 'parts' or 'ego states', we could say that for Ericksonians, every 'part' is a potential resource.

The most oft-quoted example of Erickson's utilisation approach to hypnotic induction is the case of the client who arrived for therapy in such a state of agitation that he could only pace around the room (Erickson 1959). The most obvious thing for a therapist to do would be to gently encourage the client to sit down and relax. Instead Erickson asked the man if he would continue to cooperate with him by pacing the room. Subtly, he then coupled the man's movements with indirect suggestions of calming down and relaxing. Thus, eventually the man was able to relax in the chair, and proved to be a good hypnotic subject.

THE EMPHASIS ON THE RESOLUTION PHASE

In later chapters, we shall describe how psychodynamic applications of hypnosis based on the idea of unconscious–conscious communication distinguish exploratory, uncovering and resolution phases of therapy. It is apparent in Erickson's work that he did not spend much time exploring and uncovering the causes of the client's problem. His therapeutic focus seems to have been to enable clients to find their own ways of solving their problems. In this he seemed to be able to work out just what he needed to do to help mobilise clients' strengths in such a way that they would come up with their own solution. Thus his insulting treatment of the 'proud

Prussian' was calculated to help the man harness what resources he had, notably his own anger, and to direct this to his own advantage. In order to do this, Erickson had to go against the normal convention, which would be to offer care and sympathy, or at the very least to be polite, to one who was disabled and suffering, something which may not have been particularly helpful to this man.

Another example is his therapy with a couple who had an alcohol problem (Haley 1993, p 194–195) and whose weekends were particularly miserable. The obvious course of action of the therapist would have been to suggest that they make a habit of arranging interesting things to do at the weekend. Probably they had already tried to discuss this between themselves. Indeed the outcome of therapy was that they decided to go camping at weekends, something they really enjoyed. How did Erickson help them to arrive at this solution? He instructed them to go boating at weekends, something they both disliked! To make this prescription, Erickson must have been able to secure their full compliance, and indeed sometimes he would make no bones about his being the doctor whom the client had to obey. But he must also have observed the couple very carefully and been satisfied that this intervention would bear fruit. How it came about was that eventually the couple came up with their own answer and asked Erickson permission to go camping instead of boating.

One danger of all this is that admirers of Erickson will try this method out on their next similar client. We do know of a colleague who was brave enough to tell us that he once tried Erickson's symptom-prescription approach with an overweight patient. This patient did not turn up for her next appointment. When contacted again, she reported that she had felt very depressed by the therapist's instructions. Clearly, Erickson's methods are not 'standard techniques'. One must allow for the uniqueness of each client and make a strategic intervention such as this only after a careful study of the client and the nature of his or her problem.

REFRAMING

Not dissimilar to the idea of utilisation is 'reframing' (literally to put a different frame around something). Again what is initially framed as a problem may be re-interpreted or acknowledged to be an asset or a solution to a problem. For example, overeating and smoking are acknowledged problems but both may be construed in positive ways from the client's point of view. Both may be a way that the person copes with stress and they may also be ways in which the person self-rewards. They are not the solutions that the client consciously wishes, so they may be said to be 'unconscious solutions'.

Indeed, some Ericksonian therapists consider that it is important to 'show respect' to the unconscious mind for 'looking after' the client by, for example, overeating, smoking, being afraid, being angry, or whatever. This may be acknowledged by asking the client to internally say, 'Thank you' to the unconscious mind (or the 'part that is in charge of the problem'). Having thus reframed 'the problem' as *one* choice that the unconscious mind has made in order to help the client, the next step is to increase the range of choices available. So clients do not *have* to smoke in order to achieve whatever smoking does for them; other more adaptive or less destructive solutions may be available. In other words, therapy does not take choices away from clients; it helps them to discover more choices for themselves. One ploy that has been described by Grinder & Bandler (1982) is to ask the unconscious mind (or the 'creative part of the mind') to generate one or more alternatives and to give a signal (say by raising a finger) every time a choice has been unconsciously identified. We ought to mention that some extraordinary claims have been made for this kind of 'therapy by digital levitation' but no proper evidence has been forthcoming. (Bandler and Grinder in their various books (Bandler & Grinder 1975, 1979, Grinder & Bandler 1976) claim to have been able to distil the essence of Erickson's work (and that of others) into a series of 'press button A, pull lever B' techniques. These seem to bear little resemblance to what Erickson actually did.)

TRANCE

We have discussed the Ericksonian concept of trance in Chapter 10, a crucial property being the possibility for clients to suspend their 'habitual frame of reference' and thus discover other choices. Although Ericksonians adhere to an altered-state conception of hypnosis, for them trance is nevertheless a naturally occurring phenomenon, with or without a formal induction. Thus, say, during therapy there may be times when clients naturally enter a trance – a momentary state of mind when they are particularly receptive to what the therapist is communicating. Hence, it is important that the therapist carefully observes the client's non-verbal behaviour for signs of the trance (see Ch. 6) in order to maximise the impact of a communication. Such 'moments of trance' may of course be deliberately engineered by the therapist, as when he or she throws the client 'off guard' by saying something designed to surprise or confuse the client.

ERICKSON'S IMPACT ON MODERN HYPNOSIS AND PSYCHOTHERAPY GENERALLY

Erickson was a renowned figure in the field of hypnosis during his lifetime and he became increasingly so after his death. He did not offer a structured or systematic theory of hypnosis in the same way as modern influential thinkers and researchers such as Hilgard, Barber, Spanos and Sarbin (see Ch. 4). Attempts by his followers to present a theoretical structure sit uneasily alongside current major theories (Barber 1991, Matthews et al 1993), possibly because of the strong clinical perspective.

Unlike existing theories, his ideas have not spawned a great deal of research, and some of his assertions about hypnosis – for example, concerning literalism in the hypnotic trance (Erickson 1980, Erickson & Rossi 1980) and hypnotically suggested deafness (Erickson 1938a, 1938b) – have not found support (Barber & Calverley 1964, McCue & McCue 1988, Scheibe et al 1968). He did not conduct controlled laboratory-based experiments in the conventional manner of modern psychology. He did not undertake controlled clinical trials on patients.

Even within hypnosis, people seem to have great difficulty conveying in simple language, 20 years after his death, what exactly his contributions to hypnosis were. In fact, in the scholarly *A History of Hypnotism*, by Gauld (1992), Erickson's name crops up only once in the text (p 579), amidst a list of people whose contributions the author indicates he has chosen not to divulge.

Erickson has had little influence in the broader field of psychotherapy, unlike people such as Carl Rogers, Joseph Wolpe, Aaron Beck and Albert Ellis. He has made no contribution to mainstream academic psychology or abnormal psychology.

Some writers have expressed doubts about the authenticity of Erickson's accounts of his casework. As Gibson (1984, p 255) has said, 'He is the hero of all his own stories'. These suspicions have been expressed by Masson (1988), who also questions the ethics of some of Erickson's practices. McCue (1988) draws attention to disparate verbatim accounts of his interventions in two of his cases, one being the 'proud Prussian' described above. The same author complains of the sensational claims Erickson made about hypnosis, as in the instance of two people whom he claimed had remained in a trance for 2 weeks, unknown to anyone else.

Unfortunately, it is no secret that since his death, most of the books on 'Ericksonian hypnosis and psychotherapy' and various offshoots such as 'Neurolinguistic Programming' have been less than enthusiastically received amongst those who bring a more critical attitude to this area. Within clinical hypnosis, his impact is seen in the proliferation of Ericksonian societies across the world. It also appears to be obligatory for lay hypnosis societies to feature 'Ericksonian hypnosis' as a selling point in their training programmes. Two of his own lasting achievements were the founding, in 1957, of the American Society of Clinical Hypnosis and, around the same time, the American Journal of Clinical Hypnosis, of which he was first editor. Both continue to flourish.

REFERENCES

Bandler R, Grinder J 1975 The structure of magic. Science & Behavior Books, Palo Alto
Bandler R, Grinder J 1979 Frogs into princes. Real People Press, Maob
Barber J 1991 The locksmith model: Accessing hypnotic responsiveness. In: Lynn S J, Rhue J W (eds) Theories of hypnosis: Current models and perspectives. Guilford Press, New York, ch 8, p 241
Barber T X, Calverley D S 1964 Experimental studies in 'hypnotic' behaviour: Suggested deafness evaluated by delayed auditory feedback. British Journal of Psychology 55: 439–446
Erickson M H 1938a A study of clinical and experimental findings on hypnotic deafness: I. Clinical experimentation and findings. Journal of General Psychology 19: 127–150
Erickson M H 1938b A study of clinical and experimental findings on hypnotic deafness: II. Experimental findings with a conditioned response technique. Journal of General Psychology 19: 151–167
Erickson M H 1959 Further techniques of hypnosis: Utilization techniques. American Journal of Clinical Hypnosis 2: 3–21
Erickson M H 1980 Literalness: An experimental study. In: Rossi E L (ed) The collected papers of Milton H. Erickson, vol III: Hypnotic investigation of psychodynamic processes. Irvington, New York, ch 10, p 92
Erickson M H, Rossi E L 1980 Literalness and the use of trance in neurosis. In: Rossi E L (ed) The collected papers of Milton H. Erickson, vol III: Hypnotic investigation of psychodynamic processes. Irvington, New York, ch 11, p 100
Gauld A 1992 A history of hypnotism. Cambridge University Press, Cambridge
Gibson H B 1984 Review of Rossi E L (ed) 1980 The collected papers of Milton H. Erickson, vols I–IV. International Journal of Clinical and Experimental Hypnosis 32: 254–256
Grinder J, Bandler R 1976 The structure of magic II. Science & Behavior Books, Palo Alto
Grinder J, Bandler R 1982 Trance-formations. Real People Press, Maob
Haley J 1973 Uncommon therapy: The psychiatric techniques of Milton H. Erickson, MD. Norton, New York
Haley J 1993 Jay Haley on Milton H. Erickson. Brunner/Mazel, New York
McCue P A 1988 Milton H Erickson: A critical perspective. In: Heap M (ed) Hypnosis: Current clinical, experimental and forensic practices. Croom Helm, London, ch 24, p 257
McCue P A, McCue E C 1988 Literalness: An unsuggested (spontaneous) item of hypnotic behaviour. International Journal of Clinical and Experimental Hypnosis 36: 192–197
Masson J 1988 Against therapy. Fontana/Collins, London
Matthews W J, Lankton S, Lankton C 1993 An Ericksonian model of hypnotherapy. In: Rhue J W, Lynn S J, Kirsch I (eds) Handbook of clinical hypnosis. American Psychological Association, Washington DC, ch 9, p 187
Scheibe K E, Gray A L, Keim C S 1968 Hypnotically induced deafness and delayed auditory feedback: A comparison of real and stimulating subjects. International Journal of Clinical and Experimental Hypnosis 16: 158–164

The unconscious mind and the repression of memories

INTRODUCTION

As we have seen in the previous chapters, not infrequently, the rationale for clinical hypnosis has depended very much on a simple dualistic representation of the human mind, namely the conscious and the unconscious. This remains the case despite the development of more elaborate working models such as 'parts' or 'ego states'. Let us therefore explore some current concepts of the unconscious mind from the hypnosis literature and then suggest ways of thinking about 'the unconscious' that are more consistent with cognitive psychology and may inform our understanding of hypnosis and its therapeutic practice.

SOME STATEMENTS ABOUT 'THE UNCONSCIOUS MIND' FROM THE HYPNOSIS LITERATURE

Hartland (1971)

The conscious mind is the part of the mind which thinks, feels and acts in the present … . The unconscious mind is a much greater part of the mind, and normally we are quite unaware of its existence. It is the seat of all our memories, all our past experiences, and indeed of all that we have ever learned. In this respect it resembles a large filing cabinet to which we can refer in order to refresh our memory whenever we need to do so.

(p 13)

The power of suggestion is tremendously enhanced when it acts upon the unconscious rather than the conscious mind.

(p 12)

Yapko (1990)

Because of the dual nature of the human mind (i.e. conscious and unconscious) memories and details that may have been repressed or else simply escaped detection by the conscious mind may not have escaped the unconscious mind.

(p 74)

Memories in the form of powerful learnings from the client's unconscious mind can be used skilfully to make available to the person the resources she requires to handle her life in the desired way.

(p 84)

Otani (1990)

In essence, Erickson ... viewed the interspersal technique to consist of two components: 1) fixation of attention on the conscious level, followed by 2) appropriate suggestions to the unconscious.

(p 41)

Erickson & Rossi (1979)

Erickson: Your unconscious knows how to protect you ... . Your unconscious mind knows what is right and what is good. When you need protection, it will protect you.

(p 296)

Kershaw (1994)

The healing trance is a state of focused attention in which unconscious minds meet and a more positive identity is storied by the therapist so that the patient experiences a change in belief, perspective and self-narrative.

(p 148)

ASSUMPTIONS ABOUT UNCONSCIOUS PHENOMENA

From these and other writings in the hypnosis literature emerges a kind of *topographical* model of unconscious phenomena. The unconscious mind is the larger part of the human mind, the other, much smaller part being the conscious mind, and:

- It is the agent of goal-directed action and experience: it controls and modifies activities (autonomic and central), notably those that are experienced as habitual, automatic and compulsive, and internal experiences (sensory, cognitive, emotional, etc.).
- It is a storehouse of memories, learning, skills, emotions, and so on.
- It has great knowledge and wisdom.
- It processes information in a way different to the conscious mind.
- It communicates purposefully with the person's conscious mind and to other individuals.

- It receives communications from the person's conscious mind and from other individuals.
- It has 'awareness' of undesirable and maladaptive, drives, fantasies and memories that, were they to be allowed into the conscious mind, would cause overwhelming fear and guilt.
- It protects the conscious mind: that is, it acts intentionally to promote the well-being and survival of the individual.

Again from these and other writings, it appears that the following claims are being made for hypnosis. Hypnosis facilitates the hypnotist's and subject's ability:

To communicate with the unconscious mind.
To ask or direct the unconscious mind to do certain useful things.
To receive communications from the unconscious mind.

PROBLEMS WITH THE CONCEPT OF 'THE UNCONSCIOUS MIND'

Are there any problems with all of this? There need not be, provided one important caveat is borne in mind. All of these assumptions should be considered to be working models in the sense that we have described this concept (Ch. 15). They may provide a rationale for treatment, but they are not necessarily valid explanations of the treatment. Hence, it is not unacceptable within the context of therapy to tell patients, for example, that one is 'implanting suggestions deep in your unconscious mind so that they will work immediately and effectively for you in the future'. Likewise, one may ask, 'Is Mary's unconscious mind aware of any memories that are still affecting her now and that it is important to resolve?' (It is, of course, important, that your patient can make sense of these communications – that is, that you are both 'on the same wavelength'. Also you must, as stated in Ch. 15, always be concerned to seek out any kind of evidence that the methods you are using can be demonstrated to be effective.)

You must not, however, immediately suppose that once you have left the therapeutic relationship, this working model of the mind is literally and universally accurate. That the mind is divided into these two parts, the conscious and the unconscious, is an oversimplistic and potentially very misleading idea and one that unnecessarily limits our progress in understanding human psychology and hypnosis in particular. Indeed, over 100 years ago, the philosopher and psychologist William James (1890, p 163) had this to say about the unconscious mind:

The sovereign means for believing what one likes in psychology and of turning what might become a science into a tumbling ground for whimsies.

Let us try to understand why this is so.

The problems of nominalisation and reification

When we talk of our conscious experiences, we tend to use the nominal mode, affording them a material existence beyond our immediate awareness. Thus we commonly say that we *have thoughts, ideas, memories, images, perceptions,* and so on. We say such things as 'I have just had an interesting thought'; 'I have a vivid image of this person'; and 'I have lots of happy memories of my childhood'. Even psychologists, as we ourselves do in this book, speak of *memories* that are encoded, stored and retrieved.

In reality, what we are describing are *activities* that one engages in. It is more appropriate to say that we *think* rather than that there are *things* called *thoughts* that we *have*. Likewise, we *imagine* rather than *have images*. We *remember* rather than have *things* called *memories*. When we stop remembering, the memories do not *go* anywhere. They are not stored away as files are stored in a filing cabinet.

By way of comparison, consider a physical activity, namely the action of waving one's arm. Whilst one is waving, one can say one is 'executing a wave'. One may point to 'the wave' and describe 'it' in various terms – 'a silly wave', 'a regal wave', 'a welcoming wave', 'a farewell wave', and so on. But this does not make the 'wave' any more material. When one stops waving, it makes no sense to ask where the wave has gone to and to examine the arm to see where it is stored. When one resumes waving, it is not sensible to ask whether the same wave has been retrieved, or a different wave.

Exactly the same reasoning should be applied to the activities of thinking, remembering, imagining, and so on. All of these are represented by neural activities that are, in an as yet unknown (and maybe ultimately unknowable) way, associated with the conscious experiences that we call 'having memories, thoughts, images, and so on'.

Let us examine this argument a little further. Suppose that, having decided you have done enough reading for the moment, you put this book aside. However, later on, you start to think about some of the ideas that we have been discussing. Surely you can only do this if there is some *thing*, some representation of this material – a *memory* – that exists in your mind and which you retrieve, when you decide to, as you would draw a file from a filing cabinet?

We can say that this is so 'only in a manner of speaking', but a more accurate and potentially less misleading description is to say that, as you are reading this material, neurobiochemical changes are occurring in your brain that enable you, in the future, to *engage in the activity* of recalling this material.

But do not these observable neuronal properties constitute your memory of this information? Recall again the example of waving. An anatomist may perform a careful examination of a person's arm and hand and, from its macro- and microanatomical properties, conclude that indeed the arm is designed to wave. Put energy into it and it cannot fail to wave. But nowhere in the arm will the anatomist locate 'a wave'. Likewise, perhaps it will eventually be possible for neuroanatomists to examine a neuronal network and conclude from its structure and properties that, put energy into it and it cannot but engage in recalling recent activities. Even if that is not too ambitious an expectation, what the neuroanatomists will not find is *a thought, a memory* or *an image*.

What are the implications of this for the concept of the unconscious mind? In a sentence, it is simply that the unconscious mind does not exist (or for that matter the conscious mind). And William James was right.

Let us also note that Freud himself fell into the trap of reifying the metaphorical concepts of his dynamic model of the human mind, namely the ego, superego and id, and assigning to them the property of their being agents of causality. The same fate has now befallen the concept of 'ego states' (Ch. 16). It is *as if* a part of us is still a child, *as if* we have a parent part that takes control at appropriate and inappropriate times, *as if* there is a part of us that feels the pain of rejection, and so on. And therapists can work very well with this metaphor to understand and help people in distress. But it is only a metaphor, a tool that is at the disposal of therapists, to use as and when, and if, at all, they feel it will assist their purpose.

We shall have more to say about the risks of nominalisation and reification later. It is worth recalling here what we stated in Chapter 4, namely that it is best to conceive of hypnosis itself as something that people *do*, rather than something that people are *in*, or *under*, or *come out of*, and so on. It is, as we have seen, much to do with one person's attempt to intentionally influence the conscious *activity* of another person by suggestion.

ALTERNATIVES TO 'THE UNCONSCIOUS MIND'

Our task is defined by this question: in the field of hypnosis, can we have a useful paradigm that acknowledges the importance of the conscious–unconscious distinction but which is grounded in current cognitive science rather than psychodynamics? To achieve this it may be better to start thinking more about the nature of human *consciousness*, something which cognitive scientists are becoming very interested in again, and to think of what we call 'the conscious mind' as not a part of the mind but as activity performed by the brain – remembering, thinking, imagining, perceiving, etc.

Now, one could argue that certain levels of central nervous system activity are processed in a particular way, a side effect being that they are experienced as conscious, but that such a property has no effect on the processing itself. Perhaps this is like the material that appears on the VDU of a computer; the representation on the screen plays no part in determining the processing that is going on. Thus some might say that consciousness is an epiphenomenon.

However, let us assume that consciousness itself has an adaptive purpose: it is important to the survival of the organism that certain brain activity (perceiving, thinking, imagining, remembering, etc.) must take place at a level such that it may be represented in consciousness.

Now, much brain activity and functioning, by their nature and for good reason, are not in a form that may be consciously represented. Indeed, cognitive scientists have taken to using the expression (metaphorically, we hope!) the 'cognitive unconscious'. For example, when reading, we seemingly recognise the words instantaneously; the processing that occurs between the act of looking at a word and recognising it is always at an unconscious level – indeed, we cannot help but read the word. But in addition to the 'cognitive unconscious', let us consider two ways of using the description 'unconscious'.

1. Unconscious activity in a form that can be consciously expressed

First, there are cognitive activities or processes that are already able to be expressed in conscious form at any one time and compete for the privilege of being so. That which is not conscious at any time may be described as 'unconscious' (or in Freud's terms 'preconscious'). This does not mean that those 'thoughts', 'memories', etc. literally exist somewhere in a place called 'the unconscious mind'; rather the brain is not engaging in those activities at the time in question.

The process of allocating which activities are to be expressed in consciousness is of adaptive significance but is undertaken with varying degrees of efficiency. For instance, it is important that we maintain our focus of awareness on relevant stimuli and ignore irrelevant stimuli, yet be prepared to become conscious of important stimuli that are not immediately registered at a conscious level. An example is our concentrating on a conversation at a noisy gathering, ignoring all other sounds, but being immediately aware when someone mentions our name. We also have the facility to *inhibit* the conscious expression of activity that is threatening or emotionally disturbing.

This is certainly not an all-or-none process and people differ in the degree to which they seem able to do this. We shall return to this topic later in this chapter when we mention modern cognitive interpretations of repression.

That we are not always successful at controlling what is and what is not expressed at a conscious level at any time is revealed, for example, by excessive ruminating and worrying in obsessional individuals and intrusive images and memories in patients with post-traumatic stress disorder.

Another example is when we become stuck in problem-solving. This may be illustrated by the tip-of-the-tongue experience, when although we repeatedly try, we cannot recall a word, a person's name, or a piece of music that is potentially in a form that can be clearly expressed at a conscious level. Similar processes may underlie some instances of our failure to solve a problem with repeated conscious effort. For example, consider this cross-word clue:

Clue   Sacred flower of the East (six letters).

Answer   _ A _ G _ _

If we do not immediately see the answer, then an endless struggle may ensue, as we mentally go through all the names of flowers or fit likely let-ters in the missing slots to see if any floral connections are elicited.

What often happens in all of the above examples is that when we stop thinking of the problem and do something else, later when we think of the problem again, the answer suddenly comes to mind, or new ways of approaching the problem that previously eluded us. Some people may consider that the reason for this is that the unconscious mind continues to work on the problem once the conscious mind has 'given up'. This can be a useful working model: our advice to someone who is obsessively and need-lessly churning over a problem may be, 'Put it out of your conscious mind and let your unconscious mind find the answer!' Perhaps putting the communication in this terse, concrete form can be more effective than a lengthier, more abstract piece of advice.

Despite this, a more plausible explanation may be that in some way the cognitive routes that one is pursuing each time one attempts to find the answer tend to become overlearned (as though the neural pathways are invested with excess energy) and this inhibits the activation of other pos-sible routes to the answer. The effect of stopping consciously thinking about the problem then allows the habit strength of the overactivated routes to dissipate, and this gives more chance for competing routes to be con-sciously expressed.

So when we re-consider the above crossword clue after having set it aside for a while, another possible route to follow may become activated. The sec-ond word of the clue, 'flower', may not refer to a plant at all; perhaps it is actually *flow-er*, something that flows.

2. Unconscious activity not in a form that may be consciously expressed

A second major way of using the description 'unconscious' is in relation to cognitive activity that is not in a form that allows it to be fully expressed consciously, but may be assisted in being so. Intuition (e.g. when we have a strong feeling that something is wrong but can't put our finger on why) may be an everyday example. A piece of creative work, such as a poem, in its period of incubation may be another. The conscious experiences may be vague, incoherent and fragmentary and often associated with emotion and physical feelings and activity such as 'body language' and autonomic processes. (In the case of material that may be associated with difficult emotions, the inhibitory process mentioned earlier may also be operating.)

CONSCIOUSNESS AND THE ROLE OF PSYCHOTHERAPY AND HYPNOSIS

The above working model of unconscious processes is an elaboration of the reciprocal two-stage 'unconscious-to-conscious' model that we described in Chapter 16 when we considered the rationale for non-directive psychotherapy.

Stage one

At the first stage, psychotherapy may facilitate the elaboration and expression in consciousness of cognitive activity that is either not presently in this form or, if it is so, is not presently available to consciousness. Many psychodynamic procedures probably operate at both these levels simultaneously, likewise those involving hypnosis (mental and physical relaxation and inner absorption, and procedures to be described later, such as sensory focusing, age regression, ideomotor signalling, and dream suggestion). Some forms of meditation are also claimed to facilitate this process of enhanced self-awareness.

Also, as we suggested above, in everyday life the simple act of *not* consciously thinking about a problem for a while may facilitate this. These processes allow greater availability in consciousness of information that may be more apposite to the situation, problem or task in hand than that which is habitually given priority for consciousness. Perhaps this is also related to the Ericksonian idea of 'suspending one's habitual frame of reference', and utilising other ideas, knowledge, learning, and aptitudes in solving the problem.

Conversely, some hypnotic techniques may facilitate the reverse process, namely the *exclusion* of various cognitive activities from conscious expression, as envisaged by Hilgard's neo-dissociation model (Ch. 4). In clinical practice, we may refer to the exclusion (or diminishment) of aversive activity, such as the conscious processing of pain, by a competing activity (pleasant distracting thoughts).

Stage two

Stage two is the overt communication to the therapist of conscious activity. (We could also include such methods as writing down one's thoughts, fantasies and dreams.) We have seen how this is achieved by relaxing the constraints on what is to be granted such expression at any time, the simplest way being to encourage the client to 'open up' or 'free associate'. We may also include brainstorming here.

Again, some hypnotic procedures may be assumed to facilitate this process. For example, the mere fact of encouraging clients to close their eyes and physically and mentally relax may help them communicate more openly. The technique of ideomotor signalling, to be described in Chapter 19, may also be construed along these lines.

The stage two process then facilitates stage one, and so on in reciprocal fashion. Also material, having been thus expressed more fully in conscious form, then has the opportunity for further adaptive processing to enable integration with the person's existing cognitive schemas and coping mechanisms, which includes further 'talking through' with empathic others, and making decisions and taking any necessary action on the basis of this enhanced conscious awareness.

THE CONCEPT OF RECOVERED MEMORIES

The above analysis of the concept of unconscious activity is not all that dissimilar from ideas proposed by Sigmund Freud (see Freud 1933, particularly Lecture 31). However, Freud's concept of repression has proved problematical (and indeed, as we note below, was so at the time he was developing his ideas based on his clinical work). Let us now consider in more detail the idea that important memories may be repressed from consciousness because of their distressing nature, but can be recovered by procedures such as hypnosis.

In Chapter 12, we described (and we will take this further in the following chapters) how useful it may be sometimes to ask patients to relive important memories that may have adversely affected them (or, for other purposes, that evoke strong positive feelings). Our foregoing discussion of the unconscious mind has important implications for this kind of work.

The decade up to the time of writing this book witnessed a sensational and most disturbing consequence of misinformed and ill-considered psychotherapeutic practice. Thousands of adult clients in the USA, Europe and Australia came to believe that their fathers and mothers sexually abused them as children, and sometimes openly accused them of doing so. In cases that are cited as typical, prior to therapy the clients, usually women, have no memories of their being sexually abused. Such memories only emerge during therapy. The clients are encouraged to confront their families with these revelations and effectively to disown their parents. Occasionally, parents have been arrested, tried and in some cases convicted on the basis of the evidence of recovered memories of abuse (Conway 1997, Ofshe & Watters 1994, Taub 1999).

The roots of this controversy are commonly traced back (see Ofshe & Watters 1994) to Sigmund Freud and his struggle to understand what he initially considered to be actual incestuous experiences in the lives of his young female patients, then his reformulation in terms of unconscious fantasies. Perhaps, however, there is an inevitability about what has happened, regardless of which particular individuals happen to be occupying the key roles. Civilised society has always had enormous problems with matters sexual, and sexual relationships in the family are a large part of this. Not long before the recovered memory controversy broke out, our own society adopted a position of denying the parental sexual abuse of children. In the struggle to get it right, the pendulum may swing violently one way and then another, often at the expense of fairness and justice to the innocent, the guilty and the victim alike.

There are three major concerns in all this that psychotherapists need to address. First, often the alleged incidents of abuse are extremely severe and prolonged (even over many years) and occasionally very bizarre, involving more than one abuser and even many, yet the only witness is the client and the client's recovered memory.

Second, the lack of any recollection by the client prior to therapy that he or she experienced such extensive abuse would, if it were authentic, have extraordinary repercussions for our understanding of the mechanisms and processes of human memory.

Third, the practices adopted by the therapists involved raise serious concerns. They are often clearly based on the assumption that (i) a history of child sexual abuse is very common, if not the norm, in the aetiology of mental health problems, and (ii) a host of 'symptoms' that are regularly experienced by anyone with a psychological problem or disorder are indicative of a history of child sexual abuse.

The practices adopted are, according to reports, often highly coercive and clearly designed to lead the client through the stages of considering the possibility of abuse, acknowledging that it happened, 'recalling' instances of abuse, feeling rage against the alleged abuser, confronting that person, and so on.

One complication that is sometimes a feature of the above is the diagnosing of the client with multiple personality disorder (MPD) or, in the present nomenclature, dissociative identity disorder (DID). It is considered that this disorder is associated with a childhood history of extreme physical and sexual abuse. According to reports (e.g. Piper 1994), the diagnosis is again arrived at through a psychotherapeutic process in which the client is actively groomed into the role of the MPD patient.

The present authors' knowledge of these matters is not based on any direct experience and neither of us has been engaged in the diagnosis of MPD. Although in the last quarter of the 20th century the incidence of MPD in the USA and Canada increased dramatically, in the UK, as well as some other European countries, it is considered that such a psychiatric disorder, if it exists at all, is extremely rare (Aldridge-Morris 1989). The consensus here is that it is all for the good that this shall remain the case.

The role of hypnosis in the recovery of 'repressed memories'

A common procedure used by recovered memory therapists is hypnosis and age regression. Consequently, every therapist who is going to use these methods should be aware of the risks of eliciting false memories. (By false, we mean seriously inaccurate; every act of recalling is an act of reconstruction and can never be wholly accurate or complete.) To avoid such occurrences, professional societies of hypnosis such as the American Society of Clinical Hypnosis (Hammond et al 1995) and the British Society of Experimental and Clinical Hypnosis (BSECH) have drawn up guidelines on the use of hypnosis in the recall of memories. The BSECH Guidelines can be found in Appendix 1 of this book.

We should mention one theoretical basis for the use of hypnosis in 'recovered memory therapy'. This assumes that there is some mechanism whereby the content of a traumatic memory becomes dissociated from the emotion it evokes. The content is suppressed from consciousness, but the same affect continues to be expressed, notably when the person is in situations that are reminiscent of the original event (Evans 1991). So, for example, a person who experiences severe phobic anxiety about water may, during childhood, have experienced a near-drowning incident, the memory of which is repressed because it is so distressing. However, the repression is incomplete because every time the person goes near water, for reasons that are inexplicable, she becomes terrified. The idea of encouraging the conscious recall and reliving of the original memory is therefore to re-associate the affect, currently experienced as phobic anxiety, and the content of the memory of the near-drowning experience.

This working model is adopted by some practitioners of clinical hypnosis, who regularly regress their patients. It is not too dissimilar to the ideas of 'unconscious-to-conscious expression' described above although it makes more assumptions. However, it is not generally accepted by behaviour therapists and cognitive therapists, who, while acknowledging that many phobias (to take just one disorder) are acquired as a result of one or more conditioning events (the memory of which may have faded, but the conditioned response remains), it is not important to discover what this or these were.

Whatever theoretical position is taken, the rationales and steps that we shall shortly outline for the elicitation and reliving of memories during hypnosis will still allow for the possibility that repressed traumatic memories can lie at the root of some problems. Let us, however, state our own case here. We have explained that it is more accurate to speak of the *activity* of remembering than having something called 'a memory'. Consequently, let us express ourselves in the corresponding way and say that hypnosis itself does not have any property to directly distort the process of remembering. The contributing factors are the expectation that both the therapist and the patient bring to the session and that are created within the session as the therapy unfolds. However, because hypnotic subjects are particularly sensitive to these demands and expectations, where, for example, there is an emphasis on the need to recall important events that 'lie at the root of the problem', there is a risk that patients will relax their criteria for distinguishing actual memory and fantasy.

Nevertheless, there is still no particular reason why, when asked to remember events from the remote past, hypnotic subjects should recall fictitious events of their being sexually abused. Thousands of patients, laboratory subjects and trainees on courses have experienced hypnotic regression procedures without falsely recalling such events. Again the missing ingredient is the expectation on the subjects' part that they are required to recall such memories.

Expectations that patients' problems and disorders are the result of traumatic events, the memories of which are repressed and can be 'recovered' by hypnosis, appear to be founded on simplistic thinking that again involves the reification of activities and their confusion with metaphorical concepts. Thus, it is held that the unconscious mind contains repressed memories that, were they to gain admittance to the conscious mind, would cause unbearable anxiety and guilt. Hypnosis is construed as a procedure for 'communicating with the unconscious mind' and therefore a means whereby therapist and patient may gain access to these memories.

We have already argued that there is no such entity as the unconscious mind nor do we *have* memories. It follows that we cannot *do* anything to memories. For example, we do not repress our memories and we do not *have* repressed memories. Moreover, there can be no such *thing* as repression.

When an activity or process is reified in this way, it progressively assumes the status of an overvalued idea, promoted well beyond its original range of useful application. Not only this: just like the old notion of the 'hypnotic trance', it acquires a pivotal significance in the role narratives of those therapists who are committed to its authenticity. The argument between them and their opponents is not just a matter of whether 'it exists', but whether their roles as therapists have due legitimacy.

Consider, then, these three quotations from writers hostile to the notion of 'recovered memories':

There is no controlled laboratory evidence supporting the concept of repression.
(Holmes 1990, p 96)

Laboratory studies ... have failed to demonstrate that individuals can 'repress' memories. Clinical studies ... must start with the null hypothesis: namely, repression does not occur.
(Pope & Hudson 1995, p 125)

After years of research into this issue I have yet to find even one convincing case of massive repression or massive dissociation.

(Prendergrast 1999, p 54)

Do these statements not illustrate the points we are making? Here is what happens when we reify an activity or process. Some *thing* called repression is hypothesised. And for evermore no-one will be able to agree if *it* exists or not. Some people will claim they have seen it and others will claim that what they saw was something else. It is difficult to resist making a comparison with this and claims of paranormal phenomena such as ghosts and UFOs, reported sightings of which are destined never to go away.

Instead of posing an unanswerable question, 'Is there any such *thing* as repression?' or 'Does repression exist?' we would do better to frame the question in its active form: 'In what ways can people exercise control over their conscious activity, particularly with regard to remembering?' Clearly, there is still great scope for disagreement, but perhaps it is easier for us to work together when we express the question in this active way.

Indeed, there is a literature that addresses this question and some robust findings that have important implications for psychotherapists (Brewin & Andrews 2000). For example, laboratory studies have indeed revealed that some individuals, more than others, have a coping mechanism characterised by the avoidance of cognitive activity that is threatening and anxiety provoking (Myers 2000). This does not appear to be entirely consciously directed; such individuals, termed 'repressors', adopt attentional and cognitive-processing strategies that minimise the conscious experience of negative emotion such as fear, yet this is evident at behavioural and physiological levels. They interpret personal events in an unrealistically positive way and tend to present in a socially conforming manner. They spontaneously recall fewer unhappy childhood memories than non-repressors yet on further enquiry have had unhappy experiences, notably in their relationship with their fathers. They recall fewer items having negative connotations from material presented in the laboratory (Myers 2000). Perhaps there is a relationship between repression and the concept of self-deception in some highly responsive hypnotic subjects, as envisaged by some authors (Coe & Sarbin 1991) and discussed in Chapter 4. In contrast, preconscious cognitive mechanisms for inhibiting recall during the period of suggested posthypnotic amnesia have been indicated in laboratory results obtained by Smith et al (1999).

The purposes of clinical hypnotic procedures in the elicitation and reliving of memories

There now follows our own recommendations for defining the purposes of hypnotherapeutic procedures for eliciting and reviewing significant memories. We have already asserted (Ch. 12) that there are beneficial and productive hypnotic procedures that require a patient to relive in imagination significant past events. It is important, however, that therapists understand their task in facilitating this.

1. The therapist helps the clients to identify *for themselves* whether, if they are willing to engage in this, there are any memories (presently unspecified) that it may be useful to bring to mind in order to help them with their problems. Either negative or positive memories may be sought. This may be done most often by simple discussion but may also be undertaken during hypnosis using the ideomotor signalling method (see Ch. 19).
2. The therapist helps the clients to *identify* one or more such memories. Again, this may in most cases be achieved by normal questioning or a technique such as ideomotor signalling or age regression.
3. The therapist helps the clients consciously to recall the targeted memory, with due regard to any feelings of anxiety, guilt, sadness, and so on that may inhibit this process of recall in the case of unpleasant memories. We shall later describe ploys for helping clients do this, although the therapist's reassurance and empathy may be all that is required to facilitate this.
4. Again with due regard to any distressing feelings that may inhibit this process, the therapist encourages clients to verbally communicate their recall of the events in question, and express any emotions that they arouse. Again, empathy and the non-judgemental attitude of the therapist may be all that is required here or techniques may be introduced and these will be discussed later.
5. If the previous stage is not sufficient for this, the therapist will help resolve the difficulties that this memory causes the clients or if the approach is a cognitive-behavioural one, use the memory to rehearse strategies for coping with the situation.

What the therapist should on no account do is to make the assumption that clients' problems are caused by or associated with a repressed traumatic memory and that their task is to 'go on a fishing trip' and 'uncover' the memory in question. It may be the case that clients will recall events that they afterwards describe as 'forgotten'. However, therapists need not concern themselves with what clients actually mean by this term, which people use in varied and different ways. We have indicated our dissatisfaction with the current impasse between those who believe 'repression exists' and those who do not. We acknowledge that people have the ability to regulate what is expressed at a conscious level, and that this applies to the activity of remembering or cognitively reconstructing past events. Experts in human memory can advise us on the various mechanisms that are behind these processes and whether hypnosis can play a role.

REFERENCES

Aldridge-Morris R 1989 Multiple personality disorder: An exercise in deception. Erlbaum, Hove

Brewin C R, Andrews B 2000 The example of repression. The Psychologist 13: 615–617

Coe W C, Sarbin T R 1991 Role theory: Hypnosis from a dramaturgical and narrational perspective. In: Lynn S J, Rhue J W (eds) Theories of hypnosis: Current models and perspectives. Guilford, New York, ch 10, p 303.

Conway M A (ed) 1997 Recovered memories and false memories. Oxford University Press, Oxford

Erickson M H, Rossi E L 1979 Hypnotherapy: An exploratory casebook. Irvington, New York

Evans F J 1991 Hypnotisability: Individual differences in dissociation and the flexible control of psychological processes. In: Lynn S J, Rhue J W (eds) Theories of hypnosis: Current models and perspectives. Guilford Press, New York, ch 5, p 144

Freud S 1933 New introductory lectures on psycho-analysis. Hogarth Press and The Institute of Psycho-analysis, London

Hammond D C, Garver R B, Mutter C B et al 1995 Clinical hypnosis and memory: Guidelines for clinicians and for forensic hypnosis. American Society of Clinical Hypnosis, Des Plaines

Hartland J 1971 Medical and dental hypnosis and its clinical applications, 2nd edn. Baillière Tindall, London

Holmes D S 1990 The evidence for repression: An examination of sixty years of research. In: Singer J L (ed) Repression and dissociation: Implications for personality theory, psychotherapy, and health. University of Chicago Press, Chicago, p 85

James W 1890 Principles of psychology. Holt, New York

Kershaw C J 1994 The healing power of the story. In: Lankton S R, Erickson K K (eds) Ericksonian monographs, number 9: The essence of a single-session success. Brunner/Mazel, New York, p 146

Myers L B 2000 Deceiving others or deceiving themselves? The Psychologist 13: 400–403

Ofshe R, Watters E 1994 Making monsters: False memories, psychotherapy and sexual hysteria. University of California Press, Berkeley

Otani A 1990 Structural characteristics and thematic patterns of interspersal techniques of Milton H. Erickson: A quantitative analysis of the case of Joe. In: Lankton S R (ed) Ericksonian monographs, number 7: The broader implications of Ericksonian therapy. Brunner/Mazel, New York, p 40

Piper A 1994 Multiple personality disorder. British Journal of Psychiatry 164: 600–612

Pope H G, Hudson J I 1995 Can memories of childhood abuse be repressed? Psychological Medicine 25: 121–126

Prendergrast M 1999 From Mesmer to memories. In: Taub S (ed) Recovered memories of child sexual abuse: Psychological, social and legal perspectives on a contemporary mental health controversy. Charles C Thomas, Springfield, pp 40–55

Smith C H, Morton J, Oakley D 1999 Hypnotic amnesia and the suggestibility of goal-orientated recollection: Evidence for preconscious output inhibition. Contemporary Hypnosis 16: 253–254

Taub S (ed) 1999 Recovered memories of child sexual abuse: Psychological, social and legal perspectives on a contemporary mental health controversy. Charles C Thomas, Springfield

Yapko M D 1990 Trancework: An introduction to the practice of clinical hypnosis, 2nd edn. Brunner/Mazel, New York

Hypnotic procedures in psychodynamic therapy

Chapter contents

INTRODUCTION

In this chapter, we shall be presenting hypnotic methods that may be used within a psychodynamic framework. However, as we shall see in due course, therapists who are more committed to behavioural and cognitive approaches may also find many of them useful as adjunctive procedures. They may all be understood in terms of our presentation in the previous chapter of the nature of unconscious and conscious activity. As a rule, when one is undertaking psychodynamic work using these procedures, it is natural to choose the first approach to hypnosis, described in Chapter 6. This emphasises absorption on inner experiences and thus is consistent with the ideas presented in the last chapter.

IDEOMOTOR SIGNALLING

The method of ideomotor (IMR) signalling can be a useful technique provided that it is applied selectively and strategically. It involves the use of suggestion to evoke what are ostensibly automatic or involuntary movements. (We are aware that the issue of what constitutes involuntariness is by no means clear. For a discussion of this in the context of hypnosis, see Kirsch & Lynn 1997.)

A good practical introduction to IMR signalling is by an adaptation of Chevreul's pendulum, described in Chapter 2. We suggest you practise this with some colleagues before progressing to the main procedure that we shall describe, namely IMR signals using finger movements.

IMR signalling using Chevreul's pendulum

We shall first describe this method by adopting as our working model the simple metaphor of 'the unconscious mind'. When we describe IMR finger signals, we shall present variations on how to describe the method to the subject.

Having established that your subject is responsive to suggestions of various movements of the pendulum (see Ch. 2), place a blank A4 paper underneath the pendulum. Ask the subject to fixate the bob of the pendulum and suggest that deep down in the subject's unconscious mind, he is thinking about the message 'Yes'. As the unconscious mind is thinking about the message 'Yes', it will cause the pendulum to move in a particular direction to communicate that message. Keep repeating the word 'Yes' and observe how the pendulum moves. Mark the direction with an arrow on the paper and then repeat the procedure with the message 'No'. You may also elicit a movement for the message 'I don't know', and perhaps another one, 'I don't want to tell you'.

Then proceed to interrogate your subject's 'unconscious mind' by asking questions to which the answer is 'Yes' or 'No'. For example, you might ask the questions 'Is Bill a medical doctor?'; 'Is Bill currently married?'; and 'Has Bill been to Japan?' Of course, Bill could simply answer these questions orally, but the purpose of the exercise is to familiarise you with the IMR method.

You may go on to ask about Bill's likes and dislikes. For example, you could ask, 'Does Bill like football?' You might probe a little deeper and ask questions such as, 'At the moment, does Bill enjoy his work?' Before you do this (and this illustrates one use of the IMR signalling method), you could ask Bill's unconscious mind for permission to ask this question. So the first question would be 'Is it OK if I ask Bill if at the present time he is enjoying his work?'

The pendulum method has been used in clinical work as a psychodynamic technique (Cheek & LeCron 1968). For example, we could ask more probing questions such as, 'Is Bill's unconscious mind aware of any particular memory that has a bearing on his present problems?'; or 'Are Bill's headaches associated with any particular problem in his life?' Nowadays, however, the preference is to use involuntary finger movements.

IMR signalling using finger movements

There are a number of variations on the IMR finger-signalling method. (The thumb is included as a potential signaller, while the ring finger is the least preferred for these purposes because of the difficulty of lifting it independently.) One normally uses the method when one has undertaken a hypnotic induction and deepening routine, although it is possible to use it 'cold', and some practitioners apply the method in some circumstances with the patient's eyes open.

Some practitioners stipulate one hand to work with, as with two hands there is the problem of dividing the therapist's attention. The arm(s) may be raised in the flexed position so the hand hangs loose; it may be that this facilitates the automatic quality of the movements. Otherwise the hands may rest on the lap or arms of the chair.

How you describe the method to the patient depends on your own personal style. You may refer to 'the unconscious mind' if you wish, as this makes sense to most patients; or you may talk about 'the back part of the mind', 'deep down in your mind', or whatever variation you prefer. Some practitioners communicate the suggestions and questions as if they are literally talking to a separate part of the mind, as in the illustration of Chevreul's pendulum earlier. Others prefer to address the questions in the normal way. This distinction will become clearer below.

If you wish, you can present an everyday rationale to the patient prior to eliciting the responses. You may say something like:

In everyday life, you communicate not just consciously in words, but also unconsciously by movements such as gestures of the hand, movements of your body, and facial expressions. You do these movements unconsciously, without thinking, but they communicate important messages about your feelings, ideas, wishes, and so on. For example, when you want to communicate the message 'Yes', you nod your head. When you want to convey the meaning 'No', you shake your head. You do this automatically (*or* your unconscious mind/the back part of your mind does this for you). When you don't know the answer or you don't want to say, you lift your shoulders, again quite automatically and unconsciously.

Right now, in this same way, you (*or* your unconscious mind, etc.) can choose a way of communicating the message 'Yes' by moving one of the fingers or your thumb on one of your hands (*or* your right/left hand) ... quite automatically and unconsciously. So deep down, you (*or* your unconscious mind, etc.) can be thinking of the message 'Yes' ... 'Yes' ... 'Yes' ... and one of your fingers or your thumb will lift quite naturally and automatically (*or* your unconscious mind/the back part of your mind can choose one of your fingers ... etc.) to convey that message 'Yes' ... 'Yes' ... 'Yes' ... .

Sometimes the movements are unconscious in the sense that the patient is ostensibly not simply unaware of any conscious intent to move the fingers, but is also unaware that the movements are occurring at all. Therefore you may also emphasise the idea of conscious–unconscious dissociation by saying:

You can go anywhere you like in your conscious mind now ... perhaps somewhere where you would feel very pleasant and relaxed ... and let the movements happen automatically (*or* let your unconscious mind do all the work).

If the patient is slow to respond, you may also say:

You may feel a sensation in one of your fingers or thumb – perhaps a tingling – and when this happens you can help that finger move a little.

The typical movement is a slight, hesitant lifting of the finger or thumb, often with some flickering tendency. A smooth, brisk movement is likely to be a deliberate, compliant response, unless the patient has good dissociative ability. If you suspect compliance, then it is important to repeat the procedure with a suggestion such as, 'Just let your finger move on its own', or 'Let your *unconscious* mind move that finger for you ... all on its own'.

When the 'Yes' response has been elicited say, 'Thank you, that's fine. Now this is your 'Yes' finger' and gently touch it.

Repeat this procedure for 'No' and, if you wish, 'I don't know or I don't want to say' (or you may have two separate responses for these).

Now, it may be useful to allow the patient to become accustomed to responding by IMR signalling. You can ask questions of a factual nature requiring the answer 'Yes' or 'No', as illustrated above with Chevreul's pendulum. Again, it is up to you to choose whether to address 'the unconscious mind' or 'the back part of the mind' or to put the questions directly to the patient. Before embarking on this say:

Now, I want to ask you (or the unconscious mind, etc.) some questions (about e.g. Mary). If you are (or 'If Mary's unconscious mind is') willing to do this you (or it) can signal with the 'Yes' finger and if not, with the 'No' finger.

If the answer is 'Yes', say 'Thank you. Now I'd like to ask...' and continue as with Chevreul's pendulum above. If the patient withholds permission, then this probably indicates anxieties about the method, concerns about what it may reveal, and so on, and these can be explored by normal discussion.

Our experience and that of our colleagues appear to suggest that usable responses may be elicited in around 75% of patients, so you have to be prepared to move on to something else if your patient is not proving responsive to this method.

Applications of the IMR signalling procedure

IMR signals may be used to augment other hypnotic and non-hypnotic therapeutic procedures and we shall refer to their use in other chapters. For the moment, let us summarise their major applications.

The main application of IMR signalling is as an exploratory technique in psychodynamically orientated therapy. The therapist is endeavouring to establish if, for example, it is going to be useful for patients to review any memories of events that may still have a bearing on their presenting problems. Thus the techniques may be a useful prelude to a revivification or age-regression procedure. We shall present various age-regression methods later that are augmented by IMR signals. For the moment, please bear in mind that regression methods are not just for recalling difficult memories; often we wish patients to recall a time when they were confident, happy, healthy, and so on.

Similarly, IMR signals may be used to explore whether there are any unresolved feelings or emotional conflicts that need to be addressed and which may underlie the presenting problem. For example, the patient's symptoms may be tension headaches and the therapist may suspect that these are related to interpersonal stresses in the patient's life that she is not fully acknowledging and needs to deal with. So one might ask if the headaches are caused in any way by any difficult feelings or emotions. If a 'Yes' response is given, then one might ask, 'Is it an anxious feeling?'; 'Is it an angry feeling?', etc. If further affirmative responses are elicited, one could ask, for example, 'Is this anger to do with any member of your family?'

Ultimately you are probably going to ask patients if it would be acceptable for them to think more about the material that is being explored and one can ask for permission through the IMR signals. If one is using the model of the unconscious mind, one might ask, 'Is it OK for Mary's conscious mind to become aware of all this now?' Thus we can use IMR signals to enable patients to indicate permission to proceed, or to indicate that they are not yet ready for the next step.

Some writers use the term 'IMR signal' to cover any movement that the patient is instructed to make in order to communicate with the hypnotist, for example to indicate when she is ready for some medical or dental procedure to commence. There may be occasions when it is useful for permission to be given in an unconscious manner, but unless this is so it is better not to use the term IMR to designate such a signal.

Another adjunctive use of IMR signals is 'communicating with parts'. If one is working with this metaphor, one might, for example, say to a patient suffering from bulimia, 'Is it OK for me to speak to the part of Debby that wants to keep eating?' One can then engage in a further dialogue, first continuing to use IMR signals, and then gradually encouraging the patient to communicate by speaking. We shall see later that we can use IMR signals in a similar way for exploring whether there are any problems with changing in the desired way. For example, we can ask the patient to imagine having overcome the presenting problem and then ask the question 'Is there any part that finds the change difficult to cope with?' Some therapists, notably those of an Ericksonian persuasion, ask to communicate with 'resourceful' parts, for example 'the part of you that is assertive in your job' or 'the creative part of you'.

Always bear in mind that this working model of 'parts' is only a metaphor. Used as such, it may provide a very useful means for facilitating the processes of inner communication and communication with the therapist that we have described in the previous chapters. Problems arise when the 'parts' are reified, that is given a literal status. This is one of the avenues whereby clients are coached in the role of the patient with multiple personality disorder.

Let us consider this important point further. At some stage of this discussion, readers have probably wondered what advantage there may be in obtaining the information in this convoluted way, if one could more easily ask the patient for the information in the normal face-to-face manner. Indeed, one would only use these methods if one had reason to believe that they would elicit more useful material than normal methods.

One fact readers are probably able to appreciate is how much control these methods give to the patient and therefore how useful they may be when broaching very sensitive and distressing material. Indeed, it is possible to undertake useful therapeutic work even when the patient has not disclosed to the therapist significant material that has been evoked during the session. For example, Raj, a teenager with secondary nocturnal enuresis (seen by MH) was adamant that he could think of no reason or causes for his bedwetting, yet gave a 'Yes' IMR response when the relevant question was put to him. A 'No' IMR signal was given to the question 'Is it OK for you to talk to me about this?' but he gave an affirmative response when asked to think of possible ways of dealing with these matters other than by wetting his bed. Thus, *perhaps* (we can't be sure) he was able to acknowledge and contemplate that his problem might be connected to other events in his life, by just registering this with a tiny flicker of his finger.

A rational working model for the therapeutic utility of IMR signals

There are several problems with the IMR signalling procedure that need to be addressed before we can advocate its use in therapy. The major problem is the lack of a good theoretical rationale. It is by no means unacceptable to inform patients that their unconscious mind, or the back part of their mind, can communicate information about their problems which is not available to their conscious mind. However, this can only be construed in metaphorical terms (i.e. it is *as if* such is the case). We have already declared ourselves against this idea of the unconscious mind in literal terms.

Another problem is the temptation of the therapist, and even the patient, to overvalue the IMR responses. This probably arises from the notion that they are 'messages from the unconscious mind' and are therefore more truthful than 'conscious' replies to the therapist's questions. There may be times when this is so but there is no reason to suppose that this is always the case. Unfortunately there is little systematic research exploring the nature of IMR signals.

Undue credulity on the therapist's part renders the procedure particularly vulnerable to a tendency about which we have already warned readers, namely that ideas and practices are liable to be extended into areas beyond their range of validity and applicability. Hence, some practitioners almost invariably use IMR-signalling methods regardless of the patient's problem, on the assumption that the unconscious mind always knows the cause of and means of solving the problem.

Perhaps an alternative working model for the therapeutic use of IMR signalling, one that might be developed as more acceptable than a simple model of 'the unconscious mind', can be based on the two-stage model of unconscious–conscious communication developed in Chapter 18. We can do this by drawing on two sets of ideas.

First, verbal communication allows a range of replies to a question requiring an affirmative or negative response – for example, 'No', 'I don't think so', 'I'm not sure', 'Possibly', 'I think so' and 'Yes'. An avoidant defensive mind-set would bias the responses allowed by shifting each one towards one end of the negative–affirmative continuum. For example:

Therapist	Are you aware of any memories that may still be troubling you now?
Patient	No, I can't think of any at all.

Or:

Therapist	Do you think that you have now come to terms with this?
Patient	Yes, definitely.

Or:

Therapist	Are you angry about this now?
Patient	Not at all.

However, we have a much wider repertoire of responses in non-verbal modalities – for example, body posture, head movements, facial expressions, autonomic activity (e.g. pallor and blushing) and vocal tone. These responses tend to be analogue in nature rather than discrete; for example, one can blush anywhere from very slightly to an extreme degree. So when we ask someone a question, say 'Are you feeling OK?', the non-verbal response (e.g. facial expression and voice quality) may be much more telling and convincing than the verbal answer ('Yes', 'Not too bad', 'Not really', etc.).

Indeed, sometimes there is a direct conflict between the verbal and the non-verbal response. Someone might ask us, 'Do you like my new outfit?' Our verbal response may be 'Yes' but our non-verbal language is, unfortunately, communicating something rather different.

Importantly, our non-verbal communications and the messages they are conveying vary in the level at which they are expressed in our consciousness (and in that of the person observing us). On occasions, typified by the last-mentioned example, we are usually all too aware that our body language and vocal expression are giving the game away and the answer they and we are communicating is a definite 'No!' Sometimes, however, someone asks us a question and our conscious reply is conveyed verbally while, at a below-conscious level, our non-verbal communication may be something different. 'You are not angry with me are you?' a friend may ask us. 'Not at all!' comes back our answer, genuinely expressed, at a clearly conscious level. But something in our gesture, facial expression, voice tone, etc. may be registering, 'Well, actually, I *am* a bit; and, at the same time, I am also a little anxious about being angry because you might then be angry with me; and I am feeling a little guilty because I was brought up to believe that it is usually me who is at fault; and I am also a little sad that our friendship has hit a bad patch, as I vaguely recall in the distant past more than one occasion when I lost a friend because we argued over such a little thing...'.

What it is to be human! All of this may be registered by the non-verbal behaviour yet the cognitive activity represented by these statements may be hardly expressed at a conscious level.

It requires much conscious effort to bias our non-verbal communications in the way that was earlier described for verbal communication. (For this reason, it is important always to attend to a patient's non-verbal responses in a session of therapy.)

It may be, therefore, that what we are attempting to do when setting up IMR signals is to harness the patient's non-verbal communication system by nominating a particular response, namely a slight finger movement, to convey the reply to our question. Note that the reply, rather than in analogue form, is now encoded in terms of a limited number of discrete values – 'Yes', 'No', 'I don't know' and 'I don't want to say'.

This does not, however, explain how the index responses can be nominated by the hypnotist. One possibility is that when one sets up IMR signals one is giving the patient the opportunity to take less responsibility for the answers given. In fact, some patients deny being aware of what the finger responses are; this may be because they have the facility to dissociate, that is to displace from consciousness both the awareness of the intention of raising the finger and the kinaesthetic feedback of its position and movement. Whatever the case, the response is, in a manner of speaking, 'happening somewhere else'. Thus, we have a response method that is less sensitive to defensive biasing than the normal channel of verbal communication. As such, it has the potential (i) to facilitate the conscious expression of cognitive activity not presently in this form or denied access to consciousness, and (ii) to facilitate communication by the patient of information that he or she finds difficult to convey by the usual verbal means.

IMR signalling, however, should not be construed as a revelation of 'the truth'. It simply allows the therapist and patient more leeway to explore various *possibilities*. Hence patients who give a 'Yes' signal in reply to a question they have previously given an oral reply of 'No', are not now 'confessing the truth'. They are simply indicating 'OK, I am willing to explore that possibility'.

It is worth mentioning that ideomotor responding accounts for the messages elicited by the ouija board ('Yes' or 'No') and other methods that supposedly spell out messages from the spirit world. It is also the explanation for facilitated communication (Biklen 1992), a procedure whereby autistic children and those with learning difficulties are seemingly able to use a keyboard to tap out fluent messages on a VDU display, even without having previously learned to write, so long as their hand is supported by a facilitator. Research has suggested that the information communicated actually comes from the facilitator (Mulick et al 1993). Ideomotor responding is likely to be the basis of many dowsing practices. As in many claims of psychic abilities (and, incidentally, unorthodox healing practices), the magnitude of the abilities claimed for dowsing has diminished exponentially with more stringently controlled scientific investigation (Enright 1999).

Final thoughts on ideomotor signalling

We mention all of these things in order to encourage readers to adopt the appropriate degree of caution and discretion in their approach to the technique of IMR signalling. We know of highly regarded clinicians who never use this procedure. However, IMR signalling is a method that we would wish to keep in the armamentarium of techniques at the disposal of the practitioner of clinical hypnosis. The reason for this is that many sensible, competent and experienced therapists find it extremely useful, even though we suspect that many are overcommitted to it through misplaced credulity. It seems then that in the absence of any guidance from controlled investigations, readers must decide from their own experience what the value of this procedure is in their work.

THE SENSORY-FOCUSING METHOD

The theoretical rationale for this method can be understood from the foregoing discussion and that of the previous chapter. In Chapter 6, we described a very useful preliminary to hypnotic induction that we termed 'sensory focusing'. Patients close their eyes and spend some time observing their 'inner experiences' (as opposed to external stimuli). After some time, they are asked to comment on anything particular that they notice. By way of introduction to this, one can say:

Your body communicates to you by different feelings. A particular feeling might tell you that you are hungry and that you want something to eat; another feeling may be telling you that you are thirsty and need to drink; another feeling might be telling you that you are tired and you need to rest, or that you are full of energy and want to do things. Just observe what your body is telling you now.

When clients are asked if they notice anything in particular, the most common response is that they feel very relaxed, and then you can proceed with the induction. Sometimes clients may report tension somewhere – say in the neck, head or chest – flickering of the eyelids, restlessness of the legs, and so on. Ask clients to focus on that feeling and say:

Just let it be there. Maybe it will change in some way, become more noticeable or less noticeable, spread or diminish, or change to some other kind of feeling. Just notice what happens.

After some moments, you might venture the question:

Do you understand what the tension (*specified*) is about? Can you make any sense of it?

Very often clients may say that it is to do with the situation they are in; they may say, 'I'm a bit apprehensive as I have never been hypnotised before'. Perhaps one can reassure them here that this is quite natural and they will find that as the induction proceeds, they will be able to relax and feel completely safe.

Sometimes it is important to explore the tension further. For example, the reply to the last question may be, 'Well I think it's because we were talking earlier about my mother and I am still feeling a bit upset about this'. The therapist can then encourage clients to keep thinking about that and to say a little bit more about the feeling.

Sometimes clients may have some tension somewhere but cannot make any sense out of it. One can say:

Sometimes we notice that our body is telling us we are tense, but we don't understand the message. Just keep in touch with that feeling and see what happens.

It is important to note that when using this method, the therapist is not intending to alleviate the feelings in any way. Therefore, the therapist must proceed very carefully and not subject clients to any undue distress; if it is the first session of hypnosis, there is a risk that the therapist may push clients too far and they will not return for the next session.

The key sequence of instructions is as follows:

- Keep focusing on the feeling.
- Just observe what happens.

- Can you make any sense out of that feeling?
- Is it an angry/sad/anxious/etc. feeling?

If, for example, clients say it is an angry feeling, then ask:

Did you have that anger with you when you came today, or has it come on since you arrived?
Does your anger make any sense to you?
Is it a familiar feeling? Have you had it before?

If clients talk about, for example, angry feelings concerning their parents, it is useful to encourage them to focus on a particular memory. Therefore one might say:

Is there any particular memory that is coming to mind now as you are talking about this?

Case example

Maria, a 30-year-old woman, had a lifelong problem of claustrophobia, a fear of being in the house alone and fear of the dark. This problem had become worse in recent years, probably owing to marital conflict, her husband having left her for another woman. The therapist (MH) planned several sessions of relaxation, desensitisation and anxiety management training. At her first session of hypnosis, he asked her to close her eyes and to focus inwardly, in the manner described earlier. He then noticed that her face bore a troubled expression and he asked her what feelings she noticed. She reported a tense feeling in her eyes and some flickering of the eyelids. The therapist asked her to focus on these feelings and see what happened. Gradually, the flickering of the eyelids increased and some tears were noticeable.

The therapist asked the client to continue to focus on this and then asked her what feeling she noticed. She replied that she was feeling very sad. Again the therapist asked her to stay with this feeling, and more tears were noticeable. He then asked her if she understood her sadness and she replied that she felt very guilty that she was taking up the therapist's time when he probably had patients with more serious problems. Rather than reassure her that this was not the case, the therapist asked her to keep thinking about this. He then asked her if this was a familiar feeling; was it one that she recognised? The patient replied, 'Yes, I could never go to my mother with my problems; she never wanted to know and she made me feel guilty when I did'. The therapist then encouraged her to bring to mind any particular memories of when this happened and, in ways that are to be discussed later, helped her with the distress that these memories were still causing her. (The practice of selecting a salient memory to work on was advocated in Ch. 12 as a means of helping people with very difficult feelings.)

Having done this work with this patient, the therapist proceeded with the plan of using behavioural methods to help her with her claustrophobia. It may well be that the exploratory work done initially helped her have a more profound response to hypnosis, as otherwise her guilt and unease at the attention she was receiving may have inhibited this.

The sensory-focusing method illustrates that it is more effective to start with physical feelings, then move up a stage to the affect associated with them, and then the cognitive content, rather than the other way round. For example, the therapist may initially ask the above client how she got on with her mother when she was a child. She may say, 'Fine', or even 'Well she was rather distant and I could never go to her with my problems'. However, when answering the question, she does not experience the full nature of her relationship with her mother and the very sad feelings around this. (This is of course essential from an adaptive point of view; life would be intolerable if every single time we recalled something we reacted with the associated affect.)

The following is a second case illustration with a patient (seen by MH) who had difficulty closing her eyes. As in the above example, the material elicited related to the client–therapist transference, but this is not always the case. Again we caution readers to be very careful and sensitive in using these methods.

Case example

A woman in her early 30s was referred because of her panic attacks experienced in con- fined places such as her church and restaurants. She seemed to quickly develop a dependency on her therapy; after the first session, she was literally having nightmares about arriving and finding the therapist's room empty. As in Maria's case, the plan was to use behavioural methods and in the first session of hypnosis, the sensory-focusing method was introduced.

Immediately the client opened her eyes and said, 'I don't want to do this'. However, the therapist encouraged her to 'stay with the feeling' and after several attempts she was able to keep her eyes closed. She was then asked what was happening and she seemed to be experiencing some tension. She then said that she was very conscious that the therapist was looking at her while she had her eyes closed and she opened them again. The therapist then asked her to close her eyes and to keep thinking that he was looking at her. This she did with obvious discomfort and began to cry.

Further encouragement revealed that she thought the therapist was looking at her in a critical way. The next question was 'Is this a feeling that you have experienced before?' She immediately said, 'Yes' and began crying more and she became very distressed. She then revealed that her husband was always criticising her and looking for things that were wrong with her. She said that he had a habit of coming into the room and staring at her so that she would have to ask him what was wrong. Some time was spent on this and eventually the patient was able to say how relaxed she felt and she had no desire to open her eyes. The 'safe place' deepening method was used and on alerting, the patient commented on how she felt very calm and indeed she appeared to be rather amnesic for the hypnotic procedures used. When she returned the next week, she commented that for the rest of that day she felt like she 'had taken a tranquilliser'.

It should be noted that during the assessment of this patient, when asked how she felt about her husband, she said, 'He's wonderful' and declared how much she loved him, and no doubt these were genuine expressions. As in the previous case, this method, by first encouraging the patient to become more aware of the non-verbal, out-of-conscious responses, then building up to the affect, then the content, enabled her first to focus more fully on her relationship with her husband, and second to communicate this information to the therapist. This was, in fact, a prelude to more disclosures about how she felt about her husband.

Readers may discern how the above sensory-focusing method corresponds with the two-stage model, 'unconscious-to-conscious, conscious-to-overt expression', outlined in Chapter 18, whereby activity not immediately expressed in conscious form is assisted in becoming so and then may be overtly communicated to the therapist; then the process of resolution can take place, as will be discussed later.

Stanton (1992) has described a similar method, which he terms the 'diagnostic trance'.

AGE REGRESSION

In Chapter 12, we described ways in which it may be useful to ask a patient to relive in imagination a significant memory. Age regression is really a special case of this and involves the reliving (or revivification) in imagination of memories from an earlier developmental period of one's life. It is said that true hypnotic age regression occurs when the observed responses do not occur with waking regression (see Nash 1987). However, there is a problem of definition in distinguishing 'waking' from 'hypnotic regression' and Hilgard (1986) reports that highly susceptible subjects regress without the benefit of a hypnotic induction.

In age regression, the subject, to a greater or lesser degree, *dissociates*, experiencing the imagined events as very realistic yet remaining able to respond to questions and instructions appropriate to the non-regressed state and the context (e.g. 'Now I would like you to come back to the present time'). We also noted in Chapter 4 the occurrence of 'trance logic' in some highly susceptible subjects.

Sometimes, spontaneously or under the instruction of the hypnotist, subjects dissociate in the sense of *observing* themselves as a child (rather than *being* themselves in the situation). Sometimes this may be construed as a protective device against distressing emotions and thus can be encouraged by the therapist by the adoption of one of the appropriate regression methods described below. Laurence & Perry (1981) have reported that those subjects who spontaneously retain an observing self tend to be those highly susceptible individuals who show the 'hidden observer' effect (see Ch. 4).

The regressed subject should speak of the events in the present tense, but this may not be so necessary for therapeutic work. Indeed, in a therapeutic context, a regression to childish behaviour and manner of speaking does not necessarily make for better therapy. Given the right expectations, a subject will do this (e.g. as a volunteer for a demonstration or for entertainment) but it may be more to do with role-playing skills than the intensity of the experience. When we age regress subjects, above all we are normally interested in the emotional component of the experience – what it feels like to relive that memory. The emotion experienced may be similar to the original but it will be modified by the maturational process and learning that have occurred since. So, patients may feel extreme anger when reliving the memory of their being cruelly treated, but the anger is now that of the adult rather than the child.

Early reports alleged that dramatic reinstatements of age-appropriate behaviour, thinking, feeling, physiological and neurological functioning, and so on, were elicited by age regression. More recent and better-controlled experiments have refuted these ideas. Nash (1987) reviewed the evidence and his paper is essential reading for anyone who claims any specialist knowledge of hypnosis. Variables that must be allowed for in such research include the person's existing skills and knowledge to effectively role-play, compliancy, the relaxation response, and, when experimenting on volunteers such as students, the priming of new subjects by those who have already done the experiment.

We have already discussed the matter of the validity of the content of the memories elicited by hypnosis (Ch. 18 and Appendix 1). All remembering (during hypnosis or not) is an activity of construction and is therefore inaccurate to some degree. Further distortions will occur in the subjects' account of the memory to the therapist, and the therapist's own understanding of what patients are saying. Distortions and confabulations will occur in response to implicit or explicit demands and expectations that the patient interprets from the context. The more remote the regression, the greater the tendency to distort and confabulate. For example, a regression to birth or to the womb, while possibly being an interesting and even useful fantasy for some people, is not a valid method of accessing anything the patient experienced at the time.

The conduct of a session of age regression

Most people are capable of replaying in imagination an event from their past. Hypnotic procedures will facilitate this. It is important to ask permission from the subject or patient to 'go back in time and look at some important memories' and whatever procedure is adopted, the therapist should secure the patient's consent to proceed at each stage, using normal or IMR signals.

A brief induction and deepening routine of the first kind (Ch. 6) is often sufficient, ending up with an imagery method (e.g. the 'safe place' technique). Patients will 'go deeper' as they become more involved in the experience.

A safety device can be the instruction that whenever patients need to, they can leave the memory and go back to their safe place. One can make use of the 'hidden observer' (or ego state) idea as follows:

Whenever I place my hand on your shoulder like this (demonstrated), you will immediately be the 'adult you' again and the 'adult you' will be able to talk to me about what is going on. Then, when I let go of your shoulder like this (demonstrated), you will be back as the 'child you'. This will only happen while you are having hypnosis with me.

Once regressed, initial oral commentary by patients may be difficult (e.g. because of the relaxed articulatory muscles) and they may become temporarily more alert again. As the experience develops, commentating by patients may facilitate their experience.

The therapist's interaction should be appropriate to the regressed age of the patient, who should be gently encouraged to speak in the present tense. The first question is often 'How old are you?'; then 'What do you like to be called?' It may help the patient to 'set the scene' by reference to factual information, say by asking, 'Who do you live with?'; 'Do you go to school?; and 'Can you tell me your teacher's name?' As the patient's narrative unfolds, the therapist should generally use open-ended questions (e.g. 'What's happening now?'; 'Where are you now?' and 'Who is with you?') but at times can encourage greater involvement by asking for details from different sensory modalities, such as, 'Can you see mummy?'; 'What is mummy wearing?'; 'Can you smell the cooking?'; 'What does Teddy feel like as you hold him?'; 'What is Daddy saying?'; 'How does your ice cream taste?' Encourage the patient to linger on good experiences; these may be anchored, say by a squeeze of the thumb and forefinger, and the easy retrieval of those good feelings may be suggested. Sometimes in therapy one can ask, 'What would you like to do now?' and this may be acted out in fantasy.

If patients become upset, you do not normally immediately bring them out of experience, although you may remind them of their 'safe place'. (Sometimes you may want to insist on this.) Follow the guidelines in Chapter 6.

Before de-regressing say, 'Is it all right to leave that memory now?' The therapist can then change to a more adult tone and say, 'Are you ready to come back to the present time? ... OK, take all the time you need, ... coming back into the present ... etc.'. (You could do this using the 'safe place' as a first step.) Say that the patient need only recall as much of the session as needed, just as with a dream. Remind the patient of the present date, time and place and say, 'Tell me when you are right back in the present'. Then alert in the usual way. Discuss with patients anything they feel is important and ensure they are fully debriefed.

Age regression may be contraindicated for the deeply or suicidally depressed person; depressed people have easier access to bad memories, and re-experiencing these may lower their mood even further. Paradoxically, reliving a good memory sometimes has the same effect ('I'll never be able to feel like that again') so while this suggestion can be beneficial, great care must be taken to avoid an adverse reaction.

Some patients think they *must* be regressed to overcome their problems, but ultimately the solutions lie in their present life. The manoeuvre must be part of a proper plan with some aim at resolving any traumatic kinds of memory if such are elicited. Plenty of time must be allowed in the session for this eventuality.

Methods of age regression

These are some of the common methods used.

Open-ended method

Say, for example:

In the unconscious (*or* deep) part of your mind you have many memories stored away, some of them good, some not so good, some clear and vivid, some faded and patchy. Some of them may be relevant to how you are feeling today, in your present life. Just allow yourself to drift back in time without really trying and see what the unconscious (deep) part of your mind comes up with. It might be a clear memory or something vague. Take all the time you want and when you are there just let me know (head-nod or finger signal).

Regression to a target age

You can elaborate on the above suggestions by, for example, specifying a particular age. A variant is to count down from the patient's present age to the target age and, as you are doing this, suggest that the patient is going back in time, becoming a year younger with each count. You may also suggest that as the patient is going back in time:

Your body is getting smaller and smaller. You are feeling like a little boy again. When you reach the age of (say 6), you will think like a child, act like a child, talk like a child ... *and so on.*

Using ideomotor signalling

Establish IMR signals (at least for the message 'Yes'). Then say that you are going to count down from the person's age and as you are counting, the person is getting younger and younger ... etc. When you reach the age at which some important memory occurs that is relevant to his or her problems, the 'Yes' finger will automatically lift. (You will have to count back slowly.)

A variant of this is to exclude the suggestions for regression at first and to run back through all the years, noting which ones are associated with a signal. (This is sometimes called 'the diagnostic scan'.) Then you regress the person to each of the ages. (Remember that there may have been more than one incident at a given age.) Some therapists also count back up again in the same way and then regress the patient to the ages at which an IMR signal was obtained when descending *and* ascending.

Another variant is to first establish by IMR signal if there is a memory that it is important to review now. Then establish at what age this was; this may be short-circuited by such questions as 'Was it at or before the age of 20?', etc.

Arm-lowering method

With the arm in the raised position (catalepsy may or may not have been suggested), say that as the arm is getting heavier and coming down, so patients are drifting back in time to the target age, date or relevant incident. Patients will not be there until the arm has come to settle on their lap. The advantage of this method is that it allows patients to proceed at their own pace.

The affect bridge or somatic bridge method

This is a useful method described by John Watkins (1971) and may be the preferred choice when a significant somatic component or well-circumscribed affect is expressed – for example, self-consciousness, panic or psychosomatic problem. However, it is very direct and may provoke an immediate abreaction. The physical response, feeling or affect, is used as a bridge to the cognitive content of the memory, in a manner not dissimilar to the sensory-focusing method described earlier. Remember at each stage to ask permission from the patient.

1. Elicit the relevant affect or somatic experience by asking the patient to relive in imagination a recent memory when this experience occurred.
2. Instruct the patient to let go of the content of the memory and focus on the full affect or physical feelings.
3. Ask the patient to increase the intensity of the affect or somatic experience, for example by a factor of 2 ... 3 ... 5 ... etc. (There is no need to do this if the experience is already quite strong.)
4. Suggest (with the patient's permission) that the patient is going back in time, taking these feelings along too (using, if desired, the image of a bridge, shrouded in mist, etc.) to the first time these feelings were experienced.
5. Resolve the memory (see later).
6. Check if there are any earlier (or later) memories.
7. Now return to the recent memory that was first elicited and ensure that the patient now feels better about it in some important way (e.g. that he or she can now cope with the same situation).

Screen methods

These methods are useful with patients who have extremely traumatic memories. They purposely aim to protect patients from the emotional experience, which would otherwise be so severe that they may be at risk from being further traumatised or would block recall altogether. It is suggested to patients that they are in a safe place, viewing the memory as one would a video recording, and they can turn the recording off, switch channels, or control the image in some other way (e.g. blurring the focus or moving the screen further away).

As these procedures are especially useful for patients with post-traumatic stress disorder, they will be presented in further detail when we cover that topic later in this book (Ch. 30).

The confusion technique

This was briefly described in Chapter 10 and is considered by some as being useful with patients who are not susceptible to direct methods.

Miscellaneous methods

Therapists are at liberty to construct their own methods. Some methods identify the year first, then the month and then the date by the use of suitable imagery. For example, patients may be asked to imagine going down a corridor passing doors, the number on each door being calendar years (in descending order – e.g. 2001, 2000, 1999, 1998, etc.). It is suggested that when they reach a year in which something occurred of significance to their problems, the door will open up to another corridor in which each of 12 doors has the name of a month written on it. Again, the door bearing the month of the year during which the important event happened will open to reveal a corridor of doors numbered by the days of the month (1, 2, 3, etc.). When they reach the door corresponding to the date of the event, this will open. When they are ready, they are to enter and to relive the memory in question.

There is a similar method to this in which patients imagine being in a library; the shelves have years on them, the books on each shelf months, and the chapters dates. One could also use the idea of a video library if one were using a screen technique.

Applications of age regression or revivification

Age regression (and revivification generally) may be used as a procedure in psychodynamic, behaviour and cognitive therapy (see later chapters). Common reasons for using the technique are as follows:

1. You may wish to elicit further information about a particular event that the patient experienced. For example, in cognitive-behavioural

therapy you may be asking questions such as 'What are you feeling emotionally at this point?'; 'Where in your body are you experiencing that?'; and 'What thoughts are you having at this point?'

2. You may wish to help the patient access positive feelings and resources, as in the 'clenched fist' procedure (Ch. 12) and in certain desensitisation methods for counter-conditioning anxiety (see Ch. 20).

3. You may wish to help the patient re-experience, re-interpret or reconstruct a significant memory in a more adaptive way, or imagine more effective coping. This application was discussed in Chapter 12 and will be further explored later in this chapter.

AGE PROGRESSION

We saw in Chapter 12 that it is sometimes useful to ask patients to imagine themselves at some future point in time. The actual time may be specified (e.g. 'exactly 1 year from now', 'next Christmas', 'on your holidays next summer', or '5 years from now'). Alternatively, you may wish to specify certain key landmarks (e.g. 'Imagine yourself in the future when you no longer have this problem', or 'when you have reached your target weight', or 'when you have lost just 13 kg (2 stone)'). It is sometimes interesting to ascertain from patients how long they imagine it will be before they have overcome their problem.

As with age regression, patients may need time to mentally 'set the scene', so initially their commentary may be more of a factual nature (e.g. 'Let's see. I'll be 45 and probably have been promoted to senior level. The children will have left home – that will feel very strange ... '). As patients 'get into the part', they will become more aware of feelings associated with changes that they foresee in their life. As before, gently encourage patients to speak in the present tense and frame your questions accordingly ('What are you doing now?', etc.).

Methods of age progression

Methods of age progression are quite straightforward. Usually a simple instruction, as illustrated in the above examples, is usually sufficient. As always, ask patients' permission at each stage and ask them to signal when they are ready to describe their experience. If you wish, you may use some method of counting the years up, interspersed with suggestions of moving ahead in time. Another method is arm-lowering, described above for age regression. Lift the patient's arm into the raised position and suggest that as the arm is getting heavier and coming down, the patient is moving forward in time and that the arm will come to rest on the lap when the target date is reached. Another method is to use the image of a crystal ball. The patient imagines gazing into it and it is suggested that gradually a picture will come into focus of the patient in (say) 5 years' time. A screen technique may also be used. With such a method, at some point you can suggest that the patient steps into the screen and 'becomes the future' rather than just observes what is happening.

Applications of age progression

As with age regression, age progression may be used as a procedure within a range of different types of therapy.

We discussed future rehearsal in Chapter 12 within a cognitive-behavioural framework and we shall describe the use of anticipated benefits of changing in Chapter 20. In fact, encouraging patients to keep in mind these benefits may be a useful way of maintaining their motivation, particularly when treatment inevitably means confronting anxieties and difficulties that they have habitually avoided.

In both cognitive-behavioural and psychodynamic approaches, one can age progress to a landmark in therapy (partial or complete resolution of the problem – e.g. complete cessation of smoking) and then, using IMR signals if preferred, ask if there are any problems about changing that need to be addressed. This may be done by reference to 'parts' of the person (e.g. 'Is there any part of you that is having difficulty with this change?').

Case example

Sally, who had problems of bulimia and obesity, was age progressed by one of us (MH) to the point at which she had achieved her target weight. Using IMR signals and the idea of 'parts', she indicated that she felt very vulnerable. She related this to a fear of being hurt, and her experience of having an extramarital affair in her early 20s, as a result of which she became pregnant and had a termination. The man concerned stopped seeing her as soon as she became pregnant, and because she was unable to tell her husband or anyone else what had happened, she had to deal with the termination entirely on her own. Of course, she was able to recall all of these events before coming to therapy, but the age-progression procedure helped her become more aware of how much her experience of these events was still affecting her.

Age progression is a very useful procedure whether you are adopting a psychodynamic, cognitive-behavioural or humanistic approach. Useful clinical papers on age progression are Frederick & Phillips (1992), Phillips & Frederick (1992), Torem (1992) and Van Dyck (1988).

RESOLVING DIFFICULT MEMORIES

In previous chapters, we have stressed that whenever one is using a therapeutic technique, one should always have in mind its purpose and rationale with regard to the patient's problems and the broader therapeutic approach that one is adopting. In Chapter 15, we showed how this is addressed with reference to the concept of the working model. From this standpoint, let us give some further consideration to why one should ask a patient to relive in imagination the memory of an event that was particularly distressing.

Let us first 'play the devil's advocate' and protest at the very idea of encouraging patients to relive an unhappy memory when very often they are already distressed enough about current aspects of their life. This is a serious question and whatever answer we give should be qualified with the caveat that the reliving of an upsetting memory should only ever be undertaken with discretion and sensitivity and with a clear understanding of how it may ultimately benefit the patient. If such advice is not heeded, then the outcome may simply be a more distressed and, in some instances, a re-traumatised patient. (We do acknowledge that occasionally the memory of an unpleasant event and the distress associated with it are unexpectedly evoked in therapy.)

This applies even to patients whose main presenting problem is their inability to come to terms with painful experiences in their childhood, such as physical, sexual and emotional abuse. Therapy with these patients will be very much centred around the talking over of the experiences and the ventilation of emotion by the patient, the principal role of the therapist being to communicate warmth, empathy and unconditional support in the traditional client-centred manner. We have already (Chs 16 and 18) outlined a working model for the rationale of this approach, namely the reciprocal two-stage process of 'unconscious-to-conscious, conscious-to-overt expression'.

Of course, therapists adopting a behavioural, cognitive or gestalt approach may incorporate into therapy their own techniques aimed at facilitating this process. Likewise, the practitioner of hypnosis may incorporate, hypnotic procedures such as regression. But techniques such as these should only be applied after carefully considering how they will assist the therapeutic process and balancing this against any risks such as an unproductive session in which the patient is caused further distress. It is therefore important that this work is client-led, hence the usefulness of techniques such as IMR signalling and even the simple regular act of asking the client's permission. Ultimately, these kinds of decisions can only be made by those therapists who have proper training and experience in psychotherapy and it is not within the scope of this book to equip those who have not had this with the required expertise.

Let us also remind readers that we do not advocate the habitual use of regression purposely to locate the cause of the problem in some repressed traumatic memory (see Ch. 18). It is true that there are published case illustrations in which this appears to have happened. However, as we argued in Chapter 15, clinical anecdotes do not provide reliable support for a theory or working model.

Encouraging ventilation of feelings

The reliving of some memories will be associated with an abreaction, that is the expression of intense emotion (fear, sadness, anger, guilt, etc.). As we stated earlier, sometimes the feelings will be those appropriate to the incident but the child will not have been able to express them at the time. Sometimes they *were* expressed but in isolation of any acceptance, understanding or comfort. No-one was around or the child was made to believe that he or she was not supposed to feel this way. Very often the emotions expressed are directly linked to the memory, but in reality they will be the emotions of the adult patient reacting to the memory, and these may sometimes be very different from the original feelings.

Sometimes it is useful for patients to express their feelings about what happened, in imagination to, say, the person who was causing the distress or anger at the time. This is similar to the 'empty chair' techniques described in Chapter 16.

Very often, the ventilation of emotion is all that is required. Some practitioners consider that this 'release' of emotion is in itself therapeutic. One way of understanding this (an explanation that is commonly offered in everyday life) is a 'hydraulic model', whereby emotional pressure builds up and needs to be released. Certainly people do seem to suppress their emotions, only to occasionally 'explode' (particularly with anger or sadness) as though the pressure is too much to bear. However, we regard this only as a metaphor with a limited sphere of usefulness.

The reason why simple ventilation of feeling can be therapeutic may be partly understood in terms of the already discussed process of enhanced (unconscious-to-conscious) self-awareness. It is not uncommon, even in everyday life, for people to say, 'I didn't realise how angry (sad, etc.) I felt about this'. A change in self-perception may also occur. Whereas previously patients may have considered themselves as 'somebody who never cries (gets angry, etc.)', now they consider themselves as able to express their emotions with no adverse consequences.

Very important, however, is the fact that much therapeutic work is achieved through the patient's sharing the emotional experience with the therapist. The role of the therapist is simply to be a 'good parent', to offer support and empathy, and to allow the full expression of whatever feelings are evoked. We also discussed this in Chapter 6.

In addition, there are various procedures that one can take patients through in imagination to assist them in coming to a satisfactory resolution if this goes beyond the simple expression of emotion.

Telescoping trauma and too-late comfort

This procedure was described by Karle (1988) and is useful when the traumatic incident recalled was actually resolved satisfactorily, but it is not resolved in memory. That is, the patient's memory is, as it were, frozen at the moment of maximum distress and despair. This aspect of the memory predominates and continues to cause distress to the patient. It is as though it has become dissociated from that part of the memory that is associated with feelings of relief, safety and reassurance. For example, Karle (1988) describes how this technique may be used with patients who have bad memories of being left in hospital as children. Typically, patients recall the time when as children they were taken to hospital by their parents. The parents left them on the ward and went home, leaving them feeling that they had been completely abandoned by their parents. In fact, the parents returned later at visiting time, yet when patients recall the incident now, it is clear that they are still suffering from the distress of the sense of being abandoned. The technique involves taking patients to the point approaching maximum distress and then immediately fast-forwarding to the point at which relief is at hand. This is done several times in order to reinforce the association. (One could use an anchor here for each part of the memory to facilitate the procedure.) It is important that this procedure is continued until patients signal that the memory no longer causes them distress.

Case example

This method was used with Eva, a patient one of the authors (MH) saw. She suffered from a form of claustrophobia, which caused her to feel anxious in any situation where she felt that she 'had no choice'. For example, she was very anxious on buses because as soon as the bus would set off she would feel that she now had no choice but to stay on it. This gave her a sense of feeling trapped. She came to one appointment and described how that week she had visited the dentist and was informed that she would have to come back and have some fillings done and this would require a local anaesthetic. Up until then, she had never been afraid of the dentist, but then she started to dwell on the idea of having a local anaesthetic and this caused her to feel anxious. Her explanation was that once the anaesthetic had taken effect, she would have no choice about its being there.

This incident was used in the affect bridge procedure and the memory was elicited of her brother's locking her in a wardrobe when she was a little girl. (Apparently, he did this kind of thing on a number of occasions.) She was absolutely terrified and had a feeling that she was going to be left there for ever. However, it was not long before her mother heard her, opened the wardrobe, hugged her and reassured her that she was safe. The 'telescoping trauma and too late comfort' technique was used satisfactorily, pairing the point where she believed she was trapped for ever with her mother's appearance and comforting her. The success of this manoeuvre was then checked by asking her to imagine being at her future dental appointment and having a local anaesthetic. She actually started to lick her lips and, when asked, said she could feel the anaesthetic in her gums, but she was able to signal that she felt fine about this. Unfortunately, she defaulted on all further appointments so it is not known if, in reality, she went through with her dental treatment satisfactorily.

Counselling the 'child'

Another method is to counsel the patient during the regression as one would if the incident were really happening in the here and now. For example, Smith (1979) describes his treatment of a lady with spider phobia whom he regressed to the first time she could remember being afraid of a spider. She was in her bedroom at the time and she panicked. The therapist took her through the incident again, this time counselling the 'child' about how the spider was, in reality, a very tiny creature and was afraid of her. (One could, when using this procedure, encourage the patient to give the spider a name.) The child was then encouraged to comfort the spider and it was suggested that they were now good friends. Further examples of this use of age regression in therapy for phobias are provided by Lamb (1985).

Other examples are provided by patients who were sexually abused as children and were made to feel guilty and ashamed. While reliving this memory, the therapist may counsel 'the child', reassuring the child that what happened was not her fault. (An important message to patients who are haunted by guilt and self-recrimination over some incident is that they made the best choice available at the time from what they knew.) We shall see in Chapter 21 that a very useful concept provided by cognitive therapy is that of the 'cognitive schema'. In our formative years, we acquire certain biases in thinking about ourselves and our world. A schema is like a theory, but is less formally structured. Later on in our lives, some schemas may prove inappropriate and maladaptive, yet we persist in holding onto them. For example, a person may have a schema that says, 'When people are angry with me, it is always my fault' or, 'If I get anxious, then I can't cope'. Schemas are not usually thought of as having formed as a result of just one incident; rather they evolve as a result of habitual experiences. However, there may be one or two incidents that, for the person, are emblematic of all the ways in which he or she acquired that way of thinking. The method of counselling the 'child self' at the time of one of these 'emblematic' memories can be very useful for helping patients change their maladaptive schemas, as can the following method.

The use of 'parts' or ego states

One very effective method is to use 'parts' or ego states. A common approach is to bring 'the child' to the point of despair and then to ask the adult ego state to 'go back in time', confront the child and give the child all the comfort and reassurance that she needs in order to cope with this situation and feel better about it. The adult is also encouraged to embrace the child and this may be performed overtly in mime. Then the therapist asks to speak to the child again and asks the child if she feels better and if there is anything else that she needs in way of help. This can be done verbally or by IMR signals according to the therapist's own experience and preference. This process is continued until the child is able to say that she has everything needed from the adult part to cope with the situation.

An example of this procedure is given by Karle (1988). The memory elicited was of sexual abuse by the patient's father at the age of 6. The memory was one of running to tell her mother who informed her she had a 'filthy mind' and sent her to her room as punishment. The therapist asked the adult part to 'pick up her child self', cuddle her and give her all the comfort that she needed and to explain the truth of the situation.

Case example

This procedure was also used by one of the authors (MH) in the case of Selina, a nursery school teacher, who had a disabling lack of self-confidence. She came to her second session and described an incident when her husband's friends visited and were talking about some political issues. She realised that she had insufficient knowledge of what they were talking about to make any contribution to the conversation and she was overwhelmed with anxiety in case somebody asked her for her opinion. This incident was used by the therapist in the affect bridge procedure and, through this, the patient recalled a memory of her being at school at around the age of 7. She was asked by the teacher to spell a word and she got it wrong. The teacher called her out in front of the class and proceeded to rap her knuckles with a ruler. This was a very distressing incident for the patient to recall.

The therapist then addressed the 'adult part', reminding her that she herself was a teacher now and could understand how terribly distressing it can be for a child to be treated in this way. She was also reminded how she was able to comfort children who were upset. Then she was asked to go back in time and come face-to-face with her 'child self' and provide her with all the comfort that she needed. When the child part was able to acknowledge that she had everything she needed from this, the next stage was to move forward in time to the incident that had more recently distressed her. The purpose of this part of the procedure is to make sure that the patient is now able to cope better with the situation as an adult and if not, one can, for example, do more ego-state work.

This method can be very effective in changing the way people feel in difficult situations in their present life. In the experience of the authors, the more emotionally charged the adult–child encounter is, the more effective the manoeuvre. It is also important that the patient is judged by the therapist to have sufficient resources (ego strength) such as self-worth, to adopt the comforting parent role. Thus sometimes one has to wait until the patient has made sufficient progress in therapy before the procedure may be effectively used.

Further examples of ego-state therapy will be given in later chapters on specific problems. It is also recommended that readers consult the April (1993) issue of the *American Journal of Clinical Hypnosis* (vol 35(4)) which is devoted to articles on ego-state therapy.

Coping more effectively with the situation

This procedure involves cognitively rehearsing coping with the situation using whatever one has learned since, including what one has learned from therapy. This procedure was described in Chapter 12.

Final comments on resolving memories

Sometimes it is not possible to satisfactorily resolve a memory before the end of a session of therapy. It is important to allow patients time to 'put that memory away' with the reassurance that they will find a way of resolving it with their therapist. When this happens, it is important not to leave the next appointment too far ahead in the future, and to arrange that patients can contact you before the next session if they feel the need. If one is experienced in dream suggestion (see later), one could suggest that between now and the next session patients will have one or more dreams that will help them to understand the memory and how to come to feel better about it.

Later in the book, we shall consider other approaches that are appropriate in confronting and resolving memories associated with post-traumatic stress disorder.

MISCELLANEOUS FANTASY PROCEDURES IN PSYCHODYNAMIC THERAPY

The procedures presented in this section have two common features. They each require clients to engage in two acts of construction. First, clients are given the suggestion that they are to engage in a creative activity – a dream, fantasy, drawing or a piece of writing – and that the result will have some important bearing on their problem. Often the material elicited is in symbolic form. The second act of construction is that clients are to interpret this material in their own way with reference to their problems.

These and similar procedures are generally understood from a psychodynamic standpoint. Our own formulation is that both acts of construction allow the conscious elaboration of cognition and its associated affect as described in Chapter 18. However, in our experience, the procedures are not as widely used by practitioners of hypnosis as those that we have so far presented, and many practitioners do not use them at all. This may be partly because they lack a good theoretical model that is acceptable to therapists of a variety of persuasions. Certainly many cognitive-behavioural therapists would have difficulty accommodating them in their repertoire of techniques. They also create the expectation that a significant revelation is going to emerge – for example, a suggested dream or fantasy that will cast new light on the client's problems. This may cause anxiety in both therapist and client about the possibility that this will not happen – for example, the client will not have a dream, or the dream will prove incomprehensible. Finally, these procedures appear to require from clients a good capacity for absorption, imaginal involvement and creative thinking, and some authorities would also emphasise a capacity for dissociation. Not all clients fit this description.

Whatever the case, we advocate that only practitioners who are well experienced in psychotherapy should use these procedures and they should be considered as adjuncts to a broader programme of therapy, to be introduced according to the therapist's discretion and judgement.

For all of these procedures, the induction and deepening methods outlined in Chapter 6 (i.e. the first approach to hypnosis) are recommended.

Dream interpretation

Dreams remain a genuine mystery for psychologists and a great deal is yet to be learned about them. Nearly everybody dreams, although many people do not remember their dreams. There are various types of dream, but here we are interested in the vivid, multi-modal experiences that are associated with rapid-eye-movement (REM) sleep. People tend to have several episodes of REM sleep during the night and these become longer as the night progresses. There is some evidence that when people are deprived of dreaming, but not sleep generally, they subsequently dream more to compensate. This suggests that we need to dream. The idea has been around for some time that dreaming is a way that the brain reprocesses information that has accumulated during the day and this is of adaptive significance.

Do dreams mean anything?

Are our dreams telling us something? There is a long history of dream interpretation and some rather extraordinary ideas. Some people consider that dreams may be portents of future events and thus have a paranormal status. A famous precedent for this is the interpretation by Joseph of the dream of the Egyptian Pharaoh described in the Bible. Needless to say we do not accept these ideas.

Freud himself postulated that dreams are fantasies resulting from a 'relaxing of repression' and hence a representation of unconscious activity that is threatening to the ego (Freud 1933). The dream is still subject to censorship, hence the content is in symbolic form, relating to primitive emotional and sexual themes.

Dreams are certainly bizarre creations and it is probably true to say that we would find it difficult to consciously construct in the waking state the dreams that we have at night. They also have an absurdity, realness and spontaneity that make them different from most waking fantasies.

Although there is no shortage of popular books on dream interpretation, we see no evidence to support the idea that dreams can be understood in terms of 'If you dream about X, this means Y' kinds of explanations. Perhaps the dream itself, then, is random gibberish. This is not dissimilar to the theory that was put forward in 1917 by Poetzl (see Poetzl 1960), namely that a dream consists of information that we did not fully attend to during the day, and consequently need not be of significance. But as an act of construction by the client's mind, surely the dream should have *some* meaning of relevance to the client, just as a poem, painting or piece of music says something about the mind of the person who created it.

We cannot be absolutely sure about this. But perhaps it is not the dream itself, but how the client *interprets* the dream that is significantly revealing. Asking the client to do this may be similar to doing a projective test such as the Rorschach inkblots or the Thematic Apperception Test (TAT) (Morgan & Murray 1935). The latter consists of a series of pictures about which the respondent has to make up a story.

Case example

Eight-year-old Peter was shown (by MH) a TAT picture of a boy sitting alone on the steps of a wooden house. Peter's interpretation of this was that the boy's real mother had gone away and he was being looked after by a different mother. He did not like her and he was sitting waiting for the real mother to return. In reality, Peter had always lived with his mother, but in the past she had been physically cruel to him and the Child Guidance Unit was keeping a close eye on them. (Followers of Melanie Klein may wish to interpret Peter's story in terms of the defence of splitting.)

In recent years, projective tests have been regarded with some disfavour, and certainly the inkblot tests have not passed muster according to the stringent requirements of reliability and validity. On the other hand, it does not strain credulity to consider that projective storytelling may reveal valid information about a person's inner world, considering how much is commonly inferred from works of literature and poetry about the workings of their creator's minds. Hence, even if a dream is nonsense, the client's interpretation of it may still be of therapeutic value.

A simple method of dream analysis

Sometimes clients come to a session of therapy and spontaneously describe a dream they recently had that seemed significant in some way. Perhaps the feeling in the dream was unusually intense or the memory of the dream keeps recurring. Also, the dream itself may recur. The following is a simple method that can help clients use the dream as a means to achieve greater self-awareness along the lines we discussed in Chapter 18.

The first step is always to ask clients what sense they make of the dream. This may be all you need to do: there is not necessarily a right or wrong answer. What you should help clients achieve, however, is a simple, parsimonious interpretation that uses as little of the dream content as possible and that makes sense to them. What clients initially do is to become hooked on the specific details of the dream when, according to this method, these are not necessarily of significance. For example, a client may say, 'I can't understand why I was driving a Ford, when my car is a Volvo' or 'Why did my old school friend Ted pop up in my dream? I haven't thought about him for ages'.

It may be advantageous for clients to go through the dream in imagination, frame by frame, whilst giving a running commentary. This may elicit further content and affect, but there is a possibility that if the dream was upsetting, then the client could re-experience all the original bad feelings. This is unnecessary for present purposes. Whatever the case, you wish to know from your clients what is or are the predominant emotion or emotions in the dream.

Case example

Arthur (seen by MH) was a wealthy businessman who was receiving counselling for stress. Seven years previously, he had served a prison sentence for fraud. Since his release, he had prospered. He was married with two children and lived in a magnificent house. When seen for counselling, he reported that he had started to have bad dreams of his time in prison and being tormented by the prison officers. He would wake up sweating in a panic.

Arthur could not explain why he was having these dreams. One possibility was that he still had not got over the trauma of his imprisonment, but that did not seem to ring true with Arthur. Whatever the case, the main emotions in his dream were anger, frustration, helplessness and some fear.

The next step is to help the client express the theme of the dream in its most abstract sense, devoid of as much content as possible. This is not always easy, as clients often have difficulty leaving behind the details. In Arthur's case, the theme of his dreams was his being trapped and unable to do anything about it.

You now ask clients to put together the theme and the feelings and ask, 'In what way does this connect with anything that is happening in your life *now*?' The 'now' is important.

Case example (continued)

When Arthur was referred for counselling, his business was in trouble, but he knew that if he kept working, eventually the economic cycle would turn in his favour, his business would start to pick up again and he would be able to pay off his debts. In the meantime, he was compelled to work long hours, commute great distances each day, arrive home exhausted every night, and so on. He saw no way out as he had committed himself to a huge mortgage, was educating his children privately, and felt obliged to keep his family in the manner to which they had grown accustomed.

In this example, the meaning of the dream appears so obvious that one is entitled to ask, 'So what?' In fact, it is not unusual that when one brings clients to the point where the interpretation of the dream seems so obvious, it still seems to elude them. One way of thinking about the dream, then, is that, figuratively speaking, it is drawing clients' attention to something that they are not fully acknowledging. It is, as it were, a kind of inner communication that says, 'Please attend to this'. Sometimes, as in Arthur's case, clients are not able to do much about these matters, but the understanding and enhanced self-awareness that this kind of simple interpretation of the dream gives clients can still be very helpful.

Dream suggestion and interpretation using hypnosis

A more elaborate method is to ask clients to go through the dream during hypnosis and to make the suggestion that they will be able to interpret the dream in their own way. In this kind of analysis, the content of the dream assumes greater importance than in the former method. To start with, however, one can give clients the posthypnotic suggestion that between now and the next session they will have a dream of significance to their problem.

The mechanisms that may account for why a posthypnotic suggestion such as this should prove effective, requiring as it does a response that is not under the control of the subject, have not been adequately explicated. Degun & Degun (1988) review the experimental evidence that such a posthypnotic suggestion can be effective, but it does not appear that investigators have provided adequate controls for such things as baselines and compliance with the demands of the experimenter.

The following is a procedure used by the British clinical psychologist Marcia Degun-Mather and described in Degun & Degun (1988). Her method actually incorporates the possibility that the dream may occur during the day and may be no more than a sudden, 'out-of-the-blue' thought. Here, however, we keep to the single suggestion of a night-time dream.

First, one explains in a simple way something of the nature of dreams. For example, one can say that sometimes we are worried about something but may shelve it to the back of our mind in favour of everyday routine activities and distractions. The content of the concerns and worries may later surface in the form of dreams at night. Dreams are often illogical, and symbols and other methods of disguise are used.

One can then go on to explain that it has been shown that people can have dreams during hypnosis (we shall discuss this later) or as a result of posthypnotic suggestion. Therefore hypnosis can be useful in eliciting a dream or dreams that may reflect important aspects of the problem that can be the focus of therapy. It is also necessary to explain that even though one does not initially understand one's dreams, it is possible to make sense of them and again hypnosis may be a useful means for helping this.

Do not be put off if clients say they never remember their dreams or indeed that they do not dream. If they are hypnotisable, the hypnotic suggestions of recalling dreams seem to work for those who are highly motivated.

During hypnosis, the posthypnotic suggestion is given as follows:

Between now and your next appointment, you will have a dream which will throw light on your problems, and how you might overcome them. You will remember the dream so that you can tell me about it when you come to your next session.

Reassurance is given that once clients are able to perceive and understand the problem through the medium of the hypnotic dream, they will be able to solve it in one way or another with the therapist's help. Instruct clients to have paper and pencil at the bedside to write down the dream. Encourage them to write down anything and everything that they recall of their dream, even if it seems like nonsense.

It is often easy to assume that clients understand that dreams take disguised forms. They frequently do not understand this and think that they will dream in very concrete and specific terms about their problem, though this is very seldom the case.

When clients describe the dream do not be deterred by the fact that you yourself do not understand it. If you feel you do understand it, do not be tempted to interpret it, as the client's understanding may be quite different from what you expected.

If clients are unable to understand the dream at the next session, then hypnosis is again used and suggestions are made that they will go through the whole dream and be able to elaborate on the meaning. This can be done by using an imaginary blank screen or theatre stage with the dream projected onto it. Through relating the dream in more detail, as is often the case, a further understanding of the dream is possible. Care is taken not to impose interpretations, though questions can be asked by the therapist.

This then opens the way to making adaptive changes in thinking and behaviour as discussed in Chapter 18.

Hypnotic dreams and fantasies

Instead of a dream at night, the therapist may suggest that clients have one during the hypnotic session. The preliminaries and instructions are similar to above. One can simply say that the dream will begin when clients are given the signal and they are to signal when the dream has ended. Clients may commentate on the dream as it is unfolding, but the usual procedure is to wait until the dream has ended before asking clients to go through the dream again, in the manner described above, encouraging them to come to their own understanding.

It is useful to precede the dream suggestion with the safe place or beach or garden deepening technique. Clients are to imagine being in that place, lying down, closing the eyes, and having the dream.

A similar technique, originally described by Wolberg (1946), is to suggest that the fantasy takes place on the stage of a theatre or the screen of a cinema.

Wolberg's theatre visualisation technique

Clients are told to imagine that they are sitting in the stalls at a theatre. They are to give a signal as soon as they can picture themselves quietly sitting there looking at the closed curtains, waiting for the performance to begin. They are told that they can see a woman (or man, in the case of a male client) standing on the side of the stage, and peeping behind the closed curtains. This woman can see what is taking place on the stage behind the closed curtains and what she sees is making her look very frightened or unhappy. Clients signal when they are ready to have the curtains open and when they do so they can see what is actually causing the woman to look so unhappy or frightened. As soon as they can see the play that is occurring on the stage, they are to raise their hand. As soon as this happens, they are asked to describe the action that is taking place on stage. They are then encouraged to come to their own understanding of what the scene means in terms of their problems.

When using this and other techniques described in this chapter, occasionally the client spontaneously abreacts and this is one reason why the methods should only be used by experienced psychotherapists.

Clients are then told that they will see the curtains close. A second suggestion may then be given that the woman at the side of the stage can now see something happening on stage that is making her look extremely happy, as if her dearest wishes had been fulfilled. It is suggested that clients will be wondering what it is that is making this woman feel so happy, and when they are ready to signal for the curtains to open again, they will be able to see the action on the stage. As soon as they can see this, they are to give a signal and to describe exactly what they can see. Again, clients are encouraged to arrive at their own understanding of this scene.

The jigsaw puzzle visualisation technique

This is similar to the theatre or cinema technique described above. The suggestions are as follows:

I want you to sit upright in the chair and imagine a small table in front of you. On that table there are several coloured boxes ... red ... green ... yellow ... and blue. Each of these contains the pieces of a separate jigsaw puzzle. You will notice that there is no picture on the lid of the box. Let me know when you can picture this.

That's fine. Now I want you to choose one of those boxes – any colour that you prefer – and turn out the pieces of the jigsaw puzzle on the table and let me know when you have done this.

I don't know what picture will eventually emerge and at the moment you probably do not know yourself, but it will be the picture of a scene or incident that is closely connected with your present problems. Your unconscious mind (*or the back part of your mind*) knows and will help you to fit those pieces of the jigsaw puzzle together so that we shall be able to see what this picture is.

Now start fitting the pieces together. You will be able to do so much more quickly than when you are wide awake. Tell me what you can see as the picture gradually builds up.

In the above procedure, the kind of picture that is to be produced may be specified but this is not always necessary. It may be better first to leave the choice of the picture to clients until they have become familiar with the technique. Then, if desired, it may be suggested that the picture is one associated with some difficult feeling or with pleasure, as in the theatre technique.

It may well be that the colour of the box selected is not entirely without significance. Some therapists believe that when the red box is chosen, it not infrequently happens that the picture, together with the client's associations to it, reveals the presence of unacknowledged fears or even aggressive or sexual conflicts. The green box is often said to be associated with conflicts in which jealousy (particularly sibling rivalry) plays an important part, the yellow one with feelings of inadequacy, and the blue box with conflicts centred around problems of frigidity and lack of feeling. This is part of the folklore of analytical hypnosis and we are not aware of any controlled research on the subject.

Some clients will enact the whole process of picking up the pieces of the puzzle and fitting them together. If, at any stage, clients say they can see nothing more, they can be told that the picture is not yet complete, and that as they continue to fit more of the pieces together, they will be able to describe what else they see.

Clients may begin by describing scenes containing meadows, water, trees and houses. In that case, it may help to gently ask a question such as 'Can you see any people or children there?' At some stage, one can ask if the scene is a familiar one, what clients think is going on, what the people are doing and thinking, and so on. At this point, clients may start to free associate to the image, and this may lead to further elaboration and understanding. Sometimes, however, clients may be reluctant to disclose the material and it may be better to suggest that there is no need for them to acquaint you with the content of the picture as long as they take a good look at it themselves and work out its significance.

Automatic writing and drawing

The technique of automatic writing or drawing is undertaken by placing a pencil in the client's hand during hypnosis and suggesting that the hand and arm may behave without any conscious thought or effort on the client's part. It may be helpful to refer to common everyday examples of when this occurs. It may then be suggested that the hand will begin to write and will move along quite automatically so that the client will not be aware of what is being written. As with the other methods, it is suggested that the message will help clients understand better their problem and how they may solve it.

The product of such writing is usually quite different from clients' normal writing. It is often quite undecipherable. Letters are badly formed, words run together and sentences are incomplete and fragmented. Whenever clients are able to open their eyes without becoming fully alert again, they can be instructed to write the full meaning of the communication underneath the automatic writing. If they are unable to open the eyes in this way, they can be given the posthypnotic suggestion that the meaning of the automatic writing will be quite clear to them after they are alerted. As usual, it is always best to let clients translate it for themselves.

Rather than write, clients may either be instructed to draw whatever they like, or themes may be suggested to them by the therapist. In their drawings, clients may reveal attitudes towards members of their family, their spouses and children or even the therapist, of which they are not fully aware. One variation of this is to ask clients to make up a story about their drawing. Some therapists combine this technique with age regression, the idea being that clients may be able to more easily express in drawings, attitudes and feelings that are denied at the 'adult level'.

METHODS FOR CHILDREN AND ADOLESCENTS

All of the methods described in this chapter may be used, with suitable modifications, with children and adolescents. In addition, the following two methods have been presented by Benson (1984, 1988). The first is intended to help children broach problems in their life that may be addressed by therapy or counselling. The second is a kind of age-progression technique that may, as we have described in the earlier section on age progression, again disclose problems that need to be addressed.

The 'parcels' fantasy

This procedure is preceded by the 'tidying a desk' fantasy described in Chapter 14. It also uses the metaphor of 'the subconscious mind' described in that chapter.

Have you given that desk a good sort out? Have you found any particular problems in there that need tackling today?

If 'No' is signalled, move on to next stage of therapy. If 'Yes', then proceed as follows:

Imagine now that those problems are made up into a paper parcel. ... Each layer on that parcel is a different problem. Each layer has a big label on it. ... On one side of the label, it tells you what the problem is and on the other side of the label your subconscious mind gives you some ideas what can be done to sort it out.

The questions below are a guideline only and have to be adapted to the particular situation in which this method is being used.

Can you see the label on the top layer? Can you read what it says?

If 'No' is signalled, ask for a few clues:

Now, you don't have to tell me anything if you don't want to but if you do want to talk you can do ... quite easily and naturally. ... It won't stop you relaxing. ... Do you want to tell me what the problem is?

If this is disclosed, continue:

Now, turn the label over and see what suggestions there are for getting rid of that problem.

One then proceeds with further therapy, counselling and advice as appropriate. Then continue:

Do you think you can get rid of that problem now?

If the answer is in the negative, then ask if this is possible at some future date. If 'never', then suggest that the child will learn to cope with it and will learn not to get upset by it.

Get rid of it, then – throw it away on a bonfire and signal 'Yes' when it's gone.

Work through each problem layer until the parcel has disappeared.

The crystal ball and maze fantasies

Now I want you to imagine that you've got a crystal ball in front of you. The sort of crystal ball that fortune-tellers have to look into the future. You can't really see what's going to happen in the future but I'd like you to look into that crystal ball and get a good clear picture of how you would like your future to turn out ... when all this trouble is over and things have settled down. ... What you'll be doing ... where you'll be living ... what sort of person *you* would like to be. Signal 'Yes' when you've got a good clear picture of your future.

Await the signal, then continue:

Now imagine that the future you want for yourself is on the other side of a maze ... maybe the sort of maze you get in a comic where you have to trace a path with a pencil ... or maybe a real maze with paths and hedges. You have to find your way through the maze from where you are now to where you would like to be on the other side. It might not be easy; you might have to go over a few obstacles; you might have to go a long way round; or you might have to start again. But there *is* a way through, so you see if you can find it. If you get through without my help, signal 'Yes' to let me know. If you get really stuck somewhere, signal 'No' to let me know you need some help to get through.

If 'No' is signalled, counsel and advise as appropriate, then try again.

That's very good. You're really making plans for your future now. You know what you want and you know how you're going to get there!

Modern metaphors

As we indicated in Chapter 14, readers may wish to use more contemporary material for these kinds of fantasies. For example, in both of the above cases, computer games could be substituted, the crystal ball now being a VDU controlled by the child, likewise the maze, or the child may travel in a time-machine or space-ship.

REFERENCES

Benson G 1984 Short-term hypnotherapy with delinquent and acting-out adolescents. British Journal of Experimental and Clinical Hypnosis 1: 19–28
Benson G 1988 Hypnosis with difficult adolescents and children. In: Heap M (ed) Hypnosis: Current clinical, experimental and forensic practices. Croom Helm, London, ch 29, p 314
Biklen D 1992 Typing to talk: Facilitated communication. American Journal of Speech and Language Pathology January: 15–17, 21–22
Cheek D B, LeCron L M 1968 Clinical hypnotherapy. Grune and Stratton, New York
Degun M D, Degun G 1988 The use of hypnotic dream suggestion in psychotherapy. In: Heap M (ed) Hypnosis: Current clinical, experimental and forensic practices. Croom Helm, London, ch 21, p 221
Enright J T 1999 Testing dowsing: The failure of the Munich experiments. Skeptical Enquirer 23: 39–46
Frederick C, Phillips M 1992 The use of hypnotic age progressions as interventions with acute psychosomatic conditions. American Journal of Clinical Hypnosis 35: 89–98
Freud S 1933 New introductory lectures on psycho-analysis. Lecture XXIX: Revision of the theory of dreams. Hogarth Press and The Institute of Psycho-analysis, London
Hilgard E R 1986 Divided consciousness: Multiple controls in human thought and action. Wiley, New York
Karle H 1988 Hypnosis in analytical psychotherapy. In: Heap M (ed) Hypnosis: Current clinical, experimental and forensic practices. Croom Helm, London, ch 20, p 208
Kirsch I, Lynn S J 1997 Hypnotic involuntariness and the automaticity of everyday life. American Journal of Clinical Hypnosis 40: 329–348
Lamb V D 1985 Hypnotically-induced deconditioning: Reconstruction of memories in the treatment of phobias. American Journal of Clinical Hypnosis 28: 56–62
Laurence J-R, Perry C 1981 The 'hidden observer' phenomenon in hypnosis: Some additional findings. Journal of Abnormal Psychology 90: 334–344

Morgan C D, Murray H A 1935 A method for investigating fantasies: The Thematic Apperception Test. American Medical Association 34: 289–294

Mulick J A, Jacobson J W, Kobe F H 1993 Anguished silence and helping hands: Autism and facilitated communication. Skeptical Enquirer 17: 270–280

Nash M 1987 What, if anything, is regressed about hypnotic age regression? A review of the empirical literature. Psychological Bulletin 102: 42–52

Phillips M, Frederick C 1992 The use of hypnotic age progression as prognostic, ego-strengthening and integrating technique. American Journal of Clinical Hypnosis 35: 99–108

Poetzl O 1960 The relationship between experimentally induced dream images and indirect vision. Monograph 7. Psychological Issues 2: 41–120

Smith C S 1979 Age regression and cognitive restructuring in the treatment of a spider phobia: A brief case report. Bulletin of the British Society of Experimental and Clinical Hypnosis 2: 19–20

Stanton H 1992 Brief therapy and the diagnostic trance: Three case studies. Contemporary Hypnosis 9: 130–135

Torem M S 1992 'Back from the future': a powerful age-progression technique. American Journal of Clinical Hypnosis 35: 81–88

Van Dyck R 1988 Future oriented hypnotic imagery: Description of a method. Hypnos: Swedish Journal for Hypnosis in Psychotherapy and Psychosomatic Disorders 15: 60–67

Watkins J 1971 The affect bridge: A hypnoanalytic and counter-conditioning technique. International Journal of Clinical and Experimental Hypnosis 19: 21–27

Wolberg L R 1946 Hypnoanalysis. Heinemann, London

20

Behaviour therapy: an introduction and the application of hypnosis

INTRODUCTION

In this chapter, we shall describe how hypnotic procedures may be used to augment a course of behaviour therapy. In order to acquaint readers who are not familiar with this field, we first present a basic introduction.

THE ORIGINS AND NATURE OF BEHAVIOUR THERAPY

Within psychology, there is a history of conflict between those who believe that a science of psychology should examine mental processes and those who believe that, because these are not observable, they are not proper material for scientific investigation. The latter maintain that we can only observe behaviour, and therefore psychology should be about investigating the laws governing observable behaviour. This school of thought is termed *behaviourism*.

For practical purposes, there is no absolute dichotomy between behaviourists and non-behaviourists, rather shades of grey. However, behaviourism developed in part as a reaction in the 1920s and 1930s against introspectionism. This was an approach particularly associated with German psychologists in the later 19th and early 20th century. Subjects, and experimenters themselves, were trained to introspect when performing various mental tasks, and on the basis of their reports, various hypotheses about how the mind works were drawn up.

One of the earliest behaviourists was John B. Watson (1878–1958), a professor of psychology at Johns Hopkins University, who eventually went into advertising. His first major article on behaviourism appeared in 1913 and his major book *Psychology from the Standpoint of a Behaviourist* was published in 1919.

Much of the important work and ideas of behaviourism are based on work with *laboratory* animals (particularly rats and pigeons), in contrast to the study of behaviour characterised by the work of ethologists such as Konrad Lorenz and Nikolaas Tinbergen, who study animal behaviour in the natural environment. Also, most of the work has been on the learning of behaviour, so behaviourism gave rise to a number of influential learning theories, for example that of Clarke L. Hull (1884–1952) who developed a highly sophisticated theory of behaviour in the 1940s and 1950s. The framework of this survives but not the details. (Surprisingly, as we mentioned in Ch. 1, Hull was also interested in hypnosis, and developed ideas based on the role and influence of imagination.)

Operant conditioning or learning

Behaviourism, for obvious reasons, is often called stimulus–response (S–R) psychology, and probably the most famous S–R psychologist is B. F. Skinner (1904–1990). Skinner did not elaborate a theory of behaviour as did Hull, but he was concerned with principles that determine the occurrence of a particular behaviour. He and his followers assumed that most behaviour was learned or modified by learning and was shaped by the occurrences of reinforcing stimuli and punishing or aversive stimuli in the environment. These behaviourists studied *operant* or *instrumental* conditioning or learning. The following concepts are important.

Operant

This refers to a behaviour mediated by the skeletal somatic nervous system and is 'voluntary' (and therefore does not include reflexes). In the laboratory, the most obvious example is a rat that is pressing a lever in a cage, known as a Skinner box.

Positive reinforcement

This is a stimulus which, when contingent on a response, leads to an increase in the frequency of the response. In the last example, the pressing of the lever might result in the delivery of a food pellet, which would be the positive reinforcement or reinforcer, or in more everyday terms, the reward.

Negative reinforcement

This is commonly taken to mean punishment but the latter term is in fact used for another kind of stimulus. Negative reinforcement is said to occur when the frequency or probability of a response is increased by the removal of a stimulus. In the Skinner box, an instance of this may be when the rat has to press a lever to turn off an electric shock. In this case, the pressing of the lever is said to be 'negatively reinforced'. Notice that it would be wrong to say that the response had been punished.

In human terms, we may also extend the term to cover the alleviation of uncomfortable internal states such as anxiety. For example, when a patient leaves a supermarket because of a panic attack and then calms down, we can say that the patient's response of escaping has been negatively reinforced and is more likely to occur again because of this.

Punishment or aversion

This occurs when the stimulus contingent on a response leads to a decrease in response rate or probability. For example, if a rat in a Skinner box stepped onto an electrified grid, received a shock, and stepped off the grid, we would say that the response 'stepping on the grid' had been punished (and stepping off the grid has been negatively reinforced). Reprimanding children for naughty behaviour is normally an act of punishment. The bad behaviour may also be punished by the withdrawal of positive reinforcement, for example by taking away the child's sweets.

Pavlovian, classical or respondent conditioning or learning

Ivan Pavlov (1849–1936) was the great Russian physiologist who pioneered work on classical or respondent conditioning. A *respondent* is behaviour mediated by the autonomic nervous system and other involuntary responses such as reflexes. In his famous experiments on dogs, he conditioned the response of salivation to the sound of a bell. Initially, the *unconditioned response* (salivation) was measured on appearance of the *unconditioned stimulus* (food). On the conditioning trials, food was repeatedly presented, each time being preceded by the sound of a bell. After this stage, it was demonstrated that the bell (now the *conditioned stimulus*) could reliably elicit salivation (now the *conditioned response*).

Summary

Behaviourism assumes that most behaviours and emotional responses are learned and shaped by continuous complex patterns of operant and respondent conditioning. Behaviour therapy is different from psychodynamic therapies, which assume that the presenting problems are the expression of underlying emotional difficulties and conflicts that need to be resolved in the therapy. Behaviour therapy assumes that people's problems arise through the conditioning of maladaptive habits of responding and may be corrected by unlearning these habits (extinction) and learning adaptive habits (acquisition). However, we do not need to accept the first part of the assumption (since, for example, some would argue that certain problems are genetically or organically determined); generally, behaviour therapy is aimed at understanding how problems are *maintained* rather than how they began in the first place.

The paradigm of classical conditioning gives rise to therapeutic procedures for the treatment of emotional problems, for example anxiety and phobias.

Operant conditioning in its purest form is more applicable to behavioural problems where we wish to modify or eliminate inappropriate or maladaptive behaviour and help the person acquire better ways of responding. Nowadays, behaviour therapists are usually happy to include under the label of *operant*, cognitive activity such as obsessional ruminations and, as we shall see, to acknowledge its reinforcing and aversive properties, and its usefulness in rehearsing the acquisition of new ways of responding.

BASIC PROCEDURES IN BEHAVIOUR THERAPY AND THEIR AUGMENTATION BY HYPNOSIS

As we have said, behaviour therapy assumes that many problems people come for help with are the result of their learning maladaptive habits, and these can be unlearned and replaced with more appropriate habits. So the methods of behaviour therapy are all structured refinements of the various ways we learn to do things. (A very good book for the practitioner that describes behavioural and cognitive therapy techniques is Kanfer & Goldstein (1991).)

Overt versus covert methods

Although behaviour therapy has its roots in behaviourism and therefore would be expected to be concerned with *observable* stimuli and responses, the ideas of a 'stimulus' and a 'response' have been extended to cognitive events – that is, thoughts, images, memories, etc. So we can change both behaviour *and* cognitions by the methods of learning, such as reward, punishment and classical conditioning. We can also have the actual processes of learning take place at the cognitive level, that is, *covertly*. Clearly, it is mainly when we are doing therapy at the covert level that hypnosis is a useful adjunct.

Procedures

Verbal instruction (spoken and written)

This is a very common way of learning behavioural skills in everyday life, but it has its limitations. For example, one cannot learn to swim or ride a bicycle merely by verbal instruction. Applications in therapy are wide-ranging and our experience is that patients often make great use of the therapist's verbal instructions even when the therapist has used more elaborate methods. For example, a socially anxious person might report, 'I was feeling uneasy when I started talking to her but I remembered what you said about eye contact and I breathed slowly like you told me to … '.

Covert equivalents of this include self-instruction, self-suggestion and 'affirmations'. For example, people wishing to stop smoking might repeat, 'Nicotine is a poison' to themselves every time they feel tempted to have a cigarette.

During hypnosis, instruction is equivalent to suggestion (usually posthypnotic), which, as discussed in Chapter 11, can be used to augment all behavioural methods.

Rehearsal and practice

This is usually essential to allow learning (and unlearning) to consolidate. Again, there are many applications of this in therapy, for example phobias, assertiveness and social skills training, and sports training.

We have presented methods of covert rehearsal and practice in Chapter 12. A variant is the 'dissociation method'; clients or patients (if they can do this) imagine watching themselves rehearsing the new behaviour and even coach, encourage and reward themselves. Sports psychologists often use this technique.

Feedback

This is similar to the last process, but the person also focuses on the outcome of his or her behaviour. This is important because, in order to learn something, we need to know the relevant effect of our behaviour; the more immediate the feedback the better (e.g. we would be very limited in our ability to become a good darts player if we never knew where each dart had landed once it had left our hand).

Feedback comes up in various forms in therapy. One can ask a patient to keep a record of the occurrence of a habit such as smoking and overeating. This provides information that may be useful in controlling the habit. (In fact, a patient with compulsive hair-pulling whom one of us (MH) saw made dramatic progress when she started monitoring the occurrence of the habit.) Feedback from the therapist and from other members in group therapy is frequently helpful when, for example, the client role-plays assertiveness. We described biofeedback (which is assumed to work by operant conditioning) in Chapter 15.

An example of the use of covert feedback is when one asks a client to covertly rehearse using a new social skill or coping strategy to 'see how it feels'. We might ask, 'What happens; does it feel OK?', and so on.

Positive reinforcement

A very important principle in behaviour therapy, particularly in the management of behavioural problems, is to identify what patterns of reinforcement are maintaining the undesirable responses, to eliminate these, and to install rewards for the desirable behaviour. For example, parents may unwittingly reinforce children's bad behaviour by selectively attending to them when they are naughty (even though they are reprimanding them) and ignoring them when they are good. Therapists themselves will, of course, be concerned to offer praise to their patients and clients when they are succeeding.

Working with an individual patient, one can use *covert* reward. A common example of this is self-praise. You can, however, use covert reward more formally, as follows. First, you elicit from the patient a rewarding image. The image may be that of a pleasant experience, but it may also relate to the response you are reinforcing. For instance, suppose that patients wish to give up smoking and need to be able to refuse offers of cigarettes from their friends at work. The idea will then be to instruct them that every time they refuse a cigarette they are immediately to reward themselves by bringing to mind a pleasant scene. It makes good sense to use for this purpose a beneficial consequence identified by patients for not smoking. For example, they may have stated that they wish to use the money saved from not smoking to pay for a holiday the following year. The rewarding scene may be of the holiday destination and an enjoyable family outing on the beach.

In Chapters 11 and 12, we described hypnotic procedures for augmenting methods of self-control. In the case of covert reward, you can use a cue for the rewarding image. This could be a gesture such as a clenched fist, or a covert word; this might be 'Rhodes' in the above example, if this is where the patient wishes to take the holiday. You will use posthypnotic suggestions to set up the cue and to instruct the patient in the use of the covert reward, for example:

Each and every time someone offers you a cigarette, you will say, 'No thank you' and the word 'Rhodes' will immediately come to mind and the scene of your family enjoying themselves on the beach.

You will also ask the patient to rehearse this in imagination using scenes from real life in which he or she is offered a cigarette (see Ch. 12). These can be incorporated in the patient's self-hypnosis routine.

Covert reward is assumed to follow operant-learning principles; that is, the response increases in likelihood, the more often it is rewarded. However, there are probably cognitive influences as well. Also, once patients are experiencing the more immediate benefits of success, their use of covert rewards (and, as we shall see, punishments) tends to disappear.

Extinction

Here, an undesired behaviour is extinguished by withdrawal of reinforcement. Applications of this are in behaviour problems (withdrawal of attention), and hypochondriasis (withdrawal of reassurance by significant others). Although there are covert equivalents of this – for example, imagining that an undesirable behaviour, such as drug-taking, is not giving the usual positive effect (Cautela & McCullough 1978) – they do not appear to be much used.

Modelling or vicarious learning

Another potent way of learning how to do something is to observe someone else doing it. In behaviour therapy, the model enacts the desired behaviour (which may be rewarded) or the undesired behaviour (which may be unrewarded or punished). Strictly speaking, it is only modelling if the person also demonstrates a skill – that is, *how* to do something (or how not to do it).

Modelling is a technique used in social skills training and in treating phobias, where the therapist may demonstrate handling the feared object (say a spider) while using some anxiety management method such as controlled breathing. The therapist should try to ensure that the modelled behaviour is not beyond the patient's own capabilities.

In the case of covert modelling, one may ask patients to name as the model a person whom they admire. This technique is very suitable for children. Let us suppose that 8-year-old Jack has to have a blood test and he is very anxious. You ascertain that Jack's hero is 'X', a famous footballer. Then say:

You know, lots of people don't like having blood tests. I bet you didn't know that X doesn't like having them! He has to have a blood test now and again like everyone else and he gets really nervous about it. But he has a special way of calming himself down. Do you want to know what he does? It's his own secret way that he's invented. Shall we see how he does it?

Ask Jack to close his eyes and imagine a magic television on which he is watching a video about X. Then say:

Now, in a moment, you'll see X in the clinic at the football ground and he's with a nurse who's going to take his blood. Can you see him? Can you see how worried he looks? He really hates having to do this. But notice what he's doing now. He's telling the nurse to wait and he's closing his eyes. Now, he's breathing in a nice calm way, breathing slowly in through his nose and slowly out through his mouth. And as he's breathing out, he's imagining breathing out all that scary feeling … and thinking of feeling calm … and relaxed … . And now he's telling the nurse he's ready, but guess what he's doing now! He's not thinking about having the injection at all! He's put that right out of his mind and he's imagining the last match he was playing in. In a bit, you'll see a big smile on his face when he imagines how he scored a great goal. He doesn't even know what the nurse is doing – he's not a bit interested in that! And now the nurse is telling him she's finished, and he's feeling really good and ready to get back to his training.

Now, I bet you can use X's way of calming down. Shall we go ahead?

This can be rehearsed with lots of prompting and praise and then done with the injection.

Graded exposure or systematic desensitisation

This is also known as 'counter-conditioning' or 'reciprocal inhibition' (Wolpe 1958). It involves the repeated pairing of the feared object or situation with relaxation instructions or a positive stimulus. This is presumed to result in the classical conditioning of relaxation to the feared object, or extinction of the fear response (by preventing escape or avoidance).

The process is undertaken on a gradual basis, starting with the situation that causes the least fear and working up to the most feared one. The most common application is, of course, with phobic anxiety.

The covert equivalent of this is imaginal desensitisation and proceeds as follows

1. Train the patient in a method of deep relaxation, such as progressive muscular relaxation.
2. Establish a hierarchy of frightening situations (least to most anxiety-provoking). This can be facilitated by rating the anxiety experienced during each one on a scale from 0 (perfectly relaxed) to 100 (extreme terror). This is often known as a SUDs scale (for 'subjective feelings of distress').
3. Work through the hierarchy, from the least to most feared, each time asking the patient to imagine the item and to signal if he or she experiences any anxiety. If so, the image is 'switched off' and the patient relaxes again. It is necessary to persist with this until the image no longer elicits anxiety. Then the next item in the hierarchy is addressed.
4. Between sessions, the patient is encouraged to confront situations that have been 'passed' in the above way.

This is the traditional method. Around 20 situations would be chosen to work on, giving a smooth progression of anxiety as one ascends the hierarchy. However, it is time-consuming and is not much used in its full form these days for the following reasons.

First, the tendency now is to use in vivo exposure whenever possible. So, for example, in the case of a spider phobia one would encourage patients to gradually confront real spiders until they are able to physically handle them. Relaxation may not even be used and results may be achieved in one session, although this may last up to several hours.

Second, therapists are more likely to adopt, as the basis for the treatment, the idea of habituation or extinction of anxiety (and, in cognitive therapy terms, the refuting of irrational ideas). Therefore, one does not withdraw the object or image when the patient signals anxiety, but keeps it there until the anxiety abates.

The third point of difference is that therapists tend to use a more limited hierarchy (e.g. five items or situations) and are less concerned with having such a smooth transition between each one.

Fourth, it cannot always be guaranteed that the deconditioning achieved in imagination will generalise to real-live situations.

Finally, therapists often train patients in anxiety management techniques that they can use in difficult situations. Examples of these were presented in Chapter 12, when we described how these may be covertly rehearsed to strengthen their effect. These methods are useful when the nature of the phobia is such that it is difficult to arrange any kind of controlled exposure, as with social anxiety, thunderstorm phobia or fear of flying. In such cases, the therapist may enhance the realistic nature of the imagined scenes by playing recordings of the sounds associated with the situations (and in the case of thunderstorm phobia, the use of a flash light – see Heap (1981)).

A variant of covert systematic desensitisation is to use, instead of relaxation, counter-conditioning images of positive situations. These situations are chosen by asking the patient a question such as, 'I want you to think of some situations in which you have felt confident and in control in the same way that you want to feel in X (the feared situation)'. These are then anchored (as described in Chs 11 and 12), using the same anchor each time, such as clenching the right fist. The anchored feelings are then used (instead of relaxation) to work through several images of feared situations in ascending order of difficulty. Another variant is to work through between four and six actual situations from the past. As always, end with the covert rehearsal of an actual future situation.

Flooding

Here, patients are continuously exposed to the situation in which they experience maximum anxiety, without escape, until the anxiety diminishes. Again the applications are to phobias and severe obsessive–compulsive disorder.

Flooding in imagination is not, in our experience, much used. (We are not classifying under this heading, abreaction work with traumatic memories.) A variant of covert flooding is termed 'implosion' or 'implosive therapy' and is ascribed to T.G. Stampfl (Stampfl & Levis 1967). This technique incorporates symbolic psychoanalytic imagery in the therapist's description of the imagined scene.

Response prevention

This is related to flooding and is the treatment of choice for obsessive–compulsive disorder. It may also be used with vomiting in eating disorder. The patient is simply prevented from carrying out the compulsive behaviour, and the patient's anxiety will eventually extinguish.

The use of covert methods is considered to be limited in the behavioural treatment of obsessive–compulsive disorder (see Ch. 30). However, covert rehearsal of response prevention may lead to further exploratory work. For instance, we might ask the patient, 'Imagine *not* performing the compulsive act. How does it feel? Can I communicate with the part of you that wants to perform this act?', and so on.

Aversion therapy and sensitisation

There is a difference between these two (more theoretical than practical). Aversion therapy is the punishment of a response – for example, a loud noise when taking a puff of a cigarette – and therefore operant conditioning. Sensitisation is the pairing of a non-aversive stimulus (S1) with an aversive one (S2), leading to the classical conditioning of fear to the non-aversive stimulus. For example, an item of women's underwear (S1) may be paired with an electric shock (S2) to decondition the sexual arousal response of a fetishist. Just for the moment, to make the discussion easier, we shall use the word 'punishment' to cover both processes.

Punishment may be used in the treatment of antisocial behaviour, undesirable sexual urges, smoking, and alcohol and drug abuse. However, it does not appear to be used much these days.

As far as covert methods are concerned, a number of possibilities arise. The stimulus or response may be overt or covert, likewise the punishment. For example, an unwanted obsessional thought or urge (e.g. to have a cigarette) may be punished by the patient's snapping an elastic band on the wrist. Or the patient could be trained to bring to mind a nauseous image either to the smell of a cigarette or the act of putting a cigarette to the lips. A third example is that of a nauseous image contingent on the thought of a fetish object or an undesirable urge (e.g. to indecently exhibit oneself).

The following is a paradigm for incorporating hypnosis into a course of covert aversion therapy or sensitisation adapted from Wright & Humphreys (1984). These authors were working with two exhibitionists, one of whom also stole women's clothing.

1. Train the patient in hypnotic relaxation.
2. Identify appropriate aversive imagery. This may be a time when the person experienced nausea – for example, when he was violently sick – or it could be related to the problem, say when the person was arrested

or stood up in court to listen to the charges. The image is rehearsed in imagination until it may be readily brought to mind.

3. Establish a cue word for the aversive image (e.g. 'arrest' or 'vomit'). One might instead use a physical anchor, as described in Chapter 11. Rehearse the patient's use of the cue and give the appropriate posthypnotic suggestions about the use of the cue.

4. Identify the relevant undesired response or unconditioned stimulus. For an exhibitionist, this could be the urge to self-expose, and for a cigarette smoker, taking hold of a cigarette. In the case of a person who steals women's underwear, this would be an image of the same. (One could include the real objects or pictures of the object in the conditioning phase below.)

    A variant of the procedure is to identify a chain of responses or stimuli. For a cigarette smoker, this could be:

- taking hold of a cigarette
- putting it to the lips
- lighting it
- drawing on it.

5. Rehearse pairings of the undesired response or unconditioned stimulus with aversive imagery several times per session using the cue word. This is the conditioning phase and this proceeds until the patient experiences an immediate aversive reaction to the imagined response or to an image of the targeted stimulus.

    If you are using a chain of stimuli or responses, do around four pairings at each part of the chain, starting with the last one and working backwards.

6. An additional option is also to establish a covert positive reinforcement for not engaging in the undesired behaviour as described under 'Positive reinforcement' above.

7. Repeat posthypnotic suggestions that the cue word and aversive imagery will occur whenever the patient makes the undesired response(s) or encounters the targeted stimulus (stimuli) in real life.

8. Ask the patient to rehearse in imagination the occurrence of the aversive reaction (and, if used, the rewarding image) in future situations that he may encounter in everyday life.

9. You may encourage the patient to covertly rehearse the conditioning sequence during sessions of self-hypnosis. This could be put on an audiotape. You may find, however, that compliance will not be high and the effect of the aversive response without the guidance of a therapist will not be particularly strong.

10. With a problem such as sexual deviance, several sessions of the above will be necessary. Wright & Humphreys (1984) used six sessions (in

addition to assessment sessions) plus several booster sessions at 3-month intervals.

Also with more complex problems, you need to consider additional therapeutic strategies to address, for example, social skills deficits, anxiety management, poor self-esteem, and re-education and restructuring of sexual attitudes and beliefs.

Time out

When a person (e.g. a child) is exhibiting undesirable behaviour that is at risk of being positively reinforced, particularly by onlookers (e.g. other children's attention in the classroom), the person is temporarily removed from the situation (e.g. by being placed in an empty side room for a while).

Habit reversal

The patient practises a response incompatible with the undesired habit. For instance, in the case of a nail-biter, the incompatible response, to be executed as soon as the hands go to the mouth, may be the act of clenching the fists. The diaphragmatic breathing exercise to counteract hyperventilation, described in Chapter 12, is an example of habit reversal, as are simple physical relaxation techniques.

Thought-stopping and decentring

These may be construed as the covert equivalents of habit reversal or even time out. Although, as will be described later, cognitive therapy helps people by showing them how they can challenge unconstructive and irrational ways of thinking, it may be sometimes better to try to help the person ignore the thoughts, say by distraction. (We acknowledge that some cognitive-behavioural therapists may object to these methods on the grounds that they constitute avoidance tactics.) In the case of thought-stopping, patients close their eyes, allow their thoughts to freely wander, and as soon as they start to engage in some unwanted or obsessional thinking, they signal to the therapist who immediately bangs a hand on the table and says 'Stop!'. Patients can then use the therapist's intervention as a cue to switch to some other thoughts or imagery. Patients can practise this on their own by saying to themselves 'Stop!' and switching imagery.

Similar to these procedures is 'decentring'. Patients switch attention by scanning external objects and their appearance, and perhaps covertly naming them. One of us (MH) has described an elaboration of this method in Gibson & Heap (1991) called 'ego-shrinking'. This is appropriate for very self-conscious people, such as those who blush excessively. Such people (and indeed, to some degree, most of us) imagine that people are taking much more notice of them than in reality, for example, noticing that they are anxious and thinking they must therefore be stupid. The routine includes suggestions that patients covertly rehearse looking around them, imagining that they are having no effect at all on other people, and that everything would be just the same were they not there. They then imagine rising above themselves and looking down on the scene, seeing themselves as one normal person amongst the crowd.

Stimulus control

In order to gain control over some behaviour, one ploy is to arrange that it is only undertaken in a strictly defined situation, and other behaviours are prohibited in that situation. For example, a person with insomnia is instructed to sleep only in bed (nowhere else) and not to read, eat or listen to the radio or lie awake longer than 10 minutes in bed. (The person is to leave the bedroom if the last of these occurs.) Similarly, a person trying to lose weight must only eat in a particular place (e.g. seated at the kitchen table) and must not do anything else there (e.g. watch the television).

A covert equivalent is the 'worrying chair', whereby people who are inclined to worry excessively have 'worrying sessions' while sitting in a chair designated for that purpose. If possible, whenever they find that they cannot stop worrying, they are to go to their worrying chair and 'do it properly'.

Paradoxical injunction (or intention) and symptom prescription

We described a variant of this in Chapter 12. Patients are asked to deliberately produce the symptom (as in the 'worrying chair' technique), or deliberately maintain the problem (usually involving a response they are finding difficult to control). For example, patients with sleep-onset insomnia may be instructed to deliberately remain awake for as long as they can. In the case of functional urinary retention (the 'pee shy' syndrome or, as the Americans like to call it, the 'bashful bladder' syndrome), patients may be instructed only to use public urinals where they experience the problem, and to *deliberately* refrain from passing water at each visit. A person with a blushing phobia may be instructed to deliberately blush, and a patient with bulimia may be instructed to deliberately repeat in the week ahead all the bingeing behaviour that has been undertaken in the week that has just passed.

There are several reasons why paradoxical injunction may be effective:

1. It may promote relaxation. The patient stops 'trying hard' to achieve the desired effect (e.g. to go to sleep) or fighting the unwanted response (e.g. vomiting).
2. It may operate by desensitisation or exposure to the salient conditioned stimulus – that is, elimination of avoidance behaviour

(e.g. in functional urinary retention). We shall see in the next chapter that the effect of this may be construed in cognitive, rather than behavioural, terms.
3. It may encourage a sense of control (e.g. by deliberately vomiting, more control over the vomiting response may be achieved).
4. It may redirect resistance to the therapist (e.g. instructing bulimic patients they must overeat).

Covert applications of paradoxical injunction include asking patients to *deliberately* increase their anxiety by one point on an anxiety scale (see Ch. 12), or deliberately increase some pain they are experiencing. By doing this, we may be giving patients the message that if they can *increase* a difficult or painful experience they should therefore be able to *decrease* it.

Massed practice

This is a variant of paradoxical injunction. It is used with problems such as compulsive habits and tics. Symptom alleviation may be accomplished by asking the patient to deliberately perform the habit over and over again. One theory underlying this, at least with overt applications, uses a hypothetical construct elaborated by Hull (1943), namely reactive inhibition. Hull hypothesised that every action creates an inhibitory tendency against repeating that action. Massed practice therefore leads to a build-up in reactive inhibition. The idea of reactive inhibition has been used to explain why sometimes when one is learning a skill, one can overpractise and one's performance can even seem to deteriorate. (An alternative explanation is that inappropriate habits are being overpractised.) What is needed then is a period of abstention from practice to enable the reactive inhibition to dissipate.

INCORPORATION OF HYPNOTIC PROCEDURES

In most of the techniques above, as has been demonstrated in a number of cases, we can incorporate hypnotic procedures, the assumption being that their effectiveness is thereby strengthened. Thus hypnotic induction and deepening procedures may be used for relaxation and enhancing commitment and responsiveness to the instructions. Covert rehearsal of the techniques undertaken, using both previous and future imagined situation, may also be undertaken both in the session and by the patient during self-hypnosis. Liberal use can be made of posthypnotic suggestions, incorporating the cuing or anchoring technique (Ch. 11). Metaphorical anecdotes may be incorporated. Finally, each session may be rounded off by a suitable ego-strengthening routine.

REFERENCES

Cautela J R, McCullough L 1978 Covert conditioning: A learning-theory perspective on imagery. In: Singer J L, Pope K S (eds) The power of human imagination. Plenum Press, New York, ch. 8, p 225

Gibson H B, Heap M 1991 Hypnosis in therapy. Erlbaum, Chichester

Heap M 1981 Hypnosis and simulation techniques in the treatment of a monosymptomatic thunderstorm phobia. Bulletin of the British Society of Experimental and Clinical Hypnosis 4: 20–21

Hull C L 1943 Principles of behavior. Appleton Century–Crofts, New York

Kanfer F H, Goldstein A (eds) 1991 Helping people change, 4th edn. Pergamon Press, New York

Stampfl T, Levis D J 1967 Essentials of implosive therapy: A learning-based-psychodynamic behavioural therapy. Journal of Abnormal Psychology 72: 496–503

Wolpe J 1958 Psychotherapy by reciprocal inhibition. Stanford University Press, Stanford

Wright A D, Humphreys A 1984 The use of hypnosis to enhance covert sensitization: Two case studies. British Journal of Experimental and Clinical Hypnosis 1: 3–10

Cognitive therapy: an introduction

INTRODUCTION

Probably the most significant development over the last 25 years in the field of what we are broadly calling 'psychotherapy' has been the rise of cognitive therapy. For readers unfamiliar with cognitive therapy, we shall now provide a broad overview. At the end of this chapter, we also give a short list of recommended reading. However, there is no substitute for a course of training with one's peers from experts in the field.

Our overview of cognitive therapy is biased by our aim to develop an eclectic approach to psychotherapy, one to which the full range of hypnotic procedures that we have already presented, and shall present later, may be applied. In our opinion, the theorising that underpins cognitive therapy provides a useful basis for this project. Hence, in this chapter, we also give some thought to the question of what all the main psychotherapies have in common.

There are many first class introductory texts on cognitive therapy. We list some of these at the end of this chapter.

PROBLEMS AND THERAPIES: SOME COMMON GROUND

With such a range of methods of treatment for psychological problems (within each of which are dozens of variations and offshoots), readers may be forgiven for feeling confused as to what is the best approach for any particular patient they may be seeing. One might also ask the question, 'However different they may seem, aren't all of these approaches really achieving the same thing?'. In other words, perhaps they are different routes to the same ends. If so, what are the essential characteristics that they have in common? Let us pursue this theme as a way of introducing cognitive therapy.

Below is a list of psychological problems that are representative of those reported by clients attending for psychotherapy. We ask readers, 'What have they in common?'

- Philip has been depressed and agitated since his traumatic experiences as a soldier in Northern Ireland. He tries not to think about these memories and will not talk about them with anyone.
- Francine would like to go sunbathing on the beach but is too self-conscious to allow herself to wear a bathing costume.
- John sometimes feels annoyed with his wife but does not express this because he is afraid of hurting her feelings.
- Anna would like to go abroad on holiday but is afraid of flying.
- Delroy says he will never ask a girl for a date in case she turns him down.
- Marie won't let herself get close to anyone again since she got hurt in her last relationship.
- Mahmood forgets an appointment with a colleague; he rings the colleague up and says he is ill.
- Lydia will never look people in the eye when she is talking to them.
- Fred has not been to the supermarket since he had a panic attack there.
- Imran will not ask his employers to improve his working conditions in case they get angry and sack him.
- Mario wears a hat when he goes out because he is so embarrassed about being bald.
- Stephan has never had a close relationship. He was sexually abused as a child but he suppresses any thoughts or feelings about it and has never revealed what happened to anyone.
- Helen always checks the lights and switches in her house ten times before she retires to bed.

With the exception of one of these examples, the most obvious feature that they have in common is that the people concerned are all avoiding something, whether it be external, such as a supermarket, or internal, such as a difficult feeling, or an activity, such as asking someone for a date. The least obvious example is the last one, Helen, until we regard her problem as her avoiding remaining in bed in the company of that niggling doubt that she may not have turned off all the switches when she retired for the night.

So, perhaps what many psychological problems have in common is avoidance and, hence, the ultimate purpose of any therapy is to enable patients to confront what it is they are avoiding. This may be accomplished in a behavioural way, for example by taking Fred, in the above examples, to a supermarket and helping him cope with the panicky feelings. Or in some cases it may be achieved by 'talking therapy', as in Philip's case.

Behaviour therapy explains the process of avoidance (and escape) and the beneficial effect of exposure or confrontation, in conditioning terms. So in the case of Fred, by a process of classical conditioning he has developed a fear of being in a supermarket. (We may also extend the idea of a conditioned stimulus to internal events, e.g. we could say that Fred's fear is conditioned to the prodromal symptoms of panic, such as increased respiration and heart rate, which are thus the conditioned stimuli for further anxiety and panic.) When Fred experiences these bad feelings, he leaves the supermarket or abandons his plans to go there in the first place. This brings about a reduction in the bad feelings. Hence, each time he escapes from or avoids supermarkets, he is negatively reinforced. We can therefore understand his problem as being due to classical conditioning of fear that is maintained by the operant conditioning of escape and avoidance behaviour. If Fred were to remain in the supermarket, then his fear response would gradually extinguish and thus the stimulus of the supermarket would no longer be associated with anxiety (desensitisation).

We may understand Philip's problems in a similar way. By encouraging Philip to think about his experiences, talk about them, write about them, and visit places that remind him of them, gradually he would be desensitised to the memories of them. One may also argue that exposure enables the person to learn ways of dealing with the bad feelings that they experience, something that is prevented by their escape or avoidance.

A cognitive approach to escape and avoidance

Although the above formulation does work as a way of understanding a wide range of problems and the therapies that are used to treat them, we may be able to go further than a strict behavioural interpretation. Let us look at the list of problems again and ask the question, 'Can we advance in any way our understanding of why these people avoid the things that they do?'. One way we could do this is simply to ask them. For example, Anna may say that if she panics on an aeroplane, everyone will think she is stupid and childish. Philip may believe that the sheer emotion that he would experience if he really confronted those terrible memories would overwhelm him and 'send him mad'. Delroy may believe that if a girl turned down his offer of a date, then it would be evidence that people find him unlikeable and no girl would ever want him as a boyfriend. Helen may believe that if she did leave any switches on in the house, something terrible would happen for which she would be responsible. And so on.

Now we can see that with all of these people their avoidance is associated with fears and anxieties that appear to stem from the ways in which they are thinking. Of course, the way they are thinking may be entirely reasonable; for example, Imran, above, may be correct in assuming that were he to complain about his working conditions, then his employers would sack him. In that case, it might be better for him to keep quiet. However, it may be that many or all of the above people are thinking about their situations in a way that is unrealistic and unhelpful to them. But how are they going to find out if they do not confront those situations?

Let us study this question in more depth. Each one of us does not experience directly the 'real world'. All we ever experience is our representation of our world. We construct this from the raw data that come through our various senses and from our previous experiences that lead us to have certain expectations about the world. Our representation of the world may be compared to a map. Our map of our world tells us how we should act, what we should expect, what choices we have, what are the consequences of such choices, what is worth doing and what is best avoided, and so on. Each person's map is unique.

In Chapter 13, we presented this metaphor of a map as one way of helping people understand the difficulties that they may experience in life. We said that, just like an ordinary map, our personal map may be up-to-date and accurate, and provide us with a range of realistic choices. Conversely, if it is out of date, it may create problems and anxieties for us; it may unduly restrict the choices that are realistically available at any time.

So, our map guides us through our world. However, as a result of our behaviour and our encounters with our world (notably our social world), we should constantly be correcting our maps, enriching and updating them. In particular, as we grow up, our world changes. Importantly, the way our world (again, especially, the world of people) reacts to us and what it expects of us, also changes. As a result, our behaviour should change accordingly. In other words, we should always be learning from our experience. Hence, we have a developmental process that is cyclical in nature: our map determines or influences our behaviour and the results of our behaviour influence our map.

This is the ideal, adaptive way. Why then do we so often fail to do this? Somehow, we fear changing our maps. One reason may be that there are good adaptive reasons why we are reluctant to change our beliefs even in the face of contradictory evidence. We need predictability, consistency and familiarity. Our beliefs, opinions, attitudes and assumptions provide us with that. They enable us to view the world in a more orderly and predictable way. In that way, we are less anxious.

Consequently, we are *prejudiced*: we tend to interpret information and to behave in ways that will confirm or, at least, not disconfirm our beliefs. This is adaptive and necessary to some degree, but all too often we become stuck in this. We never discover more adaptive ways of thinking and doing; we restrict the range of adaptive choices (often to just one) that may be available to us. Consider how all the people in the list presented earlier are restricted and unable to achieve what they desire and what would be helpful to them.

A common goal of all psychotherapies?

So, without simplifying matters unduly, we can say that much psychotherapy, of whatever school, helps people achieve a realistic and adaptive representation of their world, including themselves, which they may then act on accordingly.

FUNDAMENTALS OF COGNITIVE THERAPY

Cognitive therapy represents the most explicit approach to psychotherapy based on the above conclusion. It is a direct attempt to help patients and clients to identify their irrational, unrealistic and maladaptive ways of representing their world, their selves and their future, to choose more rational, realistic and adaptive ways, and then act on these accordingly.

Cognitive therapy explicitly accepts that it is not the actual world itself but people's interpretations of it, the way they think, the assumptions they make, and the rules and beliefs they hold about the world, which determine how they feel and react. Personal effectiveness and fulfilment depend on how realistically and rationally people construe their world. Of course, people may think realistically about their world and still be afraid, unhappy, annoyed, and so on because that is the reality of their situation. Thinking realistically (and the fact that we are all human and none of us is entirely logical and rational) means that we are inevitably going to experience these difficult feelings. In general, however, psychological problems and disorders arise from *dysfunctional* thoughts and beliefs. The person's thinking generally, or in specific areas of the person's life, is unrealistic and habitually the subject of distortions such as:

- overgeneralising or catastrophising about the adverse consequences of some event
- the selective filtering out of anything positive (as in depression)
- jumping to unwarrantable conclusions of a negative consequence when other, more probable, explanations exist
- reacting to 'that which might be' as though it is 'that which is'
- assuming undue personal responsibility for events
- making unrealistic demands on the world and on oneself.

Basic procedures in cognitive therapy

Education

This includes educating the patient about the tenets of cognitive therapy, a process that is best accomplished gradually by involving patients as much as possible, rather than by lecturing them. It also includes providing patients with information about the nature of anxiety and panic, what is known about depression, and so on.

Identifying salient thoughts

In the therapy session, this is done by first focusing on a typical problem situation that is clear in the patient's memory. This is termed the activating event and is given the label 'A'. Then patients are asked to describe 'C', the consequence, namely what emotion or feeling was felt and how they behaved (e.g. returned home). Then the therapist asks patients to describe what they were thinking at the time that caused them to feel bad and act in this manner ('B' for 'beliefs'). The thinking may not be explicit (i.e. in the form of an internal commentary) and eliciting the thoughts is not as easy as it may seem. For example, a patient may say, 'I thought I was going to be sick', but the therapist still has to continue the analysis to come to a clear understanding of the consequences. For example, a patient may say, 'I imagined that people would see me and be disgusted'. Continuing in this vein may elicit the belief 'I'd lose the respect of all my friends', and so on.

Patients are also encouraged to do this whenever they are in a difficult situation. This can be done in writing using three columns for A, B and C.

Challenging the thoughts and beliefs

The kinds of questions one asks here are 'Is this realistic?', 'What evidence do you have for believing this?', 'Are there more likely interpretations?' and 'If this did happen, why would it be so awful?' It is important that the therapist does not 'do the work' for patients, but challenges them to think things out for themselves. Patients are also encouraged to do this in everyday life.

Identifying distortions

This is not always necessary but it may help patients if they are able to use a label now and again to describe their habitual ways of thinking. For example, a depressed patient may be able to say, 'I know – I'm overgeneralising again!' or someone with problems of self-consciousness may say while describing a difficult situation, 'I did it again – I was mind-reading!'

Cognitive restructuring

This is the process of substituting unrealistic thoughts with more realistic interpretations and rehearsing them. An example may be 'Because one person is annoyed with me doesn't mean everyone despises me'. Another involves estimating realistic probabilities (e.g. with a person with thunderstorm phobia, 'The chances of lightning striking me are less than my being hit by a car').

Again patients are trained and encouraged to keep doing this in their daily life.

Testing reality

It is very important to establish the various ways in which patients *behave* according to their dysfunctional thinking, and encourage them to abandon those ways and respond according to realistic thoughts. This exposure or 'reality testing' can itself be an effective way of changing dysfunctional thoughts, beliefs and feelings. Here we see how behaviour therapy and cognitive therapy may involve very similar procedures, but the underlying rationale is different. In the case of behaviour therapy, the rationale of exposure is based on conditioning theories, whereas in cognitive therapy terms, the rationale is the testing of the validity of the beliefs and assumptions that are restricting the patient. (In cognitive terms, avoidance of a situation also allows the person's imagination plenty of time to come up with more 'What if … ?' catastrophic kinds of thoughts.)

Let us consider a case example to illustrate this. Let us suppose that Fred, in the examples given earlier, avoids the supermarket, because he thinks that if he panics, eventually he will faint. Although his therapist will already have reassured him and explained how panic and fainting are unrelated, we can all understand that Fred needs to be convinced of this and the best way of doing this is for him to remain in the supermarket. In cognitive terms, this is to test the validity of his catastrophic thought. Suppose that Fred panics but does not faint. He can now change his thinking: 'Even if I panic I won't faint and the panic will eventually subside'.

Here we see that what we identified as the common feature of the problems listed previously, namely avoidance, and their treatment, namely exposure, can now be presented in much broader terms, namely 'testing the reality of one's ideas and beliefs' (both 'catastrophic' and 'rational') or, in terms of our original metaphor, testing the validity of our existing map. So, taking the example of Fred again, suppose that because of his fear that panicking will lead to fainting, he also has a habit of sucking a boiled sweet whenever he sets off from home ('To keep my sugar level up so I won't faint'). Suppose also that when he drives his car, he keeps the car radio on ('To reassure me that I'm still conscious'), and that whenever he feels anxious, he holds onto something ('To stop me falling'). Fred needs to test the reality of his catastrophic thinking about fainting in all of these instances by eliminating the behaviours in question. (These behaviours are sometimes called 'subtle avoidance strategies' but the avoidance aspect is not very clear in many cases; perhaps the more commonly used expression 'safety-seeking behaviour' is more understandable.)

Comparison with other psychotherapies

Cognitive therapy is highly structured and systematic and is adaptable to a wide range of psychological problems including affective, anxiety and even personality disorders. Its efficacy has been supported in clinical trials. In some senses, it falls between behaviour therapy and psychodynamic therapy. Like the former, it does not place much emphasis on the person's early experiences but is concerned to modify habits in the here and now. In fact, because cognitive therapy is often also concerned with the person's behaviour (as, for example, with 'reality testing'), we often speak of cognitive-behavioural therapy. However, as with psychodynamic approaches, it encourages clients to explore their habitual thoughts and feelings, which no doubt are influenced by early experiences. Also the big difference between cognitive therapy and behaviour therapy is the former's insistence that it is not events that determine how we feel but the way we interpret those events. Thus, in contrast to behaviour therapy, less emphasis is given to classical and operant conditioning in understanding patients' problems and their treatment.

Variations

There are two major pioneers of cognitive therapy – Aaron T. Beck and Albert Ellis. Both developed their ideas and approaches from a dissatisfaction with psychoanalysis. In general, Beck's approach tends to challenge the logic of people's thinking (e.g. 'Where is the evidence that people think you look unattractive?').

Ellis's system of cognitive therapy is called 'rational emotive therapy' and tends to challenge the underlying rules and beliefs (e.g. 'So you're not attractive? So what? Why *must* you be attractive?'). He is particularly concerned with unrealistic demands we make on ourselves and our world. That is, we may have (usually implicit) rules or demands such as 'I must never upset anyone'; 'People should always treat me with respect'; and 'I should never fail at anything'. Each of these is accompanied by a 'catastrophic judgement'; for example, 'If I do upset someone, then it's a total disaster'; 'If people treat me disrespectfully, then it means I'm no good'; and 'If I fail at something, then I'm a total failure'. This way of thinking is unrealistic and will cause people much difficulty in life if they really mean these things. A more realistic way of thinking is to change the demand ('I must/mustn't/should/ought/... etc.') into a preference ('I would prefer ... etc.') and the catastrophic judgement into a realistic appraisal ('If not, then I shall be disappointed/annoyed/fed up/etc.'). The latter feelings are not reasons to seek therapy.

A useful developmental model

There is one final component of cognitive therapy that is very useful for our quest for a model for eclectic psychotherapy. Our presentation of this reflects our own ideas and purpose, and may not accurately represent

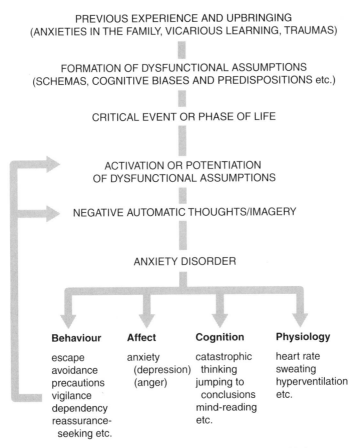

PREVIOUS EXPERIENCE AND UPBRINGING
(ANXIETIES IN THE FAMILY, VICARIOUS LEARNING, TRAUMAS)

FORMATION OF DYSFUNCTIONAL ASSUMPTIONS
(SCHEMAS, COGNITIVE BIASES AND PREDISPOSITIONS etc.)

CRITICAL EVENT OR PHASE OF LIFE

ACTIVATION OR POTENTIATION
OF DYSFUNCTIONAL ASSUMPTIONS

NEGATIVE AUTOMATIC THOUGHTS/IMAGERY

ANXIETY DISORDER

Behaviour	Affect	Cognition	Physiology
escape	anxiety	catastrophic	heart rate
avoidance	(depression)	thinking	sweating
precautions	(anger)	jumping to	hyperventilation
vigilance		conclusions	etc.
dependency		mind-reading	
reassurance-		etc.	
seeking etc.			

Figure 21.1 Cognitive model for anxiety (adapted, with the kind permission of the author, from Salkovskis P 1989 Obsessions and compulsions. In: Scott J, Williams J M G, Beck A T (eds) Cognitive therapy in practice: An illustrative casebook. Routledge, London, ch 3, p 50).

mainstream ideas in cognitive therapy. This is the developmental model that is outlined in Figure 21.1. It is one of a family of similar schematic representations of the possible aetiologies of common psychological disorders. The one given is for anxiety; others may be for depression, hypochondriasis and obsessive–compulsive disorder.

We have stated that both behaviour therapy and (at least until recently) cognitive therapy are not particularly concerned to look at early experiences. However, the developmental model of psychological disorder, represented in Figure 21.1, does acknowledge the importance of early events and upbringing. (We could also include such influences as hereditary and perinatal factors here.) These early formative experiences, notably those involving significant people in the child's life, create certain biases in important ways in which clients view the world and themselves in it. These biases are termed 'schemas' or 'schemata' and are rather fixed, general beliefs, rules, or sets of assumptions that may or may not be problematical. For example, a schema that 'If someone disapproves of something I do, then I am worthless' is likely to cause problems later when the person has to assume adult autonomy. If people are lucky in life, perhaps no ill-effects will be experienced. However, they may encounter events or pass through periods of life when the salience of such a schema is thrust to the fore (e.g. a relationship comes to an end or work pressures start to mount). The dysfunctional schema then generates the kind of distorted ideas and thoughts that we have discussed earlier. These can be considered to be 'automatic' – so habitual that they may not be fully represented in consciousness. (Thus we move nearer the 'psychodynamic' way of thinking, and therapies have indeed been developed under the label 'cognitive-analytical'.)

As we have seen, these distorted ways of thinking can lead to difficult emotional states such as depression or acute or chronic anxiety. These experiences may then provide the stimulus ('A', the activating event) for further distorted thinking (e.g. 'I'm depressed again; I'll always be depressed'; or 'I'm anxious; I'll not be able to control myself; people are noticing what I'm going through').

While the focus of cognitive therapy has been on the here and now, and thus endeavours to break this vicious circle of negative thinking and affect, in recent years cognitive therapists have shown more interest in working with the patient's cognitive schemas. (Probably Ellis's approach is more schema-focused.)

Some hypnotic procedures lend themselves very well to schema-based therapy. We mentioned in Chapter 19, that, except, for example with post-traumatic stress disorder, it is not usually the case that patients' problems are referable to just one critical memory. Implicit in the patients' behaving, thinking, feeling and physiological responding is the totality of their formative experiences. However, certain explicit memories may be available that serve as potent representations of the kinds of formative experiences which have resulted in the acquisition of dysfunctional schemas. Working with one or a few of these may be of great assistance in correcting distorted ways of thinking that restrict patients in their current life.

APPLICATION OF HYPNOSIS

The applications of hypnosis within cognitive therapy will become apparent in the next chapter, when we discuss how the developmental model presented in Figure 21.1 may provide a useful basis for an eclectic approach to psychotherapy, particularly where hypnotic procedures are used in an adjunctive manner.

RECOMMENDED READING

A good introduction to the practice of cognitive therapy is the following:

Beck J S 1995 Cognitive therapy: Basics and beyond. Guilford Press, New York

A more recent introduction is:

Neenan M, Dryden W 2000 Essential cognitive therapy. Whurr, London

Others are:

Greenberger D, Padesky C A 1995 Mind over mood: A step-by-step cognitive therapy guide to changing your emotions. Guilford Press, New York
Padesky C A, Greenberger D 1995 Clinician's guide to mind over mood. Guilford Press, New York
Salkovskis P (ed) 1996 Frontiers of cognitive therapy. Guilford Press, Hove

For an introduction to Ellis's rational emotive therapy, we recommend:

Neenan M, Dryden W 2000 Essential rational emotive therapy. Whurr, London

22

An eclectic approach to psychotherapy augmented by hypnosis

INTRODUCTION

We have now reached the end of our overview of the common psychotherapeutic approaches. Readers may already be experienced in and committed to one particular school of therapy, in which case their use of hypnotherapeutic procedures will be constrained by that therapeutic approach. Other readers may be eclectic and work at different levels, using a number of different therapeutic approaches. In that case, they may not be 'experts' in any particular approach.

If you do work eclectically, then you need a framework for determining what approach and what level to focus on with any given patient at any given time. Therapy may lose impact if it does not follow a theme or themes in a coherent manner. Let us now address this matter.

THE AIMS AND RATIONALE OF ECLECTIC PSYCHOTHERAPY

From our discussions in the previous chapter of the common aspects of the various systems and schools of psychotherapy we can suggest that one rationale for psychotherapy is that patients and clients are restricted to maladaptive ways of feeling, thinking and behaving in certain aspects of their lives (which may be general, as in depression, or specific, as in certain phobias and bad habits). Therapy therefore aims to enable people, where possible, to be less restricted in the above ways and thus to have more choices available to them. This may be achieved in the following overlapping ways:

1. By the use of methods of learning and conditioning, therapy may directly change the way patients or clients respond physiologically and behaviourally to those situations in which they are limited to

maladaptive ways of responding. (Examples: desensitisation, aversion therapy, assertiveness training and anxiety management training.)

2. Therapy may identify, explore, and challenge dysfunctional patterns of thinking that patients and clients habitually adopt concerning themselves, their problems, and their world, and offer the means for acquiring more realistic and adaptive ways of thinking. (Examples: cognitive therapy, including cognitive restructuring and education.)

3. Therapy may encourage, in an adaptive way, confrontation with aspects of the patients' or clients' internal and external world that they are avoiding. (Examples: psychoanalysis, cognitive-behavioural therapy, non-directive psychotherapy.)

Hypnosis may be used in all of the above, with a view to enhancing effectiveness.

A FRAMEWORK FOR THE APPLICATION OF HYPNOSIS TO ECLECTIC PSYCHOTHERAPY

It is customary to say that hypnotic procedures are best considered as adjuncts to therapy. But what do we mean by this? One interpretation is that the hypnotic procedures that we have described form but one component of the sum total of therapy undertaken with the patient. Yet we shall see that sometimes – for example, for smoking cessation and psychosomatic problems – the entire treatment may consist of one or more sessions of therapy in which hypnotic procedures are used throughout. In other words, therapy starts with the preparation and induction and ends with alerting the patient (and may include self-hypnosis).

Another interpretation is that the adjunctive component is the hypnotic induction and deepening routine. We could still administer all the procedures without this, but we assume that it augments the therapy, rendering it more effective.

Yet another interpretation is based on the argument that for a procedure to be defined as 'hypnotic', it has to discriminate amongst subjects of high and low hypnotic susceptibility. Within any session of therapeutic hypnosis, there will be techniques that do this and others that do not. The more the outcome of the therapy depends on the former, the more it may be validly described as 'hypnotherapy'. Hence, one might use the description 'adjunctive' in that sense.

Whatever interpretation readers favour, it is certainly the case that 'hypnotic' procedures can provide the cement for the structure of an eclectic programme of therapy, allowing one to move fluently between the different levels – cognitive, behavioural, emotional and physiological. The framework for this is provided by Figure 21.1 (p. 279). Using this framework, the plan for a course of hypnotically augmented therapy can proceed as follows:

1. Assessment

Prior to any therapy you will, as is usual in psychological treatment, conduct a careful *assessment* of the patient and the presenting problems. This will enable you to make a *formulation* of the problem (i.e. what it is and why the patient has this problem) and to establish a *working model* of how your therapy generally, and hypnosis particularly, may alleviate the problem. We have described above a general working model and this can form the basis of the particular working model that you adopt for your patient. This allows you to plan the procedures and techniques you are going to use.

2. Preparation and preliminaries

Your working model will influence the way you *prepare* the patient for hypnosis and your choice of approach as described in Chapters 6 and 7, which then determines the kinds of *preliminaries* you undertake with the patient.

3. Induction and deepening

Your choice of induction and deepening methods will again be determined by your working model and your choice of approach to hypnosis.

You are now ready to begin the main part of your hypnotherapeutic work. The following is a rough guide to the various stages that you might work through. Please note, however, that a course of therapy does not necessarily run along smooth lines and no session will include all of these stages. As we have already stated, age regression (as opposed to the recall of more recent memories) is to be used with discretion as often it proves unnecessary to review remote memories.

4. Cognitive rehearsal of problem situations

The aim at this stage is to identify salient triggers, namely external and internal stimuli, such as palpitations in the case of panic disorder, and the cognitions associated with them.

5. Regression

From the above stage, one may explore with the patient (by normal enquiry or IMR signalling) if there are any important memories related to the above problem situation. If so, one can use regression by the affect bridge to elicit these early relevant memories. Some of these may encapsulate the schemas that developed in formative years – for example, family problems, times of feeling rejected, traumas, physical and sexual abuse, and bullying at school. These may be resolved by counselling the 'child', the use of adult–child ego state therapy, and so on (see Ch. 19).

6. Miscellaneous therapeutic methods

One may then introduce hypnotic or non-hypnotic procedures specifically for changing the maladaptive ways of reacting to the problem situations.

7. Cognitive rehearsal of previous situations

One can then suggest cognitive rehearsal of coping with previous situations using these new ways of behaving and thinking introduced at Stage 6. Occasionally this work may elicit additional areas of difficulty that can be addressed by further schema-focused work using regression, thus looping back to Stage 5.

8. Age progression or future rehearsal

Age progression may be used for cognitively rehearsing coping with future problem situations, and imagining life without the presenting problem. Areas of difficulty may be identified (perhaps by using IMR signalling). This may indicate the necessity for further work requiring the therapist to loop back to Stages 5 or 6.

9. Metaphors and anecdotes

10. Posthypnotic suggestions

11. Ego-strengthening

12. Instructions for self-hypnosis

13. Alerting

14. Instructions for assignments between sessions

These may relate to confronting problem situations.

Other psychodynamic methods may be incorporated into this framework – for example, dream suggestion may be used when the therapy seems to 'get stuck'.

This plan covers a wide range of problems but it is not appropriate for all of them. The skilled practitioner will judge when it may be fruitful to use hypnosis and when this is likely to be unnecessary or unhelpful.

23

Risks, precautions and contraindications

INTRODUCTION

The next section of this book is devoted to the application of hypnosis to specific problems and disorders in medicine, psychiatry and psychotherapy. The reader will discern that hypnosis has a very wide range of application and it is difficult to identify in categorical terms any condition or disorder for which hypnosis should never be used. We shall however attempt to provide some guidance for assisting therapists in their decision whether or not to use hypnosis for any given problem. First, we shall discuss potential adverse effects, and some precautions and contraindications. The final section of this book is also very relevant to these matters.

GENERAL

It is our opinion that hypnosis is a comparatively safe procedure and that where adverse reactions have occurred these are usually not due to some special property of hypnosis, but are explicable in terms of more general effects. However, the potential for adverse effects should be taken very seriously and we shall now explore these more fully.

Does hypnosis itself, regardless of the context in which it is practised, have some special property or properties that are inherently harmful in themselves? Some people, usually those who support a strong 'trance' model of hypnosis, consider that there are (Gruzelier 2000). These writers contend that hypnosis is an altered state of consciousness involving certain neurophysiological changes that mean that the subject is vulnerable both to beneficial and to harmful influences. Thus some researchers claim to have demonstrated that following a session of neutral hypnosis or a routine non-clinical procedure such as a hypnotic susceptibility scale, certain individuals have unpleasant after-effects including headaches, panicky feelings and confusion (Crawford et al 1982, Page & Handley 1990). Some people consider that subjects may be at risk if they are 'not taken out of their trance properly' or if the suggestions given during hypnosis 'are not properly cancelled'. Barber (1999) has suggested there is a small minority of individuals who experience some degree of confusion for a period after hypnosis; these are probably what others would term as having high dissociative capacity, although Barber prefers the expression 'amnesia prone'.

Some authorities believe that these side effects are no different than those that have been reported for other relaxation and imaginative procedures such as meditation and guided fantasy (Brentar & Lynn 1989, Coe & Ryken 1979, Conn 1972, Lynn et al 1996, Lynn et al 2000).

Whether or not there are properties intrinsic to hypnosis that may have adverse consequences, anyone using hypnosis, for whatever purpose, can expect that very occasionally subjects will become upset for reasons that are difficult to predict. Sometimes this may be simply because individuals have anxieties about 'being out of control', even though they may have been assured that during hypnosis subjects are still 'in control'. In Chapter 6, we outlined ways in which the hypnotist should respond to unexpected signs of distress. Also, very occasionally we have heard of individuals who, having been hypnotised, then worry that something unusual has happened to them, for example because their mind has been controlled. We stress that these incidents seem to be rare but may arise because hypnosis does have 'spooky' connotations associated with mind control and there are a few individuals who ruminate about this afterwards. It is likely that such individuals have problems of psychological adjustment that require psychiatric help if their worries surrounding hypnosis prove persistent.

Whatever the case, many reported ill-effects caused by hypnosis are likely to arise from the way it has been used. These issues are discussed further in Chapter 33.

THE IMPORTANCE OF A THOROUGH ASSESSMENT

When hypnosis is being used to treat medical problems and pain, it is essential that patients have had a thorough medical examination, that their medical condition is appropriately monitored, and that they continue to receive the relevant medical treatment. Similarly, where patients are being treated for a psychiatric disorder (e.g. depression, anxiety disorder or eating disorder), then therapy should be informed by a thorough mental state examination, and patients should have access to the recommended psychiatric treatment (although we acknowledge that some patients choose not to take medication).

REGRESSION AND ABREACTION

On several occasions in this book, we caution that the use of direct methods of regression and the deliberate provocation of abreaction should be undertaken only with a careful assessment of how these procedures are intended to help clients or patients with their presenting problems. The therapist engaged in such procedures should have undertaken professional training and qualifications in the psychological understanding and treatment of people with emotional disorders, independent of training and qualifications in hypnosis.

In fact, modern practice appears to favour procedures that involve more gradual exposure to traumatic memories, thus avoiding severe abreactions. There are risks of further traumatising the patient with post-traumatic stress if an abreaction is not satisfactorily resolved. Readers are referred to Putnam (1992) for a thorough discussion of this subject. Similar concerns apply to the technique of flooding in imagination.

All practitioners using revivification and regression methods must be aware of the risks that memories thus elicited may be unreliable or false. This matter has been more thoroughly discussed in Chapter 18 and guidelines are given in the Appendix of this book.

CONSIDERATIONS WHEN USING GROUP HYPNOSIS

When carrying out group hypnosis, it is not recommended that any regression work be attempted. This is because of the risk of distress, as occasionally sad memories are stirred up even when the instruction is to bring to mind a happy memory. Because there are other people present, individuals may have no opportunity to talk over their experience with the therapist. It is true that some hypnotic susceptibility scales that are used in groups do have a regression item, but this is short and well structured. Even so, whether the context is the laboratory or the clinic, when conducting group hypnosis, it is recommended that the hypnotist is available for a sufficient length of time after the session to talk over any difficulties that any members of the group may have experienced during the session. Some practitioners are able to bring along a colleague or colleagues for this purpose.

SOME PROBLEMS THAT REQUIRE PARTICULAR CONSIDERATION AND CARE

If nothing else, one consequence of using hypnosis inappropriately is that it may be a waste of time. It is not easy to predict how successful a hypnotherapeutic approach will prove to be or whether its adjunctive use will enhance the effectiveness of therapy. One guide is the available research evidence on what problems and disorders appear to respond to hypnosis. This literature is reviewed in Chapter 33.

Although hypnosis is commonly used in the treatment of anxiety disorders, cognitive-behavioural therapists will be mindful of the priority given in their approach to eliminating avoidance and safety-seeking behaviours, and encouraging in vivo exposure. The use of hypnosis may actually delay this process, and the practitioner should be alert to this possibility. This caveat pertains in particular to therapy for phobias and obsessive–compulsive disorder.

Contrary to earlier accounts, hypnosis is not contraindicated in the psychological treatment of depression (see Ch. 31). However, there are now well-structured cognitive-behavioural treatments of proven efficacy for the treatment of depressive illness and, as yet, there is insufficient evidence that hypnotic procedures improve on this. Accordingly therapists treating depression should satisfy themselves that the inclusion of hypnosis in treatment has a good chance of improving outcome, and is not simply a waste of time and effort. Care should be exercised to avoid exacerbating the depressed mood by, for example, the use of regression procedures that involve the reliving of unhappy memories. As in non-hypnotic therapy, suicidal risk should be monitored.

There have been reports in the literature of the adjunctive use of hypnosis in the treatment of people who have psychotic illnesses or who are prone to psychotic-like episodes (e.g. borderline personality disorder) by practitioners who are highly skilled in psychotherapy with these patients. Without such expertise, this is not advisable; procedures that involve absorption in imagery and fantasy may further weaken the already tenuous grasp of reality on the part of such patients. Similarly, involvement in hallucinatory symptoms may be amplified. Hypnotists may risk their becoming part of the delusional system of a patient with paranoid schizophrenia, mania or a delusional state. This does not entirely rule out the use of hypnosis, say, to assist the dental treatment of an anxious psychotic patient whose illness is well controlled by medication. In such cases, the dentist should consult the patient's psychiatrist for advice and guidance.

In the USA, Canada and some other countries, the diagnosis of multiple personality disorder (MPD) or dissociative identity disorder (DID) is frequently made with the assistance of hypnotic procedures (see Ch. 18). In other countries, including the authors' own, the consensus in the mental health services is that MPD, if it exists at all as a psychiatric disorder, is extremely rare. The consensus further regards the increasing incidence of MPD in North America over the last 20 years as an iatrogenic phenomenon, although it is not disputed that the patients so diagnosed are suffering from psychiatric disturbances and are in need of treatment. The present authors strongly discourage the use of hypnotic procedures as a means by which the diagnosis of MPD or DID is made.

We contend that there is no property specific to hypnosis that has adverse physical effects. The safeguards for patients with life-threatening conditions are the same as those for non-hypnotic treatment and should be in place during a session of hypnosis. For example, any emergency medication such as asthma inhalers or anti-anginal sprays should be immediately available, and the practitioner must make it clear that patients may halt the proceedings at any time to use their medication. Severe abreactions should be avoided in any patients who are advised against sudden excessive exercise. Although hypnosis has been shown to be beneficial in the treatment of asthma, some concern has been expressed about the use of direct symptom-control methods that may reduce the patient's respiratory drive below a safe level (see Ch. 25).

REFERENCES

Barber T X 1999 A comprehensive three-dimensional theory of hypnosis. In: Kirsch I, Capafons A, Cardeña-Buelna E, Amigó S (eds) Clinical hypnosis and self-regulation: Cognitive-behavioural perspectives. American Psychological Association, Washington DC, ch 1, p 21

Brentar J, Lynn S J 1989 'Negative' effects and hypnosis: A critical review. British Journal of Experimental and Clinical Hypnosis 6: 75–84

Coe W C, Ryken K 1979 Hypnosis and risks to human subjects. American Psychologist 34: 673–681

Conn J H 1972 Is hypnosis really dangerous? International Journal of Clinical and Experimental Hypnosis 20: 61–79

Crawford H J, Hilgard J R, Macdonald H 1982 Transient experiences following hypnotic testing and special termination procedures. International Journal of Clinical and Experimental Hypnosis 26: 117–126

Gruzelier J 2000 A review of the adverse effects of experimental, clinical and stage hypnosis. Contemporary Hypnosis 17: 163–193

Lynn S J, Martin D J, Frauman D C 1996 Does hypnosis pose special risks for negative effects? International Journal of Clinical and Experimental Hypnosis 44: 7–19

Lynn S J, Myer E, Mackillop J 2000 The systematic study of negative post-hypnotic effects: Research hypnosis, clinical hypnosis and stage hypnosis. Contemporary Hypnosis 17: 127–131

Page R A, Handley G W 1990 Psychogenic and physiological sequelae to hypnosis: Two case reports. American Journal of Clinical Hypnosis 32: 250–256

Putnam F W 1992 Using hypnosis for therapeutic abreactions. Psychiatric Medicine 10: 51–65

The application of hypnosis to specific medical, dental and psychological problems

The hypnotic procedures that we have so far described may be applied to a considerable range of problems that are encountered in psychotherapeutic, medical and dental practice. In the present section, we examine common problems in which hypnosis is considered to have the potential to play an effective role. In each case practitioners are urged always to consider, for any patient and any given problem, what 'working model' they are adopting. Relevant to this are the assumptions concerning the purpose of hypnosis, including the hypnotic induction and deepening procedures, and for this we return to our earlier distinction of 'suggestion' and 'trance'. With some problems, such as smoking or being overweight, the emphasis will be on maximising responsiveness to suggestion and the expectation of a successful outcome, and the preparation and induction will reflect this. For others, such as insomnia, the aim will be absorption and detachment from the immediate environment and ongoing concerns. In some cases, such as psychosomatic problems or pain, the choice will vary according to circumstances, and sometimes a combination of approaches is appropriate. In all of the problems considered in this section, behavioural and cognitive methods tend to be favoured, but we also illustrate the advantages of a flexible, eclectic approach and the usefulness of psychodynamic procedures when these appear to be indicated.

24

Hypnosis for smoking cessation, weight reduction and insomnia

INTRODUCTION

The three problems considered in this chapter are common concerns in everyday general medical practice. Hypnosis has a proven track record in each of these and is a safe and inexpensive procedure that empowers individuals with the ability to take responsibility for overcoming their problem.

SMOKING CESSATION

There is a vast literature on smoking and its ill-effects, and strategies and treatments for quitting. A review of this literature is well beyond the scope of this chapter. Hypnosis is just one method and a course of hypnotic treatment may incorporate non-hypnotic techniques, including ploys from cognitive-behavioural therapy.

The medical risks of smoking are extensive and widely documented and, for the purposes of educating patients and clients, easy-to-read leaflets are readily available in clinics and GP surgeries and from health information services. Nowadays, we must not forget that other great reservoir of information (and misinformation) – the Internet.

The information available from all of these sources includes advice for people who wish to break the smoking habit. Self-help books are also available. For those who are not too averse to pop psychology, a recent one is *Smoke Free and No Buts!* (Ibbotson & Williamson 1998). The authors are medical doctors experienced in hypnosis, and their programme includes instructions in self-hypnosis.

Commercially available self-help audio- and videocassettes are available for the aspiring non-smoker, but, although some users will certainly stop smoking for one reason or another, we confess to having little confidence in these. We make the same judgement on subliminal tapes. On the other hand, nicotine patches and chewing gum are now available as proven aids to smoking cessation.

All of the above resources may be incorporated into a programme of therapy for those who seek help to break the smoking habit.

General considerations

Hypnosis and smoking cessation are commonly linked in the public mind, and many smokers seeking help to overcome their habit will no doubt wonder if it is worthwhile going to a hypnotist. Is it? The news on this is both good and bad. The good news is that treatments that include hypnosis compare favourably in efficacy and efficiency with a considerable range of other methods. The bad news is that it is very difficult to help many people to stop smoking when, as is most often the case, they have already tried their best without success. (Perhaps it is becoming easier with greater publicity of the ill-effects of smoking, the spiralling cost of cigarettes and the prohibition of smoking in many places.)

Expected outcome

It is not uncommon to hear of hypnotherapists who boast that they cure, say, 95% of their clients of the smoking habit. Unless they inform us about the methods they use to gather their data and how they define and assess abstention, then such claims are about as meaningful as Mark Twain's assertion that he found it very easy to give up smoking and in fact he did it all the time.

Even in the learned literature, there is almost as wide a range as is possible for the claimed effectiveness of hypnosis in smoking cessation – namely 0 to 88% (Green & Lynn 2000). If the editors of the journals in which these papers appear had adopted more stringent standards for the quality of the evidence being offered, then the upper limits of the claimed abstention rate would fall below 50%. We suggest that if you can demonstrate convincingly a continuous period of abstention of 1 year following your intervention in one-third of your clients (retaining in your figures those who fail to respond to your request for follow-up details), then you are doing very well. Single-session hypnotic treatments with no follow-up support achieve an abstention rate of between 20–25% (Ahijevych et al 2000). The baseline rate for successful abstention without external assistance is around 5–6% (American Psychiatric Association 1994, Viswesvaran & Schmidt 1992) and 15% for self-help programmes (Viswesvaran & Schmidt 1992).

One reason for the differences in outcome is that more effective interventions provide the client with support after the 'quitting session' in the form of extra appointments to deal with problems that arise. They also incorporate additional non-hypnotic ploys, notably to forestall relapse. There is also variability in the abstention period reported (e.g. 3–24 months). Accounts differ as to whether or not success is defined as continuous abstention over the reported period and whether or not dropouts and non-responders to requests for follow-up information are included in the calculation of abstention rate.

The motivation of the client is an important factor in outcome. Hence, those clients, who spontaneously decide for themselves that they really want and need to stop smoking and are prepared to pay a hefty fee, are likely to do better than those who are urged by someone else, such as their doctor or partner, or who volunteer for a clinical trial and may not be charged a fee of any significance. Finally, to be really sure of the accuracy of treatment success, it is necessary to have objective tests of abstention such as plasma thiocynate levels. This is because clients may exaggerate the degree of abstention to please the therapist.

Immediate vs gradual abstention

Some programmes, including of course single-session treatments, require the client to stop smoking immediately, while others aim for a gradual withdrawal. There is no good evidence to favour either, although gradual withdrawal guarantees more therapist–client interaction than a single-session approach, and specific problems may be addressed as they arise – for example, the cigarettes that are the most difficult to give up, such as the one smoked first thing in the morning. A gradual withdrawal must be undertaken in a disciplined way, with a specified, 'quitting day', otherwise the client will procrastinate.

Single-session vs multiple-session treatments

There are in the literature indications that the single-session approach with no further contact is likely to be less successful than one with two or more sessions or at least the opportunity for telephone support or a booster session.

If you have in your practice only a limited number of sessions that you wish to allocate to this kind of problem, then you will need to decide which of two outcomes you prefer – a higher success rate or a lower success rate with more people successfully treated. For example, a single-session, individual approach allows you to see 100 clients in 100 sessions. If your success rate is 20%, then you will have 20 new non-smokers. If you use a two-session, individual treatment, you can only see 50 clients in your 100 sessions. Your success rate may move up to 30%, but the outcome will now only be around 13–15 new non-smokers. Which do you prefer?

Individual vs group treatment

Again it is difficult to provide firm support for preferring either individual or group treatments, although we can apply the above mathematics to clarify the choice. On the basis that treatments that are tailored to the individual's needs and personality are the most successful, then we should expect one-to-one programmes to be more effective than group methods. On the other hand, with the latter, one is able to exploit the group effects such as the members' mutual understanding and support, which, if this is acceptable to clients, can operate between sessions. What is important is that the therapist endeavours to establish a good professional relationship and rapport with each group member. For this reason, we do not advocate public 'mass hypnosis' sessions for smokers; the experiences of colleagues and our students suggest that these are not particularly effective.

Cutting down vs complete abstention

With certain habit problems such as alcohol and gambling, treatments may aim at control of the habit rather than complete elimination. There is an overwhelming consensus that this is not a useful treatment option for smoking.

Assessing clients

Many smoking-cessation programmes do not include an extensive assessment phase, but it is worthwhile giving time to a number of important considerations. A crucial one is whether it is the best time for clients to stop. For example, if they are having to deal with a stressful life event, (e.g. moving house or changing jobs) or are going through an untypical period (e.g. Christmas or a holiday), then it may be better to wait until life returns to normal once again (although it might be that a 'new start' facilitates abstention). Similarly, if the client has a mental health problem such as depression or an anxiety or eating disorder, then it is usually advisable to give priority to treating this before addressing the smoking habit. Even if no psychological problem is present, if you assess the role of smoking in the client's life, you may uncover evidence that cigarettes are an important prop that ameliorates catastrophic reactions such as acute anxiety attacks or violent outbursts of anger. Again, you ought to think about addressing these problems first. You may therefore consider asking clients to keep a smoking diary, say in the fortnight leading up to their first (and possibly only) treatment session. This should include a note of the time and place of each cigarette, the triggers (internal and external) for deciding to have a cigarette, and the effect of the cigarette on how the client felt.

It is also useful to have some feel for the client's motivation, since this a key factor in success. For example, it does not bode well if clients say that they are giving up at somebody else's request (e.g. their doctor or spouse). There may be other more subtle tell-tale signs. Would you feel confident, for instance, about clients who complained that they could not afford the fee you are charging, if this were equivalent to the cost of 2–3 weeks' smoking? Whatever the case, many treatment approaches require you to identify the client's own reasons for wanting to stop smoking, in order to address these in the hypnosis script.

Finally, for clinical purposes, we do not think it is necessary to assess hypnotic susceptibility.

Hypnotic procedures for smoking cessation

It is not our intention to provide readers with a standard hypnotic protocol for smoking cessation. Instead, we shall summarise a number of techniques and ploys that have been described in the literature. We advise readers to put together their own protocol that best suits their own style and approach. We do advise that this should be flexible enough to accommodate the differing needs, lifestyles and personalities of the clients who come for help. We also recommend that the therapist uses a range of techniques (hypnotic and non-hypnotic) with any one client and offers some follow-up support, which should be limited rather than completely open-ended. We advocate the charging of a reasonable, non-refundable fee as a test of motivation; even if clients only stop smoking for a few weeks or cut down, it is likely that they will more than recover the fee charged.

Basic procedure

The most basic procedure, one on which you can build your own approach, involves a hypnotic induction and deepening routine, followed by suggestions that from now on the client will be a non-smoker and have no desire to smoke ever again. This approach is unlikely to yield an abstention rate (continuous over, say, 1 year) that is much above the 5–7% rate achieved by those smokers who spontaneously decide to quit (see above).

As we have stated, the charging of a fee and the provision of an extra session or two, or some form of follow-up support, should improve on this outcome, but there is a range of additional techniques and ploys that may add to the effectiveness of your treatment.

Choice of induction and deepening methods

For smoking withdrawal, we recommend the second approach to hypnosis, described in Chapter 7. The reason for this is that you will want to maximise the impact of your suggestions and posthypnotic suggestions by enhancing the client's expectation of a successful outcome. So you will include the preliminary suggestions described in Chapter 7.

Emphasising the dangers of smoking and the advantages of not smoking

In many approaches during hypnosis, the therapist describes as vividly as possible the dire consequences of continuing to smoke and the great benefits of quitting. The following are some hints for designing a script for an individual client and are based on a 2-hour, single-session approach described by Elliott (1988). Elliott, incidentally, prefers the term 'free breather' to 'non-smoker', as the latter term sounds rather negative.

1. While it is good to include in your script the known consequences of smoking, e.g. a shorter life, poorer health and less stamina, it is considered better to lay more emphasis on what the client has told you are personal reasons for wanting to stop. Often these are more immediate than known health risks such as heart disease or cancer in 30 years' time. Negative consequences for clients may include the stale smell of cigarettes on their breath and clothing, ugly nicotine stains on their fingers and teeth, the drain on their financial resources, which prevents them gaining things that they would really like, and the worry that it causes their family.

2. There is an impression that it is better to be as positive as possible and to emphasise the *benefits* of not smoking rather than the bad effects of smoking. One oft-cited reason for this is that too much anxiety and worry on the client's part can be counter-productive.

3. When describing the consequences of continuing to smoke and of stopping smoking, you should try to be vivid, personal and concrete, appealing to the client's imagination and emotions, and using all sensory modalities. For example, instead of saying, 'As a result of being a non-smoker you will feel healthier, fitter and stronger', say something like this:

Imagine you are on holiday in Corfu, on that lovely beach with little Tommy and Louise. Notice how you have lots of breath and energy to play with the children and race them to the sea. As you are doing this, with each breath you can smell the healthy tang of the sea. You can hear Tommy and Louise laughing and you are thinking how good it is for them that you are fit and healthy and can have lots of fun with them.

Or, if the client enjoys good food, do not simply make the bland statement that from now on the client will be able to appreciate the taste of good food, say, for example:

Now you are eating at Luigi's restaurant with your husband David, having one of your favourite pizzas. Notice how much more tasty and delicious each mouthful is ...

When you give these kinds of very specific and personal suggestions be mindful of two important considerations. First, you have to make absolutely sure (from the personal history you have taken of the client) that all the details in your suggestion are correct. So, in the first example, you must be sure that little Tommy and Louise enjoy playing on the beach. It is likely to seriously weaken the impact of your suggestion if, in reality, they much prefer to go off to the children's activity park than remain with their parents on the beach.

Second, remember what we said in Chapter 10 about how it can be better to help clients find their own ways of creating good feelings, for example excitement, rather than to try hard to 'whip up' the feelings for them. We suggested that going into indirect mode might sometimes help this process. So in the second example, we might instead say:

Now you are eating at Luigi's restaurant with your husband David. ... I wonder if you have chosen something very special on this occasion. And as you are enjoying your meal, can you imagine for yourself how different the food tastes now that you no longer smoke?

Age progression

In the above scripts, you can explicitly progress the client in imagination to a specified date or event. For example:

Now let's go forward in time to around I year from now. You are on your holidays on that beautiful beach in Corfu with Tommy and Louise ... etc.

At some point, you can then introduce this suggestion:

You now bring to mind that it has been a year since you decided to give up smoking. You look back on that year with a sense of pride and achievement. And suddenly you realise something that astonishes you. It is so amazing you find it difficult to believe. In that year, by not smoking, you have now saved ...

Prior to this, you will have calculated how much a year's cigarettes have been costing your client. This is often between £1000 and £2000.

You may also use age progression to identify any problems that may occur as a result of not smoking. Weight gain may be one that the client says has occurred during previous abstention periods. Tension and withdrawal symptoms are others. You can still adopt a positive approach with these, as follows:

As you look back over the year, perhaps you are thinking that there have been times when not smoking hasn't been easy, but you have managed to overcome these problems. If any such difficulties come to mind now, let me know.

You can then review with the client (still in the age-progressed mode) how the client managed to deal with such problems, or you can help the client rehearse ways of coping (see below).

After you have done this work, bring the client back to the original scene of the age progression, reinforcing the idea that the client has been able to handle any such difficulties that have arisen. (You may wish to check with the client how confident he or she feels in doing this.)

Self-control techniques

If clients use cigarettes to cope with everyday tension and stress (or experience these as withdrawal effects), then you can teach them one of the self-control procedures outlined in Chapter 11. A variation of the clenched fist procedure may be particularly appropriate.

Affirmations

Some standard protocols incorporate affirmations that serve to remind clients why they are no longer smoking. Clients repeat these at regular intervals during the day (with or without self-hypnosis), especially when they feel tempted to smoke. Affirmations may also be written on a cue card, which clients carry around and pin up in the home or workplace. For example, Spiegel (1970) teaches the following three affirmations:

For my body smoking is a poison.
I need my body to live.
I owe my body this respect and protection.

There may be something to be said for helping clients choose their own affirmations.

Covert reinforcement

This procedure, described in Chapter 20, may be useful for relapse prevention. Many clients state that they wish to stop smoking for financial reasons, perhaps in order to save up to buy a car. Ask them to picture the desired car in their mind, then follow the directions in Chapter 20, reinforcing the technique with cues, future rehearsal and posthypnotic suggestions. For example, if they have difficulty refusing a cigarette at work, they are to imagine the next time they are there and a colleague proffers a cigarette. They say, 'No thanks', then covertly reinforce the response with, say, an image of collecting the new car from the dealer at some point in the future.

Covert aversion or sensitisation

Aversive methods are not popular these days, but they may have a place. The protocol described in Chapter 20 gives all the necessary details.

Covert rehearsal

As well as covert rehearsal of self-control methods and covert reinforcement, clients are asked to rehearse in imagination everyday situations in which they would normally light up a cigarette, but no longer do so, and that they are feeling the better for it.

Self-hypnosis

Many approaches encourage the client to use self-hypnosis regularly, although Holroyd (1980) in her review did not consider this added to treatment efficacy. It may be useful for the client to use short self-hypnosis routines several times in the day (see Ch. 9) for tension reduction, rehearsal of covert reinforcement and affirmations, and so on.

Hypnosis tape

Especially if you are using a single session approach for immediate cessation, you might consider recording the session for the client's use at home.

Non-hypnotic techniques and ploys for smoking cessation

Some therapists (e.g. Crasilneck 1990) have augmented their approach with a nicotine substitute for smoking – for example, nicotine gum or patches. This should be seen as a 'stepping stone' to complete abstinence. Crasilneck (1990) also advocates the use of a cinnamon stick in the withdrawal period. Sucking a clove could also serve the same purpose. These are preferable to sucking mints, as this is bad for the teeth and may lead to weight gain.

Some practitioners precede the hypnosis session with the technique of 'rapid smoking' in which clients chain-smoke until they experience distaste for the next cigarette. This method can be very unpleasant.

Whatever approach is used, it is always very helpful if clients are able to recruit the assistance of family and friends for their support and understanding, otherwise they may sabotage the clients' best efforts to abstain.

Conclusions

In the meta-analyses presented by Viswesvaran & Schmidt (1992) and Law & Tang (1995), mean abstention rates for hypnosis treatment were 36% and 23% respectively. (The lower figure may represent the use of stricter criteria for inclusion in the analysis.) The previously mentioned problem of the authenticity of the client's self-report should be borne in mind here. The studies reviewed were very mixed in their methodology and many of them incorporated non-hypnotic, cognitive-behavioural methods. This has led

Green & Lynn (2000) to conclude that, so far, there is insufficient evidence that hypnosis itself is an active ingredient in smoking-cessation treatment.

Success rates as low as those quoted above may dissuade some practitioners from including smokers in their caseload. Nevertheless, they compare well with other approaches, and the benefits for every client who does quit, in terms of improvements in health, finance and self-esteem, are immeasurable.

WEIGHT REDUCTION

It does not seem possible for anyone to broach the topic of weight reduction with heartfelt optimism, given the oft-quoted statistic that around 95% or more of all diets fail and even result in an eventual net gain in weight. It is no help that more and more people, children as well as adults, are overweight and obese and that this trend is likely to continue in the years to come, with its attendant health problems. This is a feature of much of the developed Western world, yet within these societies it is not merely a problem of affluence. Indeed, obesity is something that affects poorer people as well. Nor is the problem simply that people are eating more food. It is true that there is an abundance of 'snacking-type' food with a high calorie-to-nutritional-value ratio. It seems, however, that an increasingly underactive lifestyle in which the expenditure of any physical effort at all, even walking to the television set or winding down the car window, is perceived as a problem for technology to solve on behalf of the consumer. It may not fire the enthusiasm of readers to apply their therapeutic skills to the 'battle of the bulge' when collectively we are conspiring to lose it. Perhaps the ultimate answer lies with the experts in medicine, surgery and genetics. But doesn't this mean that responsibility and ownership of yet another chunk of our lives have been taken over by the medical industry? Is there still a place for a philosophy that calls upon professional therapists to join people in their struggle, rather than take the struggle away from them?

In this chapter, we shall present some rules and guidance for a behavioural programme for weight loss and how this may be augmented by hypnosis. We shall observe towards the end of this chapter that we have reason to be confident that hypnosis does enhance the effectiveness of weight-reduction programmes.

General considerations

An effective programme for weight reduction requires that clients reduce their net intake of calories over a time period, the duration of which depends upon the amount of weight to be shed. Thereafter they must maintain their healthy weight by avoiding a calorie intake that leads to weight gain.

The recommended rate of weight loss is no more than about 1 kg (2 lb) per week. Rates above this may be achieved, particularly in the initial stages, but they require considerable effort and will be difficult to sustain, the risk being complete relapse.

This rate of weight loss is achieved by reducing the calorific value of food consumed and accelerating the rate of conversion of calories to energy by increasing activity. To achieve a consistent weight loss at this rate requires some experimentation with diet and exercise, but a general rule is to aim for a net reduction of 500 calories per day. Changes in diet and activity should be planned in such a way as to cause as little hindrance to the person's everyday essential activities, otherwise these new habits will be over-ridden by existing ones.

Healthy eating

Many clients who come for help for weight reduction are already experts in dieting and know by heart the calorific value of common items of food and drink. They may in fact have a preferred plan for weight loss and need your help in adhering to this. Whatever the case, as the therapist you will need your own guidelines on the calorific value of common consumables and what constitutes healthy eating habits. Such information is widely available through clinics, health advisory services, bookshops, the Internet, and so on.

As a rule, the more complicated and restrictive an eating plan is, the more effort it will demand from the client and the more difficult it will be to accommodate into the client's daily life. Hence, the client will be less likely to adhere to it in the long-term. Also, eating plans that involve long lists of prohibited food items create undue anxiety (rather like avoidance behaviour). Moreover, should the client succumb to temptation – for example, eating a prohibited biscuit – a risk is that he or she will be overwhelmed with guilt and self-recrimination, or may decide to 'put the diet on hold' and 'have a fresh start tomorrow'. Either way, the net result is often the consumption of the remaining biscuits in the packet.

It is much more sensible to have some general rules for healthy eating that allow as wide a range of food items as possible, including 'a little of what you fancy'. The person should eat regular meals and not go hungry, since hunger increases the risk that eating will 'go out of control'.

Exercise

Some similar advice pertains to planning an increase in physical activity. There are two areas of daily life to consider. The first is the expenditure of energy in the undertaking of one's routine daily activities. As we stated earlier, the modern trend is to reduce as much as possible the expenditure of any physical effort in everyday life by means of labour-saving and time-saving machinery and gadgetry. Hence, one way of increasing energy expenditure is to forego technology and to revert to older ways of doing things. The most obvious candidate is the activity of walking rather than being passively transported and this includes walking up and down stairs rather than taking a lift or elevator.

The second area of life is leisure time and the regular engagement in some form of exercise such as a sport or games. Certain activities are recommended as especially appropriate for a person who wishes to lose weight. These involve a sustained period (e.g. 20 minutes) of a high level of activity such as brisk walking, running, cycling, swimming or structured aerobic exercises.

Some exercise is easier to accommodate into one's everyday life than other forms; for example, going for a cycle ride, taking a walk or gardening involves less planning and arranging than going to the gymnasium or swimming pool. The easier it is to arrange, the more likely the habit will be maintained. However, to keep up the habit, it is better that it is enjoyable. Different people enjoy different things: for many, the thrills of the exercise bicycle and the jogging machine prove quite elusive and they prefer engaging in such activities in a natural setting, or at least making use of their personal stereos.

It goes without saying that clients who are embarking on a course of exercise after a period of abstaining from such should be advised by their doctor or a suitable specialist. Clients who are grossly overweight face difficulties when planning appropriate exercise and some may have medical problems, such as disabling orthopaedic and rheumatological conditions. They are often caught in a 'Catch 22' bind: their specialist informs them that their condition will only improve (or an operation can only be performed) if they lose weight, but their disability makes weight loss a difficult goal. For them, specialised advice and guidance are important, but the practitioner of hypnosis may play an adjunctive role. Elderly overweight people face similar difficulties. In fact, it may be that as one becomes older, the exercise required for a weight-reduction programme (or simply to maintain a constant weight) increases.

Non-hypnotic techniques and ploys for weight reduction

The following are some of the more important non-hypnotic techniques and ploys that are used in a behavioural programme for weight reduction.

Weighing

The standard advice is that it is not a good idea for clients to be constantly weighing themselves, or conversely, to avoid weighing. Too frequent weighings may result in clients being too controlled by the movements of the needle on the weighing scales, which will rise and fall according to natural fluctuations in weight during the day, week, month, and so on. However, not weighing at all may be construed as avoidance behaviour that may raise the clients' anxiety about their weight. Also, weighing provides feedback about the effectiveness of the clients' weight-loss programme and serves to reward or penalise appropriate or inappropriate behaviour respectively.

It is therefore recommended that clients weigh themselves once a week and always at the same time on the same day, using the same scales.

Some clients value keeping a graph of their progress, plotting weight against date (at weekly intervals). The ideal plot (a linear negative slope representing the agreed rate of weight loss per week, starting with the initial weight) can be drawn on the chart so that clients can check if they are on target.

There is an argument (and maybe some clients will prefer this) for dispensing with weighing altogether on the basis that the sole aim is a healthier lifestyle with good food and exercise, and if this is achieved, body weight will take care of itself.

Eating and exercise records

We shall discuss the use of an eating and exercise diary for assessment purposes in due course. Some weight-reduction programmes advocate the regular logging of all foods eaten and their calorific value, likewise exercise, for the duration of the therapy. Successful programmes for normalising eating patterns in bulimia nervosa have also included monitoring of food intake (e.g. Fairburn 1985). Hence, in severe cases of obesity and overeating, this may be warranted, but otherwise clients may find it an unwelcome chore. The therapist and client should use their collective judgement on how long a time it is useful to monitor food intake and exercise.

Control of availability of food

As with smoking cessation, it is important that people close to clients are recruited to assist them in their aims to lose weight. It helps considerably if the client is supported by people, especially family members, who are themselves committed to a healthy lifestyle. A key person is the one who is most responsible for the availability of food in the home. This may be the client, the client's partner, a parent, and so on. The same may be said of whoever prepares the meals. Not unlike Oscar Wilde, the majority of us find that the most difficult thing to resist is temptation itself. Hence, it is best that clients are able to arrange (on their own initiative or with the assistance of others) that problem foods, such as sweets, chocolates, crisps, biscuits and cakes, are not constantly within easy reach. Unfortunately (for present purposes), the fridge, and even the freezer, ensure that, unlike for much of the history of humankind, foods of all description are constantly accessible. It is helpful if the supply of the aforementioned food items and similar consumables is restricted in the home and that healthy, low-calorie items, such as fresh fruit and vegetables are made more available.

Alternative activities

For clients who engage in periodic episodes of overeating or bingeing, one ploy is to keep a record of when and where these occur and thus identify what might be appropriate triggers. Being in the house alone in the afternoon may be one such situation, or the interval between deciding to retire for the night and going up to the bedroom. The client makes a list of (preferably) pleasurable and easy-to-perform available activities that, if carried out, would make eating difficult or impossible. This is a kind of habit reversal method as described in Chapter 20. Examples are to go for a walk, do some gardening, have a bath, wash one's hair, phone a friend or go to the library. The list is pinned up somewhere within easy view, and whenever the triggers are present, or imminent, the client arranges to fill the time with one or more of these activities.

Miscellaneous ploys

We have not exhausted all the behavioural techniques that therapists employ for a weight-reduction programme. For example, the stimulus control paradigm discussed in Chapter 20 may be brought into play so that the times and places of eating are defined (e.g. sitting on a chair at the dining table at breakfast time). No other activity is permitted in that location and no activity (e.g. reading or watching television) is allowed while eating. It may be difficult for the client to adhere consistently to this regime for any length of time, but components of it (e.g. not doing anything else while eating) may be included.

Our advice is that more serious eating problems, such as actual eating disorders, to be discussed in Chapter 31, may require a wide range of procedures and techniques (as in Fairburn's (1985) cognitive-behavioural therapy programme for bulimia nervosa). However, for problems of excess weight and obesity that are not at the level of an eating disorder, the rule may be only to make the programme as complex as it need be.

Psychotherapy to address more general psychological problems

Unlike most smokers, it is not unusual for clients seeking to lose weight to experience associated psychological problems such as low self-esteem, lack of confidence with others, relationship and sexual problems, and more general anxiety and low mood, that may have to be addressed in therapy. Some of these problems may result from their being overweight, but some may be present anyway, and underlie the eating difficulties. These problems may be addressed within a broader programme of psychotherapy.

Assessment

You will, of course, initially ascertain that clients are indeed overweight (by reference to standard tables) and if such is not the case, decline to offer therapy (or offer to help clients with any problems they may be manifesting, say with their body image).

You will conduct an assessment of patients in general terms, including their mental state, with particular reference to mood, anxiety, current stresses, and self-confidence and self-esteem. You may augment this assessment with formal questionnaire measures (see Ch. 25), which you may repeat at intervals, including at follow-up appointments, since your clients' emotional well-being and contentment with life are important outcomes of your therapy.

You will then concentrate on assessing the presenting problem, its history, the reasons for it, the impact on the clients' life, reasons why clients want to lose weight, how they believe that their life will change as a result, reasons for the difficulties in achieving this, the attitudes of significant others (notably the spouse, whom it will be useful to involve in therapy at some stage), history of attempts to lose weight, and so on. You will also want to know the significant aspects of the medical history. If you are not medically qualified, or have any doubts or concerns about any possible adverse impact of a weight-reduction programme on a client's health, the client's GP should be only too pleased to advise. This is especially so if the client has a medical condition that has dietary implications, in which case a medical dietician will probably be able to offer guidance.

In the weeks approaching the first appointment, and in the weeks following it, it is helpful for clients to keep a diary of all food and drink taken (with an indication as to quantity), when and where, accompanying persons, and any other relevant information (such as mood and anxiety level). Exercise (formal and informal) may also be included. Some clients will be experts at calorie counting and will be able to compute their calorie consumption with ease. Whatever the case, you will need to calculate your client's average daily and weekly calorie consumption. As was earlier stated, if the client's weight is stable, then it is recommended that the client aims to reduce net calorie intake by 500 per day by attention to eating and exercise. It may take you and the client some weeks of experimentation to establish a set of rules for eating and exercise that achieve the recommended rate of weight loss. We discussed earlier the issue of the length of time a client should maintain the eating and exercise log.

How many sessions you plan for and how you distribute the sessions (and follow-ups) are decided by a combination of many factors and need to be negotiated between you and your client.

At some point, you will need to decide on the goals of treatment. The ideal goal will be something such as 'For the client to achieve and maintain the recommended body weight in ways that are consistent with a healthy lifestyle, both physically and psychologically'. However, we have to accept the fact that for people who are significantly overweight or technically obese, the accomplishment of this aim is very much the exception than the rule, so much so that you and your client may need to think of a more realistic aim. Also bear in mind that the above goal will be months or (allowing for relapses and periods of no progress) years ahead for some clients. Accordingly, it is advisable that you and your client agree on a goal for weight loss that you both feel is realistic and achievable within an estimated time-scale. For example, for an obese client with mobility problems and weighing 140 kg (22 stone), you may decide that 127 kg (20 stone) is a realistic target over a period of 25 weeks. This may not be the final goal. Should the client be on or close to target at the end of this period, you may negotiate the next phase of therapy with a new goal and time period in mind. One possibility is that the client at that stage feels confident to proceed alone for the time being and will report back on an agreed date (or after an appropriate time interval).

Hypnotic procedures in a weight-reduction programme

These procedures should be perceived as augmenting a programme for weight reduction. Hence, you will already have put together a treatment programme that incorporates some or all of the behavioural procedures discussed earlier. Some of the procedures discussed for smoking cessation also lend themselves well to present purposes.

Basic procedure

The most basic way of augmenting a programme of weight reduction with hypnosis is to use hypnotic induction and deepening methods and then to remind clients of the benefits of losing weight and take them through all the instructions for following the programme. You will, however, wish to elaborate on this approach, and the following are recommendations for doing so.

Induction and deepening approach

As with smoking cessation, we advocate the second approach to hypnosis outlined in Chapter 7 that emphasises suggestibility. Although there is reason to believe that hypnotic susceptibility itself is not a reliable predictor of outcome, convincing clients that they are responsive subjects may facilitate therapy. Accordingly we do not consider that there are good clinical reasons for assessing hypnotic susceptibility using standard scales.

Imagining the personal benefits of healthy eating and exercise

All the advice that we gave concerning the use of this method for smoking cessation applies here. It is important to personalise the script and to draw upon the client's capacity for imagery in all modalities.

Affirmations

As with smokers, the client may regularly rehearse suitable affirmations, either during self-hypnosis or otherwise (particularly when tempted to overindulge). The affirmations may be constructed by the client with the assistance of the therapist. Some therapists use standard affirmations. For example, Spiegel & Spiegel (1987) recommend the following:

For my body over-eating is a poison.
I need my body to live.
I owe my body this respect and attention.

Age progression

Here you help clients to choose an image or images that signify that they have attained their goal (either their recommended weight, or the weight that has been targeted). This may simply be 'stepping on your weighing scales and seeing the reading at 101 kg (16 stones)'. However, it could be a reward that the client has planned and that may or may not be directly weight-related. An example may be wearing a new outfit. One woman chose a visit to the opera; she estimated that on achieving her target weight, she could at long last be accommodated in reasonable comfort in a theatre seat. Age progression may also be used to anticipate problems and how they may be resolved. (See the section on age progression for smoking cessation – p. 301.)

Self-hypnosis and self-control techniques

Self-hypnosis and self-control techniques, as described in Chapters 9 and 12, may be used by those clients for whom eating is a way of coping with tension, or who are generally anxious. It may be used to rehearse the benefits of adhering to a healthy eating and exercise plan, and so on. Some clients will value an audiotape of this routine.

Covert reinforcement

As with smoking, clients may use a positive image of the consequences of successfully attaining their target weight as a covert reward for appropriate behaviour (e.g. refusing a cream cake at lunchtime). The image may be anchored and the procedure rehearsed and augmented with posthypnotic suggestions in the usual way (Ch. 20).

Metaphor

There may be very apposite metaphorical stories that one may incorporate into a session of hypnosis. In Chapter 13, we described the metaphor of a journey that is particularly symbolic for patients striving to reduce their excess weight.

Ego-strengthening

The ego-strengthening routine should be tailored to the client's needs and aspirations and address concerns relating, for example, to self-esteem, appearance, undue self-consciousness, being in control (of eating) and expectations of a successful outcome.

Active–alert methods

This approach can be used by clients who have an exercise bicycle or rowing or jogging machine. The therapist prepares an audiotape with an alert induction and alert imagery and fantasy (Ch. 10). An appropriate one for an exercise bicycle would be riding through the countryside, feeling healthy and full of energy and power, enjoying the beautiful scenery, breathing in the clean, invigorating country air, and so on. Suggestions and imagery relating to healthy eating and exercise and the benefits to be gained, ego-strengthening, and future images of success, may then be given.

Psychodynamic methods

Some clients readily admit that their being overweight arises from more deep-seated, emotional problems. Others may not make any such connection, but give one the impression that the problem is not simply one of acquiring new habits. For example, not uncommonly, a client with a chronic weight problem and a history of constant, unsuccessful dieting, will say, 'I always manage to get down to 75 kg (12 stone) and then I start to panic and put it all back on again'. These clients may describe a feeling of 'being vulnerable' when they reach a certain stage in their weight-loss programme, their large size and shape seeming to offer some protection from difficult conflicts or emotions. Perhaps also they start to notice problems in their relationship with their partner at that point; this may well indicate that partners may have their own problems.

Where you, and perhaps also your client, suspect that this may be the case, do not immediately dive in with psychodynamic techniques such as IMR signalling or age regression. Establish the behavioural plan for your client and see how things proceed. If there are some underlying emotional problems the client may not lose weight at all, or the client will begin to lose weight and this, metaphorically speaking, will bring any emotional problems nearer to the surface where they may be easier to address than at the outset of therapy. Two methods of doing this can be particularly productive.

The first method is age progression to when the client is at the recommended weight or target weight, or the weight at which relapses tend to recur. One can then explore with the client what is happening to cause any feelings of anxiety or vulnerability. One way is (perhaps using IMR signals) to use 'parts' or ego-state therapy. For example, the therapist can ask for a signal to the question, 'Is there any part of Mary that is anxious or has any difficulty coping with this?' If a 'Yes' signal is given, then one can proceed with 'Can I speak with that part?' and then encourage the patient to explore what problems there may be. One may also encourage a dialogue between say, 'the part that is panicky' and 'the part that wants to lose weight', asking the client to 'be each part' in turn. Outside of hypnosis, one could use the gestalt technique of the 'empty chair' (Ch. 16).

When using such techniques, always emphasise that you are speaking metaphorically rather than literally. For example, you may say, 'It's as though part of you wants to lose weight and part of you is afraid of this. Let's imagine that I am now talking to the part of you that is afraid. Can you be that part now?'

Material elicited in this way may relate to earlier life experiences. (One might elicit if this is so by asking 'the part that panics', 'How old is this part?') Accordingly age regression, say by using the elicited affect as a bridge to a significant memory, may then be undertaken.

The second, similar, approach may be used when the client reports that there has been a session of comfort eating or bingeing since the last appointment. The client can be asked to relive the experience, and 'parts' therapy and regression work may be undertaken as above, to help resolve whatever conflicts are emerging.

Sometimes these difficulties are more in the here and now, say in the client's current relationship, in which case regression work may not be immediately helpful.

Group work

Except for the kind of individual psychodynamic work just outlined, the hypnotic procedures described above may be adapted and incorporated into a group treatment approach to weight loss.

Follow-up and support

Once you and your client have decided that you have come to the end of your core treatment (at least for the time being), then it is advisable to agree on some kind of follow-up appointment (which may signal a further course of therapy). You may do this formally by specifying a date (e.g. in 3 or 6 months' time) or leaving it to the client to contact you at an appropriate time, in which case it is a good idea to inform the client that you will be in touch if you do not hear from him or her within a certain time. It is always useful for you to have feedback about how your clients fare in the long-term.

Conclusions

Our impression is that seeing clients for weight reduction is not a favourite clinical activity of many practitioners of hypnosis, and not infrequently we hear colleagues lament that 'they (i.e. the clients) want magic'. Certainly it is hard not to feel that with such clients one is 'up against it' ('it' probably referring to life itself). It may also be that some practitioners do not want to appear tarred by the same brush as the huge and notorious slimming industry, an industry that takes proportionately far more than it gives. Little wonder that some overweight people find the whole enterprise devaluing and demeaning, declaring that they have had enough of it and are reclaiming their identity as one for which body weight is an irrelevance. Readers will no doubt have their own opinion on the matter.

In Chapter 22, we said that the aim of therapy may be construed as helping clients and patients have more choices. One grossly overweight and out-of-work patient described what a miserable time she had had in previous jobs because of the offensive remarks of customers. She was desperate to lose weight. After several weeks of counselling (by MH), she came to her appointment excited and smiling. She had lost not one ounce, but had taken the plunge and enrolled for a training course in a new career. She had gone to a party for the new intake of trainees and felt totally accepted for who she was. She said that she did not feel that her weight was something she needed to be focusing on, at least for the time being.

Was this success or failure? Therapy is only the art of the possible, and that might mean settling for an option that is less than the ideal. At least the above patient was able to have the choice 'I can be overweight and contented'.

As with smoking cessation, we do not wish to underestimate the difficulties that face the therapist and client in successfully achieving the agreed goals. The research literature appears to indicate that augmenting cognitive-behavioural therapy for weight reduction with hypnosis significantly enhances outcome. Some authorities (e.g. Kirsch 1996) believe that the reason for this is that hypnosis enhances the expectation of a successful response to treatment on the part of the client. This may be so, but we would like to feel that the procedures that we have outlined in themselves actively enhance the likelihood of a successful outcome.

INSOMNIA

Hypnosis and relaxation procedures are of proven benefit for insomnia. In this chapter, we mainly have in mind sleep-onset insomnia, but some patients complain of a failure to maintain sleep; that is, they wake up during the night and are unable to return to sleep. The methods described here may be applied to that problem. Of less concern here is early morning wakening associated with depression. However, one may target sleep as a component of a treatment programme in say, general anxiety disorder, depression or stress. Nightmares will be discussed in Chapter 30.

General considerations

It is always important for the therapist to decide if it is better to view sleep impairment as a symptom of more general problems, and, if so, the focus of therapy will be on helping patients cope with their daytime problems. For example, patients may lie awake at night worrying about their work performance, their self-image, aspects of their life which cause anger, and so on. It may also be that patients are unduly stressed during the day, work long hours and do not take enough breaks. It is therefore important that the therapist's assessment is thorough enough to enable the drawing-up of the most appropriate plan of therapy, which may or may not include specific attention to sleep.

Defining insomnia

Parkes (1985) gives an average number of hours of sleep as 16 out of 24 for neonates, 8 for 12-year-olds, 7 for adults and 6 in old age. However, people vary in the amount of sleep that they require, and duration of sleep may be influenced by habit so that, for example, people may find that they manage on less sleep after an imposed period of reduction in sleeping time. According to Horne (1992) over several days, healthy adults may adapt without difficulty to up to 2 hours' less sleep.

Complainers of sleep-onset insomnia habitually overestimate the time they take to fall asleep (Franklin 1981). In a study by Stepanski et al (1988), the total monitored night-time sleep in patients complaining of insomnia was 364 minutes, compared with 419 minutes for people not complaining of insomnia. Therefore, many of the people complaining of insomnia may still have sufficient sleep. Moreover, daytime EEG monitoring revealed that sleepiness in the complainers was no higher than in the non-complainers. However, complainers of insomnia usually report feeling drained and fatigued during the day, and rather than loss of sleep, this may involve anxiety and depression (which may include anxiety about not sleeping sufficiently).

Hence, insomniacs may underestimate the time they are asleep. (This is something that nurses on night shifts often notice with patients who complain that they are having little sleep.) Nevertheless, it is possible that sleep quality is poorer in complainers of insomnia, with more periods of restlessness and troubled dreams.

Whatever the case, psychological factors such as stress, anxiety and tension appear to be inextricably linked with complaints of poor sleep. According to Horne (1992), psychological factors play some role in as many as 80% of all insomnia cases.

Circadian and ultradian rhythms

During a period of sleep, there are several stages that occur in periodic fashion and are distinguished by various physiological changes, including EEG pattern. The main cycle is the change from non-REM to REM sleep and back that occurs several times in the night with the REM periods becoming longer. REM stands for 'rapid eye movements', lateral movements of the eyes that accompany dreaming. Non-REM sleep is also broken down into stages 1 to 4. As one ages, stages 3 and 4 gradually fade.

There are in fact more than 100 biological functions that have been found to have maximum and minimum values over a 24-hour period. The sleep–wake cycle is normally 24 hours, but with no environmental cues it changes to a 25-hour cycle. The REM–non-REM cycle is another, and may be related to a general basic-rest–activity cycle (BRAC) which is associated with a range of physiological, cognitive and behavioural changes. So it may be important for times of retiring to bed and rising to coincide with these cycles, with sleep being easier at the onset of the next phase of rest.

Cycles are disrupted or over-ridden by stress and concentrated activity. Major depression is associated with the earlier appearance of REM sleep, and some antidepressants severely reduce REM sleep, which then rebounds on withdrawal of medication (Parkes 1985).

Sleep deprivation

Psychological and physical effects of sleep restriction and deprivation have been widely studied. Generally, the effects on performance of a night without sleep are greatest the following afternoon and evening, and slightly greater in older people. There is a slight depressant effect, but paradoxically, patients with major depression may experience a transient antidepressant effect after a total night's sleep deprivation.

General advice for insomnia

People who seek treatment for insomnia are usually well appraised of the rules and ploys for maximising the likelihood of a good night's sleep.

Obvious requirements are a comfortable bed and a dark, quiet environment that is neither cold nor overly stuffy. Avoidance of any central nervous system stimulants in the hours before retiring is commonly advised, with tea and coffee particularly in mind. On the other hand, it is considered that a warm milky drink may be of benefit. Alcohol may facilitate sleep onset but cause waking later in the night, so is not usually advised. Poor sleepers sleep even more poorly if the period immediately prior to retiring is spent studying. Conversely, many people find that light reading or an easy-to-watch television programme is of assistance (see Horne 1992, Parkes 1985). However, we shall see that the stimulus control method specifically proscribes any activity other than sleep in the bedroom. A heavy meal, taken soon before retiring, or vigorous exercise, is not recommended. There is an idea, however, that regular exercise does promote good sleep. It may be the case that this is more to do with establishing a regular, healthy routine of work, rest, play and eating. Too restrictive a diet and hunger exacerbate insomnia.

If possible, times of retiring to bed and rising in the morning should be fixed, although lie-ins are fine at weekends and during holiday breaks. Daily naps are not precluded although it is better that these are taken at a fixed time of the day. Around 20 minutes should not pose a problem. However, in the initial stages of treating insomnia, it is a good idea to prohibit napping until the sleeping pattern has been restored. We are aware of a recommendation that a nap should not extend into dream sleep, on the grounds that this will interfere with night-time sleep, but we have not located any supporting evidence.

There are special recommendations for people whose employment requires a shift rota. We will not be covering these here.

Many patients will be taking night-time sedation and may have done so for some considerable time, maybe months and even years. Nowadays, however, doctors are much more reluctant to allow repeat prescriptions of sleeping tablets, except perhaps in the elderly. Sleeping tablets can be helpful for short-term insomnia (up to 4 weeks). Thereafter, patients find that when they try to do without them, the insomnia returns, sometimes with a vengeance. It is difficult for many patients to go 'cold turkey', so a period of gradual withdrawal, in tandem with a psychological approach, is recommended. Some doctors consider that the withdrawal of medication may be facilitated by substituting the existing prescription with a longer-acting tranquilliser such as diazepam.

Assessment

As with other problems such as pain and psychosomatic disorders, a general assessment of mental states augmented by one or more of the scales recommended in Chapter 25, can be very informative.

Assessment of insomnia itself may be augmented by a sleep questionnaire such as that described by Monroe (1967). It may be useful to ask patients to keep a sleep diary that records times of retiring, use of night sedation, how long it took to get off to sleep, the restfulness of sleep, how many times they woke up in the night and what they did, time of waking up in the morning, time of rising, energy during the day, and so on.

Psychological treatments for insomnia

Three main psychological approaches for alleviating insomnia have been investigated by well-conducted clinical trials that have incorporated plausible placebo controls. These approaches are stimulus control, paradoxical intention, and relaxation (including hypnosis). All appear equally effective, although relaxation methods may yield subjective ratings of more restful sleep (Espie et al 1989, Turner & Ascher 1979). It is important to remember that all three methods involve the gradual breaking down of the habit of lying awake, and the re-installation of a regular sleeping pattern. This can only take place over a period of time. You must explain this to patients, particularly if they say, 'Oh! I tried that method once and it didn't work'.

The stimulus control method

Patients are instructed to go to bed only when sleepy and not to attempt to obtain more sleep by retiring early. They must not read, watch television or eat in bed. (We have yet to discover whether any prohibition is recommended on the remaining popular activity that normally takes place in bed.) If patients are unable to fall asleep after 10 minutes, they must get up immediately, do something else, and return to bed when sleepy. They must set the alarm clock and get up at the same time every morning, irrespective of how much sleep was obtained during the night. There must be no napping during the day.

In our experience, many patients find this method difficult. It is true that patients, if they have been awake for a long time, often do get up, say to have a cup of tea, but many find the prospect of having to keep getting up to a dark and lonely house too difficult to contemplate. Also some patients protest that it disturbs their partner.

Paradoxical intention

The instruction here is simply to deliberately lie in bed awake with the eyes open as long as possible. Again, retiring and rising times are fixed and no napping is permitted during the day.

Relaxation and self-hypnosis

The simplest approach is to teach the patient a series of relaxation techniques for the purposes of self-hypnosis, as described in Chapter 6 (i.e. the first approach to hypnosis) and Chapter 9. It is appropriate that that last one in the series involves imagery, for example, the 'safe place' technique. The patient practises this method and uses it on going to bed. Some patients like to have it on tape, provided that they have a machine that switches itself off, or a partner who is able to do this.

Most people with insomnia complain that what keeps them awake is their overactive mind, which 'churns over' things that have happened during the day, often of trivial significance. Spiegel & Spiegel (1987) have devised a method that is designed to help people with this particular problem, although it does require a good capacity for imagery. There are a number of versions of this method, but they all involve projecting one's thoughts in the form of images, or possibly even words, onto an imaginary screen. As the thoughts collect on the screen, one can then imagine those that are unwanted drifting off to the left, out of view. Either one just focuses on the ones that are remaining, or before doing so, one can imagine them separating off to the right.

Adjusting times of retiring and rising

An extra ploy to consider in any psychological approach is to ask the patient to retire later than usual (say 30 minutes to 1 hour) and get up a little earlier (say 30 minutes) before normal waking time. Again no napping is allowed. If a patient is able to do this, it may help in shifting the natural rest–activity cycle so that the time of going to bed coincides with the rest phase. In more simple terms, it may ensure that the patient is more tired on retiring. Once adequate sleep is restored, the patient may gradually resume the preferred times for retiring and rising.

Case example

Leila was a young woman in her 20s who had post-traumatic stress after a car accident 18 months prior to the start of her therapy. She had three problems – anxiety about travelling by car, uncontrollable outbursts of temper and sleep-onset insomnia. Fortunately, she was working. She would retire to bed at 11 p.m. but she would remain wide-awake and vigilant to 3 a.m. and then sleep through until 7 a.m. On waking, she would 'catnap' as long as she was able without being late for work. This was to around 7.35 a.m.

The prescription for her insomnia was as follows. It was agreed that she would continue to retire to bed at 11 p.m. as that was when her partner also retired but to rise at 7 a.m., thus eliminating the 35 minutes of catnapping. She was given the instructions to deliberately remain awake until 3 a.m. but to practise a method of relaxation. She was also instructed to count down in threes from a high number (say 1000). Each count was to occur on the outward breath and she was to visualise the number as well as hear it spoken in her head. This is a very useful ploy when one is using the paradoxical intention method for insomnia, since it helps to distract the person from worrying thoughts. (One chooses a counting task that sufficiently occupies the attention of patients, while not imposing any undue stress on them, as some people have an aversion to arithmetic.)

(continued)

Case example (*continued*)

As usual, she was advised not to nap during the day. After 1 week, there was a significant improvement and her sleep was normal after 2 weeks.

This patient's anxiety about travelling by car responded well to eye movement desensitisation and reprocessing (EMDR), a method that has now become popular for treating post-traumatic stress (see Ch. 30). The temper tantrums were not a focus of therapy because they resolved themselves when the patient realised that her anger preceded her accident and was much to do with her relationship with her father. She was able to sort this out herself.

Conclusions

One can use relaxation and self-hypnosis for insomnia in the knowledge that they are of proven value, and your patient stands a good chance of significantly benefiting (Anderson et al 1979, Becker 1993, Stanton 1989). However, insomnia is not always an easy problem to treat. The most difficult patients to help are those who, through their being unemployed and perhaps single, fall into the habit of lying in bed until the latter part of the morning and beyond, have little daily routine activity, and retire to bed in the early hours of the morning, only to lie awake for a further few hours. For them the omission of a whole night's sleep followed by a return to normal hours of retiring and rising (with no napping in the interim period) may be one answer. Insomnia in the elderly is also a difficult problem and is complicated by physical problems, life circumstances such as bereavement and loneliness, lack of stimulation, irregular sleeping habits, and so on.

Whatever the case, if one can help people to feel more relaxed in bed, to worry less about 'the need for a good night's sleep' and perhaps to think about how to be less anxious about aspects of their day-to-day life, then one has achieved something of undoubted value.

REFERENCES

SMOKING CESSATION
Ahijevych K, Yerardi R, Nedilsky N 2000 Descriptive outcomes of the American Lung Association of Ohio hypnotherapy smoking cessation program. International Journal of Clinical and Experimental Hypnosis 48: 374–387

American Psychiatric Association 1994 Diagnostic and statistical manual of mental disorders, 4th edn. American Psychiatric Association, Washington DC

Crasilneck H B 1990 Hypnotic techniques for smoking and psychogenic impotence. American Journal of Clinical Hypnosis 32: 147–153

Elliott J 1988 Hypnotherapy for compulsive smokers. Hypnos: Swedish Journal for Hypnosis in Psychotherapy and Psychosomatic Disorders 15: 87–92

Green J P, Lynn S J 2000 Hypnosis and suggestion-based approaches to smoking cessation: An examination of the evidence. International Journal of Clinical and Experimental Hypnosis 48: 195–224

Holroyd J 1980 Hypnosis treatment for smoking: An evaluative review. International Journal of Clinical and Experimental Hypnosis 28: 341–357

Ibbotson G, Williamson A 1998 Smoke free and no buts! Crown House Publishing, Carmarthen

Law M, Tang J L 1995 An analysis of the effectiveness of interventions intended to help people stop smoking. Archives of Internal Medicine 155: 1933–1941

Spiegel H S 1970 A single-session method to stop smoking using ancillary self-hypnosis. International Journal of Clinical and Experimental Hypnosis 18: 235–250

Viswesvaran C, Schmidt F 1992 A meta-analytic comparison of the effectiveness of smoking cessation methods. Journal of Applied Psychology 77: 554–561

Additional papers
The following are individual, single-session approaches:

Stanton H E 1978 A single-session approach modifying smoking behavior. International Journal of Clinical and Experimental Hypnosis 26: 22–29

Wester W C, Robinson J A 1991 Hypnotic techniques for smoking cessation: A personalised approach. Hypnos: Swedish Journal for Hypnosis in Psychotherapy and Psychosomatic Disorders 18: 98–106

The following is an individual, multi-session approach:

Watkins H H 1975 Hypnosis and smoking: A five-session approach. International Journal of Clinical and Experimental Hypnosis 26: 381–390

The following is a group, single-session approach:

Neufeld V, Lynn S J 1988 A single-session group self-hypnosis smoking cessation treatment. International Journal of Clinical and Experimental Hypnosis 36: 75–89

The following is a group, two-session approach:

Lynn S J, Neufield V, Rhue J et al 1993 Hypnosis and smoking cessation: A cognitive-behavioral treatment. In: Rhue J W, Lynn S J, Kirsch I (eds) Handbook of clinical hypnosis. American Psychological Association, Washington DC, ch 26, p 555

WEIGHT REDUCTION
Fairburn C G 1985 Cognitive-behavioural treatment for bulimia. In: Garner D M, Garfinkel P E (eds) Handbook of psychotherapy for anorexia nervosa and bulimia. Guilford Press, New York, ch 8

Kirsch I 1996 Hypnosis in psychotherapy: Efficacy and mechanisms. Contemporary Hypnosis 13: 109–114

Spiegel H S, Spiegel D 1987 Trance and treatment. Basic Books, New York

Additional papers
Cochrane G J 1987 Hypnotherapy in weight-loss treatment: Case illustrations. American Journal of Clinical Hypnosis 30: 20–27

Cochrane G 1992 Hypnosis and weight reduction: Which is the cart and which is the horse? American Journal of Clinical Hypnosis 35: 109–118

Cochrane G J, Friesen J 1986 Hypnotherapy in weight loss. Journal of Counselling and Clinical Psychology 54: 489–492

Levitt E E 1993 Hypnosis in the treatment of obesity. In: Rhue J W, Lynn S J, Kirsch I (eds) Handbook of clinical hypnosis. American Psychological Association, Washington DC, ch 25, p 533

Stanton H E 1976 Fee paying and weight loss: Evidence for an interesting interaction. American Journal of Clinical Hypnosis 19: 47–49

Vanderlinden J, Vandereycken W 1994 The (limited) possibilities of hypnotherapy in the treatment of obesity. American Journal of Clinical Hypnosis 36: 248–257

INSOMNIA
Anderson J A D, Dalton E R, Basker M A 1979 Insomnia and hypnotherapy. Journal of the Royal Society of Medicine 72: 734–739

Becker P M 1993 Chronic insomnia: Outcome of hypnotherapeutic intervention in six cases. American Journal of Clinical Hypnosis 36: 98–105

Espie C, Lindsay W R, Brooks D N et al 1989 A controlled comparative investigation of psychological treatments for chronic sleep-onset insomnia. Behaviour Research and Therapy 27: 79–88

Franklin J 1981 The measurement of sleep-onset insomnia. Behaviour Research and Therapy 19: 547–549

Horne J 1992 Insomnia. The Psychologist 5: 216–218

Monroe L J 1967 Psychological and physiological differences between good and poor sleepers. Journal of Abnormal Psychology 72: 225–264

Parkes J D 1985 Sleep and its disorders. Saunders, London

Spiegel H S, Spiegel D 1987 Trance and treatment. Basic Books, New York

Stanton H E 1989 Hypnotic relaxation and insomnia: A simple solution? Hypnos: Swedish Journal for Hypnosis in Psychotherapy and Psychosomatic Disorders 16: 98–103

Stepanski E, Zoric F, Roehrs T et al 1988 Daytime alertness in patients with chronic insomnia compared with asymptomatic control patients. Sleep 11: 54–60

Turner R M, Ascher L M 1979 Controlled comparison of progressive relaxation, stimulus control and paradoxical intention therapies for insomnia. Journal of Consulting and Clinical Psychology 47: 500–508

Hypnosis in the treatment of psychosomatic problems

Chapter contents

INTRODUCTION

In this chapter, we illustrate how hypnotherapeutic procedures may be used in the alleviation of psychosomatic complaints. By this term, we mean those conditions which have a primarily somatic presentation but which may be triggered or exacerbated by psychological factors, notably psychosocial stress. We shall limit our presentation to those disorders that are comparatively well represented in the clinical hypnosis literature. We should also remind readers that for many of these conditions there exists a literature on other psychological treatments such as cognitive-behavioural interventions. A good reference book for these is Baum et al (1997).

GENERAL CONSIDERATIONS

There is reasonable support for the efficacy of hypnotherapeutic procedures for these kinds of conditions in the form of clinical trials. We shall summarise some of this evidence in Chapter 33. There is also evidence that hypnosis is an active therapeutic ingredient and that hypnotic susceptibility may be related to outcome. Despite this, it is better to avoid the idea that one is 'curing' the patient. Some patients do indeed appear to be completely symptom-free after treatment, but it is best to speak of 'alleviating the symptoms' or 'coping with the problem', rather than 'curing the illness'.

General and specific effects of treatment

The therapist should always be aware of the likelihood that there are important non-specific effects in any treatment for these disorders. This is probably the reason why there appears to be such a multitude of treatments available for psychosomatic problems. (Many of these treatments come under the heading of 'alternative medicine' and have no rational basis.) It is therefore important for the therapist to capitalise on this by ensuring the presence of good rapport and instilling a sense of hope and confidence on the patient's part. The best doctors obtain a good placebo response, but not *only* a placebo response.

Most of the problems that we are referring to are associated in some way with the activity of the autonomic nervous system, and hypnotic suggestions and imagery may affect this at a general level. Hence, the methods that we shall present emphasise relaxation and coping with stress and tension. This requires the regular practice of self-hypnosis or some other self-control technique.

Is there anything more that hypnosis adds to the psychological treatment of these disorders? It is asserted, with some evidence, that in addition to non-specific effects such as placebo and the more general effects of relaxation and stress control, hypnotic suggestions and imagery may target the functioning of the particular system or part of the body that is associated with the disorder. These include blood flow (Barabasz & McGeorge 1978, Dikel & Olness 1980) and gastro-intestinal activity (Eichhorn & Tracktir 1955, Klein & Spiegel 1989, Whorwell et al 1992), and those who treat asthma with hypnosis assert that hypnotic suggestion may specifically alter bronchial reactivity (Ben-Zvi et al 1982, Isenberg et al 1992). Another obvious one is salivation.

These claims raise the question as to how specifically one can target a physiological process with a hypnotic suggestion. We shall not linger on this question but, as a taster, refer to some work by Olness et al (1989). These investigators found that children could increase salivary levels of immunoglobulin A by self-suggestion and imagery, to a greater degree than a relaxation control group and an untrained group. The reader may also be reminded of visualisation techniques in the treatment of cancer.

Whatever the case, underlying many of the methods presented in this chapter is the assumption that in addition to the general effects of relaxation and ego-strengthening, there is the specific effect of suggestion on the functioning of the organ or system concerned.

Assessment procedures

Patients whom you are seeing will (and, if not, should) have already been given a thorough medical examination and their medical status will be monitored in the usual way. It is a good idea, however, to undertake your own form of assessment, which you can refer to as you observe progress and evaluate the final outcome of treatment. We recommend two forms of assessment.

The first form is a general assessment of the patient's mental state, particularly with reference to mood and anxiety level. At the very least, you could do some simple scales (say a rating of mood from 0 to 10, likewise anxiety level), but there are available simple questionnaire methods that yield reliable scores, such as the Hospital Anxiety and Depression (HAD) Scale (Snaith & Zigmond 1983) and the Beck Depression Inventory (BDI) (Beck 1988). Psychologists may use an instrument such as the General Health Questionnaire (GHQ) (Goldberg 1978) or the Symptom Checklist (SCL-90-R; Derogatis 1983), which yields scores on a range of scales as well as overall scores of psychological stress. This assessment will allow you to decide if there are significant psychological problems that need to be addressed and would otherwise compromise your treatment. Generally speaking, a moderate degree of psychological symptomatology does not contraindicate the kind of symptom-oriented approach that we are advocating here, and some of this may well be secondary to the patient's psychosomatic problem. However, the presence of significant levels of clinical anxiety or mood disturbance may jeopardise your treatment. In that case, you need to decide if it is not better to move the focus of your therapy to address these problems, to refer the patient to a psychiatrist or clinical psychologist for treatment, or to consider prescribing anxiolytic or antidepressant medication and observing the patient's response to this before embarking on treating the patient's psychosomatic symptoms.

Second, we recommend that you devise some form of assessing and monitoring the patient's symptoms. Some years ago, the authors ran a small clinic for psychosomatic problems (Heap et al 1994) and we devised a means of monitoring symptoms associated with a range of disorders. This consisted of three 8-point scales ranging from 0 to 7. Patients rated at the end of the day how severe their symptoms had been, how frequently they had occurred, and how troubled they had been by them. The patients also recorded the use of medication and added any comments, such as the occurrence of any stress that day. Sometimes, during the night, patients would be symptom-free, but if this was not the case, then the form allowed patients to give ratings of how they had been during the night.

Such a form can be kept by the patient's bedside and only takes a few seconds to complete each time. Patients can be very absentminded when they are asked to complete records like this, but our experience was that this procedure presented few problems relating to patient cooperation.

This kind of form is not appropriate for many problems that we are discussing, so therapists will have to adapt it to suit the particular condition being treated. The advantage of an assessment and monitoring procedure that is adaptable to a range of problems is that it enables therapists to prepare audit data on the outcome of treatment for psychosomatic problems generally in their clinic.

The more general assessment of mood and anxiety need only be done at the first session, at the end of the main phase of treatment, and at follow-ups. The symptom record form is filled in continuously during treatment and for a period, decided by the therapist and patient, in the follow-up phase.

Assessing the patients' general mental state and asking them to record to what extent their symptoms bother them are important because they allow for one frequently observed outcome of treatment. One major problem is not so much the severity of the symptoms but how patients cope with them and are affected by them in their daily life. Patients can become very preoccupied and worried by their symptoms and may fear the worst, such as that they are developing cancer or some other life-threatening disease. Sometimes the symptoms may unnecessarily disable the patient. For example, although many patients with irritable bowel syndrome manage to continue with their everyday life in the normal way, others become so preoccupied by the symptoms and so worried, say about not having immediate access to a toilet, that they have to give up valued activities, even their employment. They may also become very dependent on their spouses and other members of their family. At the end of treatment, it may be evident that there has been little change in patients' actual symptoms, but they may report feeling less worried about them and less disabled by them. This constitutes a good outcome of therapy.

Should one formally assess hypnotic susceptibility? As we have already said, there is evidence of a relationship between susceptibility and outcome in those conditions that have a somatic component (Wadden & Anderton 1982) but the relationship is perhaps not strong enough to warrant the use of a scale of susceptibility as a screening device in normal practice. (Wickramasekera (1993), in his treatment of somatisation disorder, assesses, amongst other attributes, hypnotic susceptibility as a means of determining treatment, which may involve hypnosis or biofeedback. We have also remarked (see Ch. 3) that in some states of the USA, the use of hypnosis may have certain legal consequences and the measurement of hypnotic susceptibility may be justified on these grounds.)

These considerations aside, we have found that the Creative Imagination Scale (see Ch. 3) is a useful preliminary in the hypnotic treatment of these problems. It is a non-threatening introduction to hypnosis and allows one to judge in which sensory modalities the patient might be more responsive to suggestion and gives an overall measure of general susceptibility. When patients score low on this scale, it does not mean that they should automatically be deselected for hypnotic treatment, but you will probably have to put more effort into customising the images used in your treatment, and it may be that you will orient your treatment more towards general relaxation and stress management. These are our impressions only. An alternative to a formal assessment is the 'Is it possible?' technique described in the next chapter. This is considerably briefer, although is not scored in a standard manner.

Psychodynamic factors, secondary gain and motivation

The procedures outlined in this chapter may be designated as 'symptom-oriented'. That is, they do not endeavour to explore underlying psychodynamic processes or other factors that may be maintaining the symptoms at their current level of severity, such as those related to secondary gain. For example, patients' symptoms may relate in some way to their upbringing and experiences that occurred in their formative years. Similarly, they may form an important basis for their dependency on the marital partner, and this dependency may have a stabilising or binding effect on the relationship because of the psychological characteristics of the respective partners. Or the illness may protect patients from situations that they feel unable to handle, for example, entering into a relationship or holding down a job. The system of welfare payments may result in the fact that some people are better off being registered as ill and not working, rather than being well and working.

A number of patients who are referred for psychological treatment have had their problems for so long that they have become accustomed to the 'sick role' and their symptoms can come to dominate their lives and those close to them. (It is our experience, certainly of the patients who were referred by their specialists to our psychosomatic clinic, that a psychological approach to their problems was 'a last resort' and was not uncommonly preceded by a long history of repeated physical tests and investigations, an astonishing array of different medicines, and surgery, the effect of which was often non-existent and even, on the admission of the specialist, deleterious. There is no reason whatsoever why a psychological approach cannot be incorporated into treatment 'further up the line' rather than held in reserve as a last resort.)

Obviously these issues may be addressed by non-hypnotic psychotherapeutic procedures that we have discussed in earlier chapters. Also, the psychodynamically oriented hypnotic procedures that we have described in previous chapters can be used to explore the possibility of psychodynamic or other maintaining factors, and attempts can be made at resolving these. The psychodynamic technique of the somatic or affect bridge can be particularly useful in these cases.

Sometimes it will become evident to the therapist during the assessment of the patient that there are potent factors that may be maintaining the symptoms. More light may be thrown on this by adapting the symptom record form so that the patient records in much more detail the circumstances in which the symptoms occur.

Different therapists have their own ways of addressing these matters. Some will always assume that the symptoms have some psychodynamic significance and their therapeutic approach will be planned accordingly. On the other hand, most clinical trials of hypnosis have adopted a symptom-oriented approach and have demonstrated reasonably good outcomes. Readers must come to their own decision about how to approach these problems, but we recommend that, initially, symptom-oriented procedures are used. We shall see that a course of treatment of six sessions may comprise the bulk of the therapy along these lines and thereafter the therapist may decide whether further exploratory work, on cognitive-behavioural or psychodynamic lines, is warranted. Sometimes, underlying problems may be exposed as patients are making progress; it is easier to address these at that stage than at the beginning of therapy. Sometimes patients and their spouse or family have the resources to deal with these problems in their own way. Problems don't always require therapy!

Symptom substitution

In the past, some authorities have been very concerned about 'symptom substitution'. This is based on the idea that if patients have a psychological need for a symptom, then removing it may leave them defenceless and exposed to more severe psychological problems. In that case, they may present with another set of symptoms that serves the same purpose as the original. There is in fact very little evidence that this occurs, and, in our experience, if a patient needs a symptom, it will simply resist one's therapeutic endeavours.

Group treatment

If you are running a clinic that specialises in a particular type of problem, for example irritable bowel syndrome, you may consider seeing your patients in groups. So far as the evidence goes, there does not seem to be a disadvantage in this. Probably any loss of therapeutic impact in having to standardise your treatment is offset by the benefits of group dynamics and support.

Safeguards

We have discussed possible risks of hypnosis and safeguards in other chapters and there is not a great deal further we have to say here. We repeat again the importance of ensuring that patients have had all the medical attention necessary and that they continue to take the prescribed medication on the advice of their doctor or specialist. It is important to avoid equating the taking of medicine with failure on the patient's part. That is, patients must never be placed in the position of experiencing a conflict between the symptom-control methods that their therapist has taught them and the taking of prescribed medication.

Duration of treatment and follow-up

In our experience, and from our surveys of the literature, there appears to be a norm of around five or six core treatment sessions. At least by the end of that period you should have a good idea if treatment is working and where you are going to go from there. Initially, the sessions should be weekly, but by session six you may have already started to spread them out at, say, fortnightly intervals. If little or no progress has been made by then, then it is probably a case of 'going back to the drawing board' and thinking of either discharging the patient or adopting a broader approach, as discussed earlier. If good progress has been made, it may be that further sessions are judged necessary to optimise improvement, or you may well be ready to give your patient a follow-up appointment. (Although patients may not yet have reaped the full benefits of therapy, it may be that they will continue to improve under their own steam.)

The problems that we are discussing are often chronic and run a variable course, sometimes spontaneously improving for days, weeks and even months, and at other times becoming more severe over the same time-scales. For this reason, we cannot underestimate the importance of regular follow-up sessions. These allow you to monitor progress and, should the patient 'slip back', you can then offer 'booster' treatment with a view to preventing a relapse to the patient's pre-treatment level. An example of a programme of follow-up sessions would be 1 month after conclusion of the main treatment, then a 2-month follow-up period, and thereafter 3-month follow-ups for as long as is deemed necessary. These follow-ups could even be in the form of telephone contact if progress has been maintained.

Indicators for successful treatment

It is not easy to predict who will respond significantly to treatment. Generally, the best responders are predictably the younger patients and those whose condition is less chronic (and of later onset), who have no serious psychopathology or secondary gain, and who have some capacity for experiencing hypnosis.

OVERVIEW OF TECHNIQUES

The information in this section may be used to plan a session of hypnosis for a psychosomatic complaint using a behavioural or symptom-oriented approach. You would not, however, use all procedures on all occasions, and some are only appropriate for the first session of hypnosis. Some of the procedures (e.g. sensory focusing and age progression) may elicit material that requires a psychodynamic way of working. Whatever the case, the emphasis of therapy is ultimately to make *permanent* the changes that are achieved by the use of heterohypnosis; hence, the extensive use of posthypnotic suggestion, practice, self-hypnosis and future rehearsal.

Education concerning a working model of psychosomatic illness and treatment

If you are seeing patients who are referred by their doctor or specialist, then many of them not uncommonly arrive at their first session with some anxiety and misgivings. (It is different if patients come on their own initiative.) For some patients, a referral by their specialist means 'He thinks it's all in my head' or 'She has washed her hands of me'. Some patients express resentment about this. Other patients say, 'My doctor thinks my problems are all due to stress, but I don't really feel stressed and in any case I have my symptoms when I'm feeling relaxed'. They may be quite accurate when they make this observation, although some patients do deny real psychological difficulties. Undue stress may *not* be a factor, but the normal 'slings and arrows' of everyday life may nevertheless still be contributing.

Accordingly, the first task that the therapist may have is to correct misconceptions of this sort. For these purposes, for patients attending our psychosomatic medicine clinic, we devised a leaflet that we gave out at, or prior to, the first session. The text of the leaflet is given in Box 25.1 and explains the theoretical rationale or 'working model' adopted by the authors.

Assessment

We have discussed assessment procedures in the previous section, including the use of formal scales to assess general mood and anxiety levels and scales to monitor the symptoms. These are administered at the first session. As we indicated earlier, we recommend the use of the Creative Imagination Scale or the 'Is it possible?' procedure described in the next chapter.

Preparation and preliminaries

We have in previous chapters discussed two approaches to hypnosis and, for the purpose of treating psychosomatic problems, we recommend a combination of both, which will become clear as we describe the preparation and preliminaries.

The idea of 'mind–body communication'

As usual, there are a number of preliminaries that it is useful to go through prior to the actual induction of hypnosis in addition to describing hypnosis and allaying misconceptions. The first of these is to introduce the patient to

---

Box 25.1 Information leaflet for patients attending the authors' Psychosomatic Medicine Research Clinic (slightly abridged)

THE PSYCHOSOMATIC MEDICINE RESEARCH CLINIC

Information for Patients

The Psychosomatic Medicine Research Clinic is for patients with medical problems in which psychological methods of treatment may be of benefit. These include disorders and illnesses in which an organ or part of the body is not working in the right way or is oversensitive to factors such as stress, diet, and the way we feel generally, certain aspects of our environment, and even everyday events in our life. These organs or systems of organs in the body can acquire 'bad habits' or come to behave inappropriately, even when there is nothing obviously wrong with them. Such organs include those to do with breathing, digestion, and the distribution of the blood supply, as well as the heart and the skin. Medical treatments for these problems try to help these parts of your body to work in the correct way.

There are also psychological methods which can be used alongside medical treatments and which have been shown by specialists in this country and in the USA to help in relieving the symptoms of these kinds of problems. These methods involve the use of hypnosis and relaxation as well as the appropriate use of suggestion and the patient's imagination. They are able to work in this way because what we are thinking and how we react to certain situations affect the way the organs of the body respond. For example, as soon as you start to think about having something nice to eat, the glands in your mouth start to produce more saliva. Similarly, if you think about something very exciting that's going to happen, your heart starts to beat faster, the glands on your skin produce more sweat, your breathing may become a little faster, and so on. So the regular practice of hypnosis and suitable imagery can influence the way your body reacts and in this way help correct the faulty habits of the relevant organs and systems.

The treatment you will receive at the Clinic will probably consist of a number of sessions of hypnosis, and your therapist will explain to you how this is going to help your particular problem. Your first appointment will be to assess your problem, and the therapy will start at the second session. The assessment consists of taking a history and you will also be asked to imagine a number of simple scenes. We will also ask you to keep a very brief daily record of your symptoms. These kinds of assessments help us to plan the details of your treatment.

When you begin your treatment sessions, you will discover that hypnosis itself is a very pleasant experience in which you feel very relaxed and where your mind is focused on inner experiences rather than on things that are going on around you. This makes it easier for you to experience the suggestions and imagery described by your therapist, and therefore for physical changes to occur more easily. You will be fully aware of what is happening and be completely in control of what you are doing and experiencing. This aspect of your therapy will be explained to you in more detail by your therapist and you must not hesitate to ask the therapist about anything of which you feel you need to know more.

You will be asked to practise these procedures regularly on your own to strengthen the new habits. As you are also asked to monitor your symptoms daily, you will understand that this kind of treatment does mean that you yourself have quite a bit of work to do in order to gain the full benefits.

When the treatment sessions have been completed, you will be asked to attend a follow-up appointment after about 6 weeks or so. This is to check on your progress, and there may be further follow-ups every few months. If at follow-up you do not appear to be benefiting at all, we will either consider a variation of the treatment we have used, or if we feel we can't help any further, we will refer you back to your specialist with any recommendations we feel are useful.

Finally, we wish to emphasise strongly that because your problem is being treated by a psychological approach, this does not mean that there is something psychologically wrong with you. Everybody experiences psychosomatic problems, and many of these problems have been found to be helped by the application of psychological methods in addition to medical procedures.

the idea of 'mind–body communication'. This will already have been done to some extent if you have administered the Creative Imagination Scale or the 'Is it possible?' protocol. What you are trying to get across to the patient at this stage is the idea that the mind can influence a range of bodily functions and physical experiences. You can describe these to the patient – for example, how thinking of your favourite food can actually cause salivation, or thinking that people are looking at you disparagingly may cause you to blush. This is actually covered in the explanatory leaflet shown in Box 25.1. You can then take the patient through some of the preliminary suggestions outlined in Chapter 7, such as arm lowering, hands coming together and salivation. (You will already have some idea of the patient's level of suggestibility if you have administered either the Creative Imagination Scale or the 'Is it possible?' protocol.)

At this stage, you are conveying and demonstrating to the patient how thoughts, images and ideas can influence the way the body reacts, an important idea behind the treatment protocol.

The idea of 'body–mind communication'

From 'mind–body communication', we now move to 'body–mind communication'. Here your wish is to convey to the patient how the body communicates to us by different feelings; sometimes these feelings make sense, but sometimes we are not quite sure what the message is. In other words, you can administer the 'sensory-focusing' procedure we described in Chapters 6 and 19, adapting it for the treatment of psychosomatic problems. It is possible, using this method, that you will find yourself engaged in some psychodynamically oriented work with the patient, as was described in Chapter 19.

Eventually, you will ask the patient to focus on the psychosomatic symptoms. These may actually be present during the session; for example, the patient with eczema may be experiencing itchiness. More often, you will ask the patient to imagine the symptoms as if they are present in the here and now. In some cases, this may actually bring on some of the symptoms – for example, a tension headache. In order to assist patients in this task you may ask them to imagine the last time they experienced the symptoms.

You may ask the patient at this point (or during your assessment phase) 'What does it mean for you to have this problem or symptom?'. Here, you are trying to understand what meaning the symptoms have in the patient's life. With some patients, all they will be able to say is that, for example, 'Well I have this medical condition called eczema and I am hoping that you are going to be able to do something about it'. This may be as far as the patient can go, but some patients are able to be more psychologically minded. For example, people with eczema often feel self-conscious about their skin and this may make it difficult for them to 'face the world'. Particularly in younger people, a skin complaint can be a 'secret', something they do not wish to reveal to the rest of the world, even a source of shame. People with irritable bowel syndrome often raise the theme of control; they feel that their symptoms control their lives and stop them doing things that they want to do, since at any moment they may 'have an attack' and need to make a quick exit to get to a toilet. This kind of information can be used at a later stage, as we shall describe in due course.

The patient's image of the symptoms

The next step is to ask patients what kind of images they associate with the symptoms. What you are ideally looking for here is some kind of symbolism or metaphor that patients use to describe the symptoms. It is a good idea, therefore, to listen to how the patient does this spontaneously. For example, during the assessment phase, the patient might say, 'When I have one of my headaches, it's as though there's a workman with a pneumatic drill pounding away in my head'. Or, patients with a skin complaint may say that when they feel the itching, it is as though somebody with a feather is tickling their skin. If patients are able to do this, then encourage them to elaborate on the image. For example, patients with eczema could be asked whom they see holding the feather. The more symbolic or metaphorical (and even outrageous) the image, the better.

Not all patients can provide such imagery and, later in this chapter, we shall present standard imagery that has been used for different kinds of psychosomatic problem. Although we are unable to provide objective evidence for this, our impression is that it is better if patients *can* provide their own image. Obviously, their own image may make more sense to them than one offered by the therapist, but it may also be that patients thus feel more involved in the therapy and have greater sense of ownership of the solutions to their problem.

Paradoxical injunction

The next stage is the use of paradoxical injunction. That is, patients are asked to imagine the intensity of the symptom increasing. (The symptom may be a headache, itchiness, a painful or bloated feeling in the abdomen, and so on.) This can be done using the rating method. Patients first rate the intensity of the symptom (or imagined symptom), on a scale, say, from 0 to 7. (It makes sense to use the same scale as on the symptom-rating form mentioned earlier, if you are using this.) Then, patients are to try to increase the rating by just 1 point. Patients must not do anything physical (such as clenching their muscles) to aggravate the symptom but are to use 'willpower'. However, they are allowed to imagine a time when the symptoms were severe.

With most problems, it is possible to ask patients how their image of the problem will change as the symptom becomes more intense. For example, an image for irritable bowel syndrome may be that of rivers that are blocked with weeds and debris. Hence, a worsening of the symptom would be associated with increasing amounts of detritus leading to further blocking of the flow of the river. An example from actual clinical practice is that of a man with irritable bowel syndrome who imagined the gradual closing of lock gates on a canal.

Symptom-control method

When patients have signalled that they have spent enough time on this, the next instruction is to ask them to imagine that the symptom is decreasing in severity. We term this the 'symptom-control method' and we will give standard examples of this for specific problems in the next section. An example from clinical practice (seen by MH) is that given by a patient who suffered from headaches. He associated the pain of the headache with an image of a blue swimming cap that was being pulled tightly over his skull. When asked to imagine the headache easing, he pictured himself relaxing in a bath of water suffused with special, pleasantly scented herbs, so that the swimming cap became loose and wrinkled and eventually fell off. Whilst the patient is doing this, one can give suggestions of relaxation, calmness, freedom from discomfort, and so on.

Hypnotic induction and deepening

Having done this preliminary work, one is now ready to administer a hypnotic induction and deepening routine. We recommend one that emphasises relaxation and can be used for the purposes of self-hypnosis. The routines described in Chapter 6 are appropriate for this.

Imaginal rehearsal of the symptom-control method

The next step is to ask patients to rehearse in imagination the symptom-control method. They imagine the symptoms, associate them with the image established before or the standard image provided by the therapist, and then rehearse the symptom-control method. This is done several times and it is useful for this purpose to use memories of times when they experienced severe symptoms. However, this is not to say that the symptom-control method can necessarily be used at times when severe symptoms are experienced. For example, it is difficult for patients in the throes of a severe migraine, or experiencing severe abdominal pain, to alleviate the symptoms by these means. The symptom-control technique is best seen as a prophylactic device to forestall a severe attack. Consequently, it is of greatest use if patients experience any prodromol symptoms or if patients can anticipate situations and times when they are at risk from experiencing the symptoms. If this is so, then one can use future rehearsal of the symptom-control method. Patients imagine a time in the future when they are in a situation in which the symptoms could occur. They are then asked to imagine using the symptom-control method to forestall an attack of the symptoms.

Posthypnotic suggestions

Posthypnotic suggestions can then be given that patients will use and practise regularly the symptom-control method whenever they anticipate the onset of the symptoms in everyday life.

Ego-strengthening

Ego-strengthening suggestions may then be administered, and it is useful to incorporate in these the information that patients provided earlier about the meaning of the symptoms in their everyday life. For example, if patients have indicated that the symptoms prevent them from being in control of their life, then appropriate suggestions may be given that they are gradually being able to do the things that they want to do rather than being controlled by the problem. Likewise, if the symptoms cause self-consciousness and embarrassment, then suggestions may be given of growing confidence in social situations.

Self-hypnosis

Instructions then may be given for the regular practice of self-hypnosis. Readers should refer back to Chapter 9 for our recommendations about this. The self-hypnosis routine will include rehearsal of the symptom-control method, but, as was indicated under 'Posthypnotic suggestion', patients should also be encouraged to practise this on its own as often as possible, particularly in anticipation of any problems. The therapist may consider putting the self-hypnosis routine and the symptom-control method on tape, but, as we said in Chapter 9, patients should always be encouraged to use what is on the tape in their everyday life.

Practice

After alerting patients, they are encouraged to go through their self-hypnosis routine and to practise the symptom-control method under the observation of the therapist. Before the conclusion of a session, they may be reminded about regularly practising these methods and about keeping records of the symptoms.

Future sessions

This completes the first or second session depending on the availability of time, and future sessions will consist of further practice of the symptom-control method and addressing any problems patients may have encountered.

Additional techniques

There are a number of other techniques that may be incorporated into a session of hypnosis at the discretion of the therapist.

Age progression

One method is to use age progression to the time when patients are symptom-free and to ascertain what sort of things they might be doing that they are unable to do at present or find difficult. These may be incorporated into the ego-strengthening suggestions and may be used to motivate patients to regularly practise self-hypnosis and the symptom-control method. Age progression may also be used to explore the possibility of any problems that may be encountered if patients are to become symptom-free.

Age regression

Another technique that may occasionally be used is to regress patients to a time before they had the problem. This may be useful if one is adopting a psychodynamic approach, as it may be that the onset of the symptoms was associated with some significant event or period in the person's life that it is beneficial to explore. Sometimes the feelings of being strong and healthy can be anchored so that patients may access them in their present life. That is not to claim that it is thereby possible to be symptom-free; rather it is to help patients feel more positive and more in control of the symptoms.

Free metaphorical imagery

Some writers have used what we call 'free metaphorical imagery'. That is, the therapist relates an anecdote to patients or takes them on a fantasy that is metaphorically related to their problem but no connection between the two is explicitly made (see Ch. 13).

Case example

Carl, a boy of 15, was seen (by MH) for irritable bowel syndrome. His problem meant that he was always anxious in case he did not have immediate access to a toilet. He described how he once enjoyed climbing a wall in a gymnasium that was used for the purposes of training rock climbers. He was asked to imagine climbing the wall again and, as he was ascending, feeling stronger and more confident. He was then asked to imagine looking down and feeling anxious and worried that he might not be able to 'hold on'. He was instructed to imagine staying there and calming himself down using a breathing technique. It was suggested that he could trust his muscles to hold on for as long as he wanted and then to let go at the right moment to continue. He was assured that he had the choice of coming down again or carrying on, and he elected to carry on. Accordingly, he was told that his muscles would know exactly when to let go and move up and to hold on again. He could trust his muscles to do this. When he signalled that he had reached the top, he was encouraged to feel a sense of achievement, knowing that he could be fully in control even at times when he felt anxious and was not sure whether he could hold on for long enough. The association with the fantasy and his problem is fairly obvious, but the therapist did not explicitly make the connection.

SPECIFIC PROBLEMS

All the above procedures can be used in the treatment of a range of complaints that we are loosely referring to as psychosomatic. What remains to be done now is to examine the kinds of symptom-control methods that have been used for specific problems that have been reported in the literature to respond to hypnosis. In all of these problems, patients may be encouraged to develop their own symptom-control imagery as described above. We shall not attempt here a review of all the evidence, but in Chapter 33 we shall summarise some of the evidence for the efficacy of hypnosis in these problems. For ease of consultation, we have put the material to follow under headings arranged in alphabetical order, and organised the reference list likewise, after the more general references.

Asthma

The research on the use of hypnosis for asthma is surprisingly extensive relative to research on clinical hypnosis generally (see Hackman et al 2000 for a review). In our experience, however, even those medical doctors who are committed to hypnosis make little use of it for treating their asthmatic patients, except perhaps children. This is no doubt because asthma is a life-threatening illness that has been on the increase for some time (as have mortality rates) and there is a range of effective medication. Because of this, a number of hospitals in the UK have an open access policy for asthmatics.

Acute attacks of asthma are associated with marked bronchospasm, oedematous swelling of the mucosal lining and increase in the secretion of sputum. In longstanding cases, there is hypertrophy of the musculature of the walls of terminal bronchioles and this contributes to the severity of bronchospasm. Therefore, *hypnosis alone should never be used in acute attacks of asthma.* A patient who is well trained in self-hypnosis may use it as an adjunct when all appropriate medical emergency measures are in action. This can minimise the adverse effect of panic and the fear of dying, which may aggravate all three elements of asthma, thus creating a vicious cycle. Hence, an emphasis on being calm and in control helps patients to be more effective in the medical management of their asthma. Findings from clinical research suggest that improvement tends not to occur until after the first month of treatment and that patients should be monitored for up to a year (Hackman et al 2000).

The use of hypnosis for asthma was extensively investigated in Britain by the physician Dr Gilbert Maher-Loughnan and his colleagues (Maher-Loughnan 1970, 1984, Maher-Loughnan et al 1962, Maher-Loughnan & Kinsley 1968). They obtained superior results for hypnosis compared with breathing exercises aimed at relaxation. They felt that those patients who were committed to self-hypnosis improved the most, and physicians who were experienced in hypnosis also obtained the best results. They recommended weekly, then monthly sessions of heterohypnosis, noting that peak improvements tended to occur between the 7th and 12th week after the first hypnotic session. In this country also, Wilkinson (1988) reported good results for hypnosis, recommending daily practice of self-hypnosis for 3 months after peak improvement. In Australia, Collison (1975) also obtained good-to-excellent improvements in 54% of patients. This study used a range of hypnotherapeutic techniques and outcome was better for younger, less chronic patients who had some emotional concomitants, who were capable of at least 'a light state of hypnosis', and who were not heavily dependent on steroids, a finding also noted by Wilkinson (1988).

Symptom-control methods include the use of the clenched fist technique with an image of drawing all the tension from the chest. Other methods included relaxed breathing and control of hyperventilation (if this is a problem). Another symptom-control suggestion and image are that the bronchiolar linings and musculature are becoming resistant to external agents and immunological and psychological input, and that the internal bronchial muscles are relaxing sufficiently to allow the smooth passage of air.

Wilkinson (1988) counsels against the use of suggestions directly to reduce the perception of wheezing or tightness because of the risk that this will reduce the respiratory drive to a dangerously low level.

Dermatological complaints

Warts

There has been a considerable number of reports of the use of hypnosis in the alleviation of warts in various parts of the body (see Ch. 33). Ewin (1992) has described positive results using an analytical approach. However, most therapists have used direct suggestion that the warts will die. In some reports, the suggestion and image are that the circulation is being drawn to the surface of the skin, bringing a surge of white blood cells to devour the wart. Conversely, some reports have used an image of the cutting-off of the blood supply from the wart and the wart then crumbles away. DuBreuil & Spanos (1993) provide a review of methodology.

Eczema

In the case of eczema, a standard image is that of the healing rays of the sun on the patient's body. This is still acceptable for those patients who say that the sun has actually no beneficial effect on their skin, but one would not use this image for patients who say that the sun makes their skin worse. The same applies to the use of an image of going into a pool of cool, healing water. The images of the sun and healing water can be combined in a guided fantasy of, say, a walk along a beach or in a garden, followed by a dip in the sea or a lake (so long as the patient is a swimmer!). Suggestions may be given that the circulation is being drawn to the surface of the skin, bringing nourishment and healing. Conversely, patients may have their own ideas about what constitutes a good image.

Other suggestions are that of anaesthetisation of the affected part of the skin (by transfer of glove anaesthesia) to reduce itching. A posthypnotic suggestion may be given that every time the hand reaches to scratch the skin, even in sleep, some part of the patient will immediately become aware of this, withdraw the hand, and the patient will then feel a sense of relief from tension.

Reports favourable to the use of hypnosis have been provided by Stewart & Thomas (1995) for adults and children, and Sokel et al (1993) for children.

Psoriasis

There has been little systematic work on psoriasis. Price et al (1991) devised a course of therapy consisting of eight weekly 90-minute sessions of group therapy that included relaxation. A reduction in the symptoms of treated patients compared to controls was not significant, but there was a significant reduction in anxiety. More promising clinical results were obtained by Zachariae et al (1996) who used seven 90-minute sessions over a 12-week period; procedures included relaxation (taped for home practice) with pleasant imagery and suggestions of symptom control.

Urticaria

Methods similar to the above have been used with benefit in the treatment of chronic urticaria by Shertzer & Lookingbill (1987).

Dystonia and tics

These kinds of disorders are not traditionally designated 'psychosomatic'. Nevertheless, they fulfil our earlier definition in that, although the underlying pathology may be neurological or neuromuscular, their presentation may be significantly influenced by psychological factors. Treatment may incorporate any of the symptom-focused techniques described in this chapter. There are a number of accounts in the literature of the use of hypnotic procedures to assist people with dystonia (torticollis, blepharospasm, writer's cramp, etc.), tics and Tourette's syndrome.

Spasmodic torticollis, Meige's syndrome and writer's cramp

Hypnosis has been used to treat various types of dystonia using both general relaxation and relaxation of the affected muscles. These techniques may bring immediate relief, but the problem is to make this more permanent. Medd (1997) describes the treatment of four cases in which hypnosis was included as a relaxation procedure. Beneficial effects that outlasted the therapy session were reported in three of these. De Benedittis (1995, 1996) also describes four patients with spasmodic torticollis who benefited from treatment (including general relaxation, ego-strengthening, 'differential muscle retraining' and EMG biofeedback). Hoogduin & Reinders (1993) describe the treatment of Meige's syndrome and torticollis; components of treatment included self-hypnosis, habit reversal, suppression of the movement by sustained tension, practice of normal posture, and treatment for agoraphobia resulting from the torticollis. The last-mentioned problem was also the focus of treatment in a case of chronic torticollis described in Gibson & Heap (1991). When the patient was in a public place, his self-consciousness caused more tension and aggravated the spasm in his shoulder, leading to further self-consciousness, and so on. Treatment included relaxation and the ego-shrinking technique described in Chapter 20. For writer's cramp, Reinders & Hansen (1991) used relaxation and relaxing imagery associated with lightness of the hand.

Blepharospasm

Murphy & Fuller (1984) describe a single case study of the treatment of blepharospasm. Results indicated that ophthalmological treatment had a limited effect; brief hypnosis had a dramatic but short-lived effect, and biofeedback had a moderate and sustained effect.

Tics

Hypnosis can be used with these as a means of relaxation, both general and specific to the area of the body concerned (e.g. the head or shoulder). On the assumption that the tic may signify some unresolved emotional problems, some therapists have used hypnosis as part of a psychodynamic approach. For example, Spithill (1974) used both relaxation and age regression to a humiliating experience. Again, on the assumption that the tic serves some important purpose, Spiegel & Spiegel (1987) used hypnotic suggestion to displace the tic to a more discrete part of the body. The patient was a soldier with a facial tic that successfully moved down his leg to his toe.

Non-hypnotic methods for tics include EMG biofeedback, habit reversal (practising a competing habit) and massed practice.

Tourette's syndrome

Many psychological treatments, usually with a poor response, have been attempted with this disorder, which is now generally regarded as neurological in origin. One of us (MH) has given a short account (Heap 1989) of the treatment of a teenager who reported that there was a build-up of tension prior to his tics and vocalisations that was accompanied by imagery. Hypnotic induction procedures increased the tics, whereas challenging the boy with the suggestion that the therapist could 'make him tic' led to their obliteration in the therapy session. Rehearsal of counteracting imagery also reduced the tics, but there was no clear generalisation to the boy's everyday life. He was also prescribed the pharmacological treatment of choice, namely haloperidol titrated against its side effects, with little benefit. The main influence on the severity of his problem was his passage through adolescence. Now in his early 30s, he is a pleasant and friendly man, enjoying his work as a coach driver, and would probably be described as 'very fidgety'.

Some papers have reported some improvement using relaxation methods (e.g. Culbertson 1989 and Young & Montano 1988, who also used habit reversal in imagination and in vivo). Related to the methods that we have described earlier in this chapter is the use of symptom-control imagery of 'switching off the tic'. Patients can be encouraged to develop their own imagery for this, such as a 'stop sign' or a 'twitch switch'. Another ploy is to imagine that the energy of the tics is accumulating somewhere without discharge until a suitable place and time are available for this. These methods, and more, have been described in a very useful paper by Kohen (1995).

Gastro-intestinal problems

Irritable bowel syndrome

An extensive literature has accumulated on the use of symptom-control methods in the treatment of irritable bowel syndrome. In Britain this work is mainly associated with Dr Peter Whorwell in Manchester (Whorwell 1991, Whorwell et al 1984, Whorwell et al 1987). In one series of trials, he and his colleagues used seven half-hour sessions over a 3-month period with daily self-hypnosis. They claim a success rate of 80%. Patients with significant psychopathology and atypical symptoms do not do as well, neither do older patients.

Whorwell insists that targeting suggestions on gut activity yields a superior outcome to suggestions of general relaxation and ego-strengthening alone, although these are also included in the protocol. Hence, the term 'gut-directed therapy' is used to describe these procedures. The most common technique is the hand-on-abdomen method whereby patients place a hand over the abdomen and imagine that the hand is becoming warm and the circulation is being drawn to the organs there, helping them work properly. The hand may gently massage the abdomen and, if this is acceptable to the patient, the therapist can place a hand over the top of the patient's own hand, as though reinforcing the suggestions.

Standard images are the smooth passage of food and stool through the bowel with the appropriate sphincters contracting gently and securely. Common metaphorical images are rivers or canals that are blocked and then released by the hand-on-abdomen method. As suggested earlier, patients may be able to provide their own metaphorical imagery. One such image given by a patient of one of our colleagues was that of trains stuck in tunnels and being freed.

Patients with irritable bowel syndrome may develop phobic anxiety concerned with their inability to gain easy access to a toilet in time, and therefore soiling themselves. One can therefore incorporate into treatment images of coping with these situations and becoming more confident about being able to remain in control. As was stated earlier, the issue of control is extremely important for many patients with irritable bowel syndrome and this can be emphasised in treatment.

The hand-on-abdomen method can also be used for controlling feelings of nausea that may arise in some disorders or medical procedures such as chemotherapy for cancer. The patient is first asked to imagine a situation in which nausea is experienced, then practises the technique to reduce the nauseous feelings.

Ulceration

Whorwell and his colleagues (Colgan et al 1988) have also investigated the use of hypnosis in preventing relapse in duodenal ulceration. The symptom-control method used is again the hand-on-abdomen technique, with suggestions of warmth, control of gastric secretions and healing of the ulcers. In this study, all patients were taking ranitidine for 10 weeks after the ulcer had healed. They had seven sessions of hypnotic relaxation and imagery as above. At 28 weeks, 8 out of 15 patients had relapsed, compared with all patients in the group not treated with hypnosis.

Schmidt (1992) has reported using group therapy in patients with ulcerative colitis. Therapy continued for many months and included hypnotic relaxation and the use of patients' own imagery of their diseased intestine and the process of healing.

Headaches

Headaches appear to respond well to a range of relaxation techniques (Holroyd & Penzien 1990). The clenched fist technique (described in Ch. 12) for the relief of tension may be used, likewise the coloured vapour technique. In the latter case, patients are asked to imagine a headache and to describe what shape and colour they imagine it to be. The headache can then be breathed out in the form of the coloured vapour and the remaining colour can change to the colour of calmness and relaxation.

In the case of migraine headaches, imagery associated with hand-warming (or occasionally head-cooling) has been commonly used. The rationale of this was described in Chapter 15 and it also forms the basis of thermal biofeedback for migraine.

Alladin (1988) systematically investigated this method using ten individual weekly sessions with a 13-month follow-up. The patients were all asked to practise daily self-hypnosis with a tape. As well as a waiting list control group, there were four groups of patients, all of whom had relaxation and ego-strengthening. In addition, one group had suggestions and imagery of hand-warming whereas in another group it was hand-cooling. A third group had extra relaxation techniques and a fourth group were given direct suggestions that their headaches would ease. All groups improved, but the group given suggestions of hand-warming seemed to improve the fastest. Hand-cooling was the least effective method. Patients kept a headache diary and measures of outcome were duration, frequency and intensity of headaches, and use of medication. Improvements seemed to plateau at 6 weeks.

The present authors have used this method successfully with migraines. Hence, we recommend relaxation coupled with images of hand-warming, ego-strengthening and self-hypnosis as the preferred method.

Hypertension

Hypnosis and self-hypnosis may be used as part of a 'change in lifestyle' approach (which includes advice on diet, exercise and avoidance of undue stress) for the hypertensive patient. The therapeutic programme includes general suggestions of relaxation, tension control, self-hypnosis and ego-strengthening. Friedman & Taub (1977, 1978) used seven treatment sessions, and Milne (1985) between eight and 18.

Tinnitus

The approach for tinnitus is general relaxation plus some form of symptom-control image, commonly the idea of turning down or switching off the sound. For this the patient can choose an appropriate image, such as the volume control of a loudspeaker. Instructions may be put on tape for daily (Brattberg 1983) or twice-daily (Marks et al 1985) use. The latter authors found that the main improvements resulting from these procedures were in mood and attitude to the tinnitus rather than the ability to block awareness of the noise (which was claimed by only one of their patients).

Urinary incontinence (adults)

There is some evidence (Freeman & Baxby 1982) that urinary incontinence in women may be alleviated by hypnosis using a standard, symptom-oriented approach (relaxation, suggestions of symptom alleviation and ego-strengthening). In this study, the patients, who were diagnosed with detrusor instability, had 12 sessions of treatment.

Smith (unpublished work, 1998) has also obtained positive benefits using hypnosis in incontinent women with unstable bladders (see Smith et al (1998) for a summary of this work). In addition to the standard advice given to all such patients, the treated group was provided with three 1-hour sessions of therapy, which included anxiety control methods, explanation of stable bladder function, the hand-on-abdomen method, age progression, ego-strengthening and training in self-hypnosis.

REFERENCES

GENERAL
Barabasz A F, McGeorge C M 1978 Biofeedback, mediated biofeedback and hypnosis in peripheral vasodilation training. American Journal of Clinical Hypnosis 21: 28–37
Baum A, Newman S, Weinman J et al (eds) 1997 Cambridge handbook of psychology, health and medicine. Cambridge University Press, Cambridge
Beck A T 1988 Beck Depression Inventory. The Psychological Corporation, London
Ben-Zvi Z, Spohn W A, Young S H et al 1982 Hypnosis for exercise-induced asthma. American Review of Respiratory Disease 125: 392–394
Derogatis L R 1983 The Symptom Checklist-90-Revised (SCL-90-R). NCS Assessments/ Afterhurst Ltd, Hove
Dikel W, Olness K 1980 Self-hypnosis, biofeedback, and voluntary peripheral temperature control in children. Pediatrics 66: 335–340
Eichhorn R, Tracktir J 1955 The relationship between anxiety, hypnotically induced emotions, and gastric secretions. Gastroenterology 29: 422–431
Goldberg D 1978 The General Health Questionnaire. NFER–Nelson, Slough
Heap M, Aravind K K, Power-Smith P 1994 A psychosomatic research clinic. Hypnos: Swedish Journal of Hypnosis in Psychotherapy and Psychosomatic Medicine 21: 171–175
Isenberg S A, Lehrer P M, Hochron S 1992 The effects of suggestion and emotional arousal on pulmonary function in asthma: A review and a hypothesis regarding vagal mediation. Psychosomatic Medicine 54: 192–216

Klein K B, Spiegel D 1989 Modulation of gastric acid secretion by hypnosis. Gastroenterology 96: 1383–1387

Olness K N, Culbert T, Uden D L 1989 Self-regulation of salivary immunoglobulin A by children. Pediatrics 83: 66–71

Snaith R P, Zigmond A S 1983 The Hospital Anxiety and Depression Scale. Acta Psychiatrica Scandinavica 67: 361–370

Wadden T A, Anderton C H 1982 The clinical use of hypnosis. Psychological Bulletin 91: 215–243

Whorwell P J, Houghton L A, Taylor E E et al 1992 Physiological effects of emotion: Assessment by hypnosis. Lancet 340: 69–92

Wickramasekera I 1993 Assessment and treatment of somatisation disorders: The high risk model of threat perception. In: Rhue J W, Lynn S J, Kirsch I (eds) Handbook of clinical hypnosis. American Psychological Association, Washington DC, ch 27, p 587

ASTHMA

Collison D R 1975 Which asthmatic patients should be treated by hypnotherapy? Medical Journal of Australia 1: 776–781

Hackman R M, Stern J S, Gershwin M E 2000 Hypnosis and asthma: A critical review. Journal of Asthma 37: 1–15

Maher-Loughnan G P 1970 Hypnosis and autohypnosis for the treatment of asthma. International Journal of Clinical and Experimental Hypnosis 18: 1–14

Maher-Loughnan G P 1984 Timing of clinical response to hypnotherapy. Proceedings of the British Society of Medical and Dental Hypnosis. 5: 1–16

Maher-Loughnan G P, Kinsley D 1968 Hypnosis for asthma: A controlled trial. British Medical Journal 4: 71–76

Maher-Loughnan G P, Macdonald N, Mason A A et al 1962 Controlled trial of hypnosis in the symptomatic treatment of asthma. British Medical Journal 2: 371–376

Wilkinson J B 1988 Hypnosis in the treatment of asthma. In: Heap M (ed) Hypnosis: Current clinical, experimental and forensic practices. Croom Helm, London, ch 14, p 146

DERMATOLOGICAL COMPLAINTS

DuBreuil S, Spanos N P 1993 Psychological treatment of warts. In: Rhue J W, Lynn S J, Kirsch I (eds) Handbook of clinical hypnosis. American Psychological Association, Washington DC, ch 28, p 623

Ewin D M 1992 Hypnotherapy for warts (verruca vulgaris): 41 consecutive cases with 33 cures. American Journal of Clinical Hypnosis 35: 1–10

Price M L, Mottahedin I, Mayo P R 1991 Can hypnotherapy help patients with psoriasis? Clinical and Experimental Dermatology 16: 114–117

Shertzer C L, Lookingbill D P 1987 Effects of relaxation therapy and hypnotisability in chronic urticaria. Archives of Dermatology 123: 913–916

Sokel B, Christie D, Kent A et al 1993 A comparison of hypnotherapy and biofeedback in the treatment of childhood atopic eczema. Contemporary Hypnosis 10: 145–154

Stewart A, Thomas S E 1995 Hypnotherapy as a treatment for atopic eczema in adults and children. British Journal of Dermatology 132: 778–783

Zachariae R, Øster H, Bjerring P et al 1996 Effects of psychological interventions on psoriasis: A preliminary report. Journal of the American Academy of Dermatology 34: 1008–1015

DYSTONIA AND TICS

Culbertson F M 1989 A four-step hypnobehavioural model for Gilles de la Tourette's syndrome. American Journal of Clinical Hypnosis 31: 252–256

De Benedittis G 1995 Hypnosis and dystonia: Report of four cases and review of the literature. In: Burrows G D, Stanley R O (eds) Contemporary international hypnosis. Wiley, New York, ch 23, p 213

De Benedittis G 1996 Hypnosis and spasmodic torticollis: Four case reports. International Journal of Clinical and Experimental Hypnosis 44: 292–306

Gibson H B, Heap M 1991 Hypnosis in therapy. Erlbaum, Chichester

Heap M 1989 Antecedent imagery in a case of Gilles de la Tourette syndrome. British Journal of Experimental and Clinical Hypnosis 6: 55–56

Hoogduin A L, Reinders M C 1993 Hypnotherapy and dystonia. Hypnos: Swedish Journal for Hypnosis in Psychotherapy and Psychosomatic Disorders 20: 198–204

Kohen D P 1995 Ericksonian communication and hypnotic strategies in the management of tics and Tourette syndrome in children and adolescents. In: Lankton S R, Zeig J K (eds) Ericksonian monographs number 10: Difficult contexts for therapy. Brunner/Mazel, New York, p 117–142

Medd D 1997 Hypnosis and dystonia. Contemporary Hypnosis 14: 121–125

Murphy J K, Fuller K A 1984 Hypnosis and biofeedback as adjunctive therapy in blepharospasm: A case report. American Journal of Clinical Hypnosis 27: 31–37

Reinders M J, Hansen A M D 1991 Hypnosis in the treatment of writer's cramp. Hypnos: Swedish Journal for Hypnosis in Psychotherapy and Psychosomatic Disorders 18: 45–51

Spiegel H S, Spiegel D 1987 Trance and treatment. Basic Books, New York

Spithill A 1974 Treatment of a monosymptomatic tic by hypnosis: A case study. American Journal of Clinical Hypnosis 17: 88–93

Young M H, Montano R J 1988 A new hypnobehavioral method for the treatment of children with Tourette's disorder. American Journal of Clinical Hypnosis 31: 97–106

GASTRO-INTESTINAL PROBLEMS

Colgan S M, Faragher E B, Whorwell P J 1988 Controlled trial of hypnotherapy in relapse prevention of duodenal ulceration. Lancet 2: 1299–1300

Schmidt C-F 1992 Hypnotic suggestions and imaginations in the treatment of colitis ulcerosa. Hypnos: Swedish Journal of Hypnosis in Psychotherapy and Psychosomatic Medicine 19: 237–242

Whorwell P J 1991 Use of hypnotherapy in gastrointestinal disease. British Journal of Hospital Medicine 45: 27–29

Whorwell P J, Prior A, Faragher E B 1984 Controlled trial of hypnotherapy in the treatment of severe refractory irritable bowel syndrome. Lancet 2: 1232–1234

Whorwell P J, Prior A, Colgan S M 1987 Hypnotherapy in severe irritable bowel syndrome: Further experience. Gut 28: 423–425

HEADACHES

Alladin A 1988 Hypnosis in the treatment of head pain. In: Heap M (ed) Hypnosis: Current clinical, experimental and forensic practices. Croom Helm, London, ch 15, p 159

Holroyd K A, Penzien D B 1990 Pharmacological versus non-pharmacological prophylaxis of recurrent migraine headache: A meta-analytic review of clinical trials. Pain 42: 1–13

HYPERTENSION

Friedman H, Taub H A 1977 The use of hypnosis and biofeedback procedures for essential hypertension. International Journal of Clinical and Experimental Hypnosis 25: 335–347

Friedman H, Taub H A 1978 A six-month follow-up of the use of hypnosis and biofeedback procedures in essential hypertension. American Journal of Clinical Hypnosis 20: 184–188

Milne G 1985 Hypnorelaxation for essential hypertension. Australian Journal of Clinical and Experimental Hypnosis 13: 113–116

TINNITUS

Brattberg G 1983 An alternative method of treating tinnitus: Relaxation therapy primarily through the home use of a recorded audio cassette. International Journal of Clinical and Experimental Hypnosis 31: 90–97

Marks N, Karle H W A, Onisiphorou C 1985 A controlled trial of hypnotherapy in tinnitus arium. Clinical Otolaryngology 10: 43–46

URINARY INCONTINENCE (ADULTS)

Freeman R M, Baxby K 1982 Hypnotherapy for incontinence caused by unstable detrusor. British Medical Journal (Clinical Research) 284: 1831–1834

Smith N, D'Hooghe V, Duffin S et al 1998 Hypnotherapy for the unstable bladder: Four case reports (abstract). Contemporary Hypnosis 15: 253

26

Hypnosis and pain

INTRODUCTION

The use of hypnosis for pain management is one of its success stories. Here we are talking of immediate pain relief or control (e.g. in an emergency or when the patient is undergoing a surgical, medical or dental intervention) or acute pain of longer duration caused by an organic condition. Hypnosis has also a part to play in the management of the chronic pain patient, though in rather more complex ways.

Although these findings are contested by some, there is evidence that the best analgesic effects for acute experimental pain are obtained by good hypnotic subjects using hypnotic procedures rather than non-hypnotic ones (Eastwood et al 1998). Subjects low in susceptibility do not do very well with these methods and it may be better to adopt a non-hypnotic, cognitive-behavioural approach with them. However, as we shall see, some of the pain-control methods described in this chapter may be used effectively by patients with low measured susceptibility.

The implication of this is that the therapist wishing to offer pain management to a range of patients should be familiar with the methods developed from the cognitive-behavioural perspective (see Weisenberg 1998 for a review). It is not possible for us to describe these here. If readers are already using these, then we are sure that they can profitably add hypnotic procedures to their repertoire of techniques.

THEORETICAL CONSIDERATIONS

It is also not possible in this chapter to present much in the way of theory. If we assume that the experience of pain has survival value, then it is either to mobilise the organism for a fight-or-flight response in the case of an external pain-producing stimulus, or for immobility and restfulness for an internal pain or recuperation from an injury. However, severe and persistent pain, where no immediate relief is possible, is debilitating and may have consequences that compromise survival. Sometimes, the distraction of severe pain may interfere with life-protecting action, and on occasions, such as when one is receiving first aid, the fight-or-flight response has to be suppressed and the most appropriate response may actually lead to an increase in the pain. Therefore, we can argue that the ability to tolerate and manage pain, like pain itself, is of survival value.

Endogenous physiological mechanisms have been identified that modulate the pain experience, but behavioural and cognitive responses may also be acquired through operant conditioning (e.g. negative reinforcement by reduction in discomfort) and classical conditioning (e.g. with relaxation as the conditioned response in anticipation of pain).

Pain relief by hypnosis is probably achieved by a number of routes. For example, relaxation may be helpful if the patient has a habit of tensing up because of the pain, only to aggravate it. Some neurophysiological work has shown that when subjects are asked to imagine pain increasing or decreasing in unpleasantness, the activity in the area of the brain that registers the affective component of the pain (the anterior cingulate cortex) is changed accordingly, whereas activity in the somatosensory area, which registers the sensory component, is unchanged (Rainville et al 1997). On the other hand, Crawford's work (Crawford 1994) indicates that some highly trained, highly susceptible subjects, who can virtually obliterate all perception of pain, appear to be able to diminish the sensory component by a well-developed ability to absorb themselves in other cognitive activity (such as a pleasant image) and disattend completely from the ongoing noxious stimulation. Some cognitive pain-management strategies (hypnotic and non-hypnotic) may help the person have a more constructive and less catastrophic attitude to the pain.

The components of pain

This brief survey reveals how complex the experience of pain is. From the above, we can identify several related components of pain:

- *sensory component* – where the pain is, what is its quality, how much it is varying over time, and so on. In fact in our language we have many different words to describe pain and discomfort – nagging, aching, smarting, stinging, shooting, burning, throbbing, dull, etc. (In the authors' part of the world, patients use the word 'naig' to describe, for example, the residual nagging ache in the neck when they are recovering from a whiplash injury.)

- *cognitive component* – how the person interprets the pain in terms of the possible reasons for its being there, and its likely progress (eventually easing or worsening), anticipation (e.g. the expectation that the dentist's drill will find a nerve-ending in the tooth), and the attention given to the pain.
- *physiological component* – part of this is the neurophysiological processes that are associated with the sensory and affective experience of pain; another part is the adrenalin response with an increase in autonomic nervous arousal (sweating, tachycardia, etc.).
- *behavioural response* to the pain – this includes muscular tension, guarding responses, escape or avoidance, or, in contrast, quiescence (as with an injury that requires immobility to assist the recuperative process), and complex social behaviours such as deciding not to go into work and seeking medical assistance.
- *affective component* – the person's emotional reaction to the pain and how unpleasant he or she rates it.

The importance of cognitive factors

Of all components, the cognitive one is crucial for a psychological approach to pain and self-management. When we discussed psychosomatic problems in the last chapter, we said that it is important to try to understand what sense patients make of their symptoms and what meaning the symptoms have in their life. In fact, the way we experience anything at any time is unique to each one of us and is determined by the sum of our life experiences (plus whatever our genes have bestowed upon us). The totality of patients' experience of a pain-producing event can only be understood from their own personal map of their world, not just from an objective inspection of the physical source of the pain and the tissue's response to it. It is of adaptive importance (i.e. of survival value) that we all search for the reason for having any pain at any time.

Imagine that at the moment you have a throbbing pain from a bruise on your knee. Suppose that you received this bruise in some sporting activity – perhaps when you won a game or scored a winning goal or try. Now, imagine the same pain and injury, but this time it is from the kick of a mugger who stole your wallet or handbag while you were out shopping. Which experience of pain do you think you would cope with better?

Now, transfer the imaginary pain so that it is inside you somewhere – say, in your abdomen. Most people find that a more centrally located pain is more difficult to deal with.

Now, imagine that the same pain came on 5 minutes ago, the day before, or a year ago. In the first case, you may be alarmed by the pain, as you do not know what is causing it. What reasons do you immediately come up with for your pain in this case – indigestion, cramp or cancer? This search for meaning is associated with anxiety which in turn is characterised by increased vigilance and a bias to interpret other experiences in a threatening way – e.g. other 'symptoms' (see Ch. 30). Nowadays we often rely on doctors or one's own medical knowledge to provide the diagnosis. The diagnosis, in theory, should reduce our anxiety, although this may not happen if it is bad news for us. On the other hand, if no clear reason can be found, our anxiety may continue, along with greater attention to symptoms and a greater inclination to place a sinister interpretation on these. All of this is natural, and of survival value. However, some individuals may, by nature, be more anxious in this regard and become caught up in a vicious cycle in which they are obsessed with their pain and other 'symptoms'. Where the pain has been with you for a year, you may know what is causing it, but be more depressed than anxious, because you are still in pain.

Now, suppose that you know that over the next hour or so the pain is going to fade. Is it easier for you to ignore it than if you had reason to believe that the same pain is going to become progressively worse?

Consider now that you have a constant pain somewhere that stops you working. You dearly miss your job and your colleagues. Would it be easier or more difficult for you to ignore the pain than if your job was boring or stressful and you are glad to be out of it? (It is said that wounded soldiers seem to be unusually tolerant of their pain as they are carried from the battlefield.)

Consider how much an unremitting pain may affect you when you are stuck at home alone on a rainy day with nothing to do, compared to a day when an important event is happening, such as a family wedding, and your mind is occupied with a multitude of tasks.

Finally, how tolerant as a rule are you of pain, or for that matter, any noxious or adverse experience or event? Are you a stoic who accepts that suffering is a necessary part of your life, or do you think that your pain is something that shouldn't happen, perhaps yet another misfortune that life has thrown at you? Of course, your choice in this matter will be limited by the severity of the pain you are experiencing. Everyday pains such as the pain of a headache allow one the luxury of a choice of philosophical attitudes from acceptance and a search for meaning, to the attitude 'This shouldn't happen to me' and an immediate recourse to medication. Severe constant pain, say the pain of cancer, does not afford the sufferer the same range of options in the matter.

We may take the business of your attitude to pain to a deeper level and ask, 'What has been your experience of pain in the past?' As a child, when you cried in pain, were you comforted, or were you informed that you were a big baby and told to shut up? Did you have any significant formative experiences when you were in great pain? Was your early life full of pain or pain-free, and if the former, was the pain inflicted by disease, accidental injury, or the malevolence of others?

It used to be thought that the experience of pain was a matter of how strongly the signals from pain receptors were firing. But clearly there is a psychology of pain that determines how it is experienced and how it affects the person. Just as we construct our visual and auditory perceptions from the energy that impinges on our senses, and construct our memories from energised neural networks, so we construct our pain. But, just as our perceptions and memories are real experiences, so pain is real also (except, say, where a person is malingering for financial gain). This is an important message to put across to some patients, particularly those with chronic pain, as often, suggesting the idea of a psychological approach to their pain provokes the retort 'So you think I'm just imagining all this!'

ASSESSMENT, MONITORING AND EVALUATION OF PROGRESS

In this section, we are only concerned with pain management as a consequence of some medical condition, or during recovery from injury.

As with psychosomatic problems, a thorough assessment of patients is essential when one is helping them with the pain of illness or injury. It goes without saying that the causes of the pain should have been carefully investigated and all necessary medical treatment has been and is being given, likewise monitoring by the medical specialist or general practitioner. Even so, although it is usually the case that patients are referred for psychological assistance 'as a last resort' (compare with psychosomatic problems), there is really no reason that these approaches should not be considered earlier in treatment or rehabilitation.

Most patients will be taking analgesics on a regular basis, and unless the therapist is also the patient's doctor, this aspect of the patient's treatment should normally not unduly concern the therapist. In our experience, patients are usually careful about their use of analgesics and able to judge if it is sensible to reduce them when progress is under way. Leaving it to their judgement is better than putting patients into a situation in which taking medication is construed as a failure on their part.

As with psychosomatic problems, we recommend the general assessment of mental state, augmented by instruments such as the HAD, the BDI, the GHQ, or the SCL-90-R (see Ch. 25). Where anxiety or depression levels are high, the therapist should consider whether additional treatment for anxiety or depression is indicated. (Indeed, many chronic pain patients are clinically depressed and already taking antidepressants that may also assist in pain relief.) High anxiety may also indicate a focus on an approach using relaxation.

Questionnaire techniques have been developed for assessing pain in all its aspects and the McGill Pain Questionnaire (Melzack 1975) is one of the foremost of these. This may be repeated at the conclusion of the core

Box 26.1 The 'Is it possible?' protocol (Adapted, with permission, from: Clarke J C, Jackson J A 1983 Hypnosis and behavior therapy: The treatment of anxiety and phobias. Springer Publishing Company, Inc., New York 10012.)

Just sit comfortably in the chair and pay attention to what I am going to be saying to you. I am going to ask you a series of questions. Each question could be answered by 'yes' or 'no' but you will not have to say 'yes' or 'no' out loud, or even to yourself. You can let your answer to the question be whatever your internal response is. Just let yourself respond internally to whatever the particular question is. There is no right or wrong way to respond. I will ask you afterwards how you felt, and what you noticed as we went along. Are you ready? Any questions? Remember, you don't have to answer aloud or make any 'yes' or 'no' signs as we go along.

(*Allow 5-second pauses between each question.*)

Is it possible for you to allow your eyes to close?
If they are not yet closed, you may close them now.

Is it possible for you to be aware of the area of your back that is in maximum contact with the back of the chair (or with the bed)?

Is it possible for you to think of the chair (bed) as strong and let it support you?

Is it possible to feel the floor beneath your feet?

Is it possible to be aware of all the sounds that you can hear?

Is it possible to feel the coolness of air in your nose and throat as you inhale?

Is it possible to notice the settling down of your chest and upper body as you exhale?

Is it possible to notice any changes in temperature of any part of your body as you relax?

Is it possible to feel yourself floating as if on a cloud?
Or are you feeling much too heavy for that?

Is it possible to notice a warm, heavy feeling in your arms and hands?

Is it possible to feel any tingling in your hands or feet?

Is it possible to be aware of the space within your mouth?
And can you be aware of the position of your tongue inside your mouth?

Is it possible to notice patterns of light and movement behind your closed eyelids?

Is it possible to feel your face getting very soft?

Is it possible to hear the sound of music in your mind?

Is it possible to imagine a beautiful colour in the eye of your mind?

Is it possible to imagine the smell and taste of a food that you like?

Is it possible to imagine yourself in a peaceful, relaxing place? To look all around in this place and notice details of what you can see, or touch, or hear? (*Longer pause.*)

Is it possible to be aware again of your body in the chair (bed) ... your feet on the floor ... the sounds you can hear?

And is it possible to bring yourself back slowly to being awake and alert?
You can open your eyes, and then take a few more moments to give yourself time to feel completely awake, alert and refreshed, wide awake and comfortable.

Inquiry follows, regarding:
- what was noticed
- what was felt
- which questions were easiest to respond to
- which questions were least comfortable or natural to respond to
- an estimate of how much time elapsed during the exercise.

programme of therapy and at follow-up appointments, as can the general psychological assessments, to evaluate the outcome of treatment.

You may also wish to consider formally assessing the patient's strategies for coping with adversities. The Coping Strategies Questionnaire (Rosenstiel & Keefe 1983) is one such instrument, and the Ways of Coping Checklist is another (Folkman & Lazarus 1980; see Lester & Keefe 1997 for a review).

You will also do your own assessment of mental state and pain experience, and one of the key aspects of the latter is understanding the meaning and role of the patients' pain in their everyday life. What does it stop patients from doing (valued and non-valued activities)? What difference would it make to patients if they did not have the pain? What would they be doing? How does their condition affect other members of the family?

It is useful to ask patients to monitor their pain and for this purpose a pain diary is useful. This may be an adaptation of the symptom record form described in Chapter 25. You need to have more frequent ratings of the pain and you will want to include a few more details of the circumstances and the consequences of the pain. This will enable you to have a clearer picture of the occurrence of pain in the person's life, triggers for the exacerbation of the pain, consequences of the pain, and so on.

We recommend that you undertake some assessment of the patient's hypnotic susceptibility, as this has some bearing on your choice of approach. In the last chapter, the Creative Imagination Scale was recommended for its ease of application. A much shorter instrument is the 'Is it possible?' technique (Clarke & Jackson 1983), shown in Box 26.1. This is an indirect, qualitative method that enables you to determine if there are any particular kinds of suggestion and imagery to which the patient is especially responsive. The questions are read out to the patient. There is no formal scoring; instead, you go through the items afterwards with the patient and discuss his or her experience of each one.

It is also worth administering some of the preliminary suggestions recommended for the second approach to hypnosis in Chapter 7. Hand analgesia may be one of these.

SOME HYPNOTIC PROCEDURES FOR PAIN MANAGEMENT

The following are some ways in which some of the procedures we have presented in previous chapters may be used for the alleviation of pain. All of these methods will include hypnotic induction and deepening, rehearsal of the pain management procedure, posthypnotic suggestion, ego-strengthening, self-hypnosis and instructions for the rehearsal of the pain control method. The routine you develop for your patient may be recorded on tape for daily practice.

In all of these methods, we recommend the approach to hypnosis outlined in Chapter 6, although, as we state above, positive expectations may be evoked in more susceptible patients using some of the preliminary suggestions described for the second approach to hypnosis in Chapter 7.

Paradoxical injunction

Prior to a session of hypnosis for pain management, provided patients are not already in a great deal of pain, it may be useful to take them through the paradoxical injunction method described in Chapter 12, using a pain rating from, say, 1 to 10. No harm ensues if patients are unable to increase the pain, but if they are, the message is 'If you can control it in one direction, then you can control it in the other'.

Relaxation

As we pointed out earlier, undue anxiety about pain can aggravate the experience through the operation of attentional and interpretative biases (see Ch. 30). More attention than is useful may be given to the pain and other symptoms, and undue threat is assigned to them. Also, physical tension and increased sympathetic activity may exacerbate the pain. Hence, the learning of a method of relaxation may be of benefit to pain patients. The hypnotic induction and deepening routines described in Chapter 6 may be used for this. The patient can then learn self-hypnosis in the usual way. The procedure is appropriate even for patients with low measured susceptibility.

Distraction

This approach can also be used with those patients low in susceptibility. In fact, the previous method and, indeed, all of those described here have an element of distraction; that is, they require patients to engage their attention on something other than the pain. So, the safe place or magic television method is a commonly used procedure and has a wide range of applications. (Informal distraction techniques are naturally used by many medical and dental practitioners when performing anxiety-provoking or uncomfortable procedures, such as giving injections.) It is important to help patients choose distracting imagery that appeals to them. (Of course, in a pain management programme the use of distraction will be much broader than that used within hypnosis and will include activities that the patient enjoys.)

Time distortion

Time distortion can be incorporated into a relaxation or distraction method in patients with at least medium susceptibility or good capacity for absorption. This can be helpful for patients who have periods in which their pain 'flares up'. The aim is to condense the subjective experience of time so that it seems that only a short period elapses between the beginning and the end of the painful episode. Direct suggestions may be given that during hypnosis and self-hypnosis for pain relief, time will appear to pass very quickly, 1 minute seeming like a second, and so on (see Ch. 2).

Conversely, during periods when the patient is pain free, one might suggest time expansion during self-hypnosis. That is, say, 15 minutes of self-hypnosis (involving pleasant and interesting imagery) 'can seem like several hours of pleasure'.

Suggestions of numbness and insensitivity

Here, suggestions (coupled with suitable imagery) of numbness and insensitivity are given for a part of the body. A common procedure is to suggest glove anaesthesia, more accurately labelled 'hand analgesia', then transfer the analgesia to the affected part. Medium hypnotic susceptibility is usually a requirement for this.

Suggesting insensitivity directly on the targeted body part or using the hand analgesia method is a useful procedure during minor surgical, medical or dental procedures. (Some dentists successfully used the method as an alternative to local anaesthesia.) It may also be used in childbirth. It is useful at times of acute pain, particularly if the pain has a habit of suddenly flaring up.

This technique is generally a temporary measure and must never be used for the attenuation of pain that has important signal value. It can be a good way of demonstrating to the patient how hypnosis can alleviate the experience of pain, even if you are not going to use the technique for pain management with your patient.

Low susceptible patients, as expected, respond poorly to this and there are occasionally patients who, for one reason or another, do not like the idea of insensitivity in a part of their body. Even with medium and high susceptible patients, although they may respond well to the standard image of ice-cold water, it may be worth taking your time over the choice of imagery and allowing patients to develop their own. This entails being rather indirect in your suggestions. The approach requires only a brief hypnotic induction. We shall take hand analgesia as an example.

Ask your patient to focus on both hands and then proceed:

Notice the different sensations in your hands and fingers. Perhaps you notice feelings of warmth…or heaviness…or lightness…or maybe, in a while, you will notice a tingling feeling. Take your time and then tell me what you notice.

Let us suppose that the patient notices a tingling feeling. Proceed as follows:

That's fine. Just keep thinking about that tingling feeling and notice how it can change. Maybe it becomes more noticeable ... maybe less ... maybe it spreads ... or becomes more focused .... Take your time and then tell me what you notice.

Then proceed:

I wonder as you continue to think about that feeling, whether sooner or later it can start to change to a cool feeling, as though there is a breeze blowing over your hands. I don't know if this will happen to your left hand or your right hand first ... let's just wait and see. Let me know when you notice this.

When the patient has signalled, proceed as follows:

Now, I wonder how long it will take for that cool feeling to become more noticeable and for your hand to start to feel rather numb and insensitive .... Maybe you can recall a time when your hand did feel numb and insensitive .... As you are thinking about that, you might allow the image to come to mind. Maybe your hand is somewhere cold ... or perhaps there is something round your hand protecting it, so when anything touches it you don't feel anything .... Just bring whatever it is to mind and notice that as you are doing that, your hand is feeling more and more cold, more and more numb, more and more insensitive. Let me know in your own time what you notice happening.

Another method is to suggest arm levitation first. When the arm has stopped rising, say:

Now, I wonder when, as that light feeling continues, you will start to experience a kind of numb feeling ... as though the feeling in your hand is slowly draining down your forearm to your elbow. Just tell me when you notice something like that. Perhaps while you are thinking about it ... and noticing ... that numb feeling ... a picture comes into your mind of something around your hand that makes it insensitive to any feeling.

Whichever method you use, you may then demonstrate the effect by gently pinching the back of each hand in turn (with the patient's permission). Suggestions then may be given that, using the hand, patients are to transfer this numbness to a particular part of the body (e.g. the cheeks and gums) and as they do this, they feel a numbness and insensitivity penetrating that part. Patients may then practise the procedure for themselves.

Imagery techniques for relieving pain caused by medical conditions

These procedures are very similar to those described in the last chapter for psychosomatic problems. The patient focuses on the pain and an image is constructed of the pain – what it might look like, its shape and colour, and so on. As we discussed in Chapter 25, the patient may describe a symbolic or metaphorical image of the pain and what is causing it. For example, a patient with arthritic joint pain may talk of 'grating cogwheels'.

With just an image of the shape and colour of the pain, one may use the coloured vapour technique described in Chapter 12 to suggest pain relief. Or one may use an image provided by the patient and modify it for the experience of pain relief. For example, the patient who imagines 'grating cogwheels' in the joints may imagine oil being squirted on them, freeing up the mechanism.

A basis for pain relief imagery is provided by Melzack and Wall's Gate Control Theory (Melzack & Wall 1965, Wall 1978, 1999). It is only necessary to provide the patient with the main details of this. Neural impulses from the pain receptors are carried along two types of fibre, large diameter and small diameter. Both types of fibre stimulate transmission cells in the dorsal horn of the spinal cord, and these instigate the required action. There is, however, a gating mechanism whereby small fibre stimulation tends to open the gate (excitatory action). Thus the pain impulses reach the centres of the brain that mediate the experience of pain. Large fibre stimulation has an inhibitory action (closing the gate). (It may be that these fibres are stimulated when one rubs the part of the body in pain and gains some relief.) Also some large fibres bypass the gate and project directly to the brain. The opening and closing action of the gate can then be influenced by efferent impulses, that is, more central processes.

The therapist can draw a simple diagram of this for the patient, choosing an appropriate analogy, for example a telephone network, or (for children) the control panel of a space ship. The idea of a dimmer switch, rather than a simple on–off switch, may be more realistic. The key action of this is that the large fibres 'tell the brain about the pain' and then send messages to the switchboard, which cuts down the messages that are coming up from the site of the pain.

Other standard methods are adaptations of the clenched fist procedure for tension relief (Ch. 12) and the hand-on-abdomen method (Ch. 25), which can be useful for abdominal pain such as that caused by menstruation problems. Rather than cold and numbness, some patients prefer warmth to ease constant pain. Suitable imagery (e.g. bathing in warm water) may be chosen. A favourite of some patients is the wrapping up of the affected part in warm, soft cottonwool-type material.

Displacement

A more ambitious ploy, only appropriate for some medium and high hypnotically susceptible patients, is to suggest that the pain is moving to another part of the body that can tolerate it more easily. Earlier, we stated that a peripheral pain (e.g. in the toes) is more bearable than a centrally located pain (e.g. in the abdomen or head).

Reinterpretation

Some patients find it easier to distract themselves from the pain than others. Some seem to need to 'stay with the pain'. These patients may be taught to reinterpret the sensory aspects of the pain so it is more bearable. For example, by suggestion and imagery the pain may be converted to warmth, pressure or itching.

The meaning of the pain may also be reinterpreted. Although one should not suppose that patients are actually able to delude themselves on this count, one can train some patients to imagine that when they are experiencing the pain, it is a result of some valued activity, such as sport or recreation. (Our impression is that a pain is more unbearable if it was caused by another person's negligence or vindictiveness. What this method may accomplish in the patient's mind in such cases is to take the pain out of that context.)

Dissociation

This is for patients who are on the high side of hypnotic susceptibility (or have a good capacity for dissociation). One method is to suggest that the pain and the part affected are being separated. The pain is 'somewhere else', say in another part of the room. (This is reminiscent of the 'hidden observer' described in Ch. 4.) Or it may be suggested that the affected part of the body itself is dissociated. This experience may be summed up by a multiple sclerosis sufferer who said, 'I know my left leg is burning with pain. If I want to, I can feel it, but at the moment it is somewhere else'. In some cases of severe widespread pain, some patients may be able to imagine leaving their body. (These kinds of out-of-body experiences have also been reported by patients during cardiac resuscitation.) The patient may 'go to the other side of the room' (say to a chair) or go on a fantasy trip.

APPLICATIONS

Hypnotic pain management methods may be used in the following medical contexts.

Cancer

Cancer patients have a range of needs that may draw upon the expertise of the practitioner of hypnosis. Pain relief is foremost amongst these and there is a wide selection of literature on the application of hypnosis (see Ch. 27).

Uncomfortable or painful medical and minor surgical procedures

Specific applications, reported in the literature, have included injections and blood taking, minor surgery, including suturing and the removal of sutures, reduction of minor fractures, dressing of burns, ophthalmic surgery, endoscopy, bone marrow (and other) aspiration, liposuction, and removal of drain tubes. The aim is to minimise the patient's experience of pain, and to maximise comfort and relaxation. Any of the hypnotic procedures described in this chapter may be used, notably relaxation and pleasant distracting imagery.

General surgery

There are occasional reports that entire operations, such as dermabrasion of the face, rhinoplasty, cholecystectomy, caesarean section, and leg lengthening, have been undertaken with hypnosis as the only method of analgesia and with excellent control of bleeding. However, the more routine use of hypnosis is in *facilitating* major surgery and general anaesthesia. Applications include relaxing the patient in the preoperative period, thus reducing preoperative sedation, muscle relaxants, and general anaesthetic requirements, and facilitating intubation (Kessler 1997, Kessler & Dane 1996). Preoperative sessions of hypnosis may instil confidence in the patient with suggestions of a successful outcome in all relevant aspects. Thus Blankfield (1991), in a review of the literature, reports shorter stays in hospital, reduction in postoperative pain and anxiety, a reduction in the use of narcotics for analgesia, lowered blood loss, and earlier return of gastrointestinal functioning (see also Benson 1971, Hart 1980). Earlier mobility and more rapid healing are also evident when patients are well trained in hypnotic imagery rehearsal, as described in Chapter 28 on the use of hypnosis in childbirth.

The imagery chosen may incorporate a wide range of metaphors appropriate to each requirement. For example, in bleeding control one may use the image of the blood vessels tied with a magic thread even before patients enter the operating theatre, so that when the surgeon puts the knife on them there is 'nothing to bleed'; or in the case of dissection of a tumour, one may think of the tumour as being wrapped up in cellophane so that it will be 'easily shelled out'.

The major benefit of this kind of approach may be that patients can develop the idea that they are in control and are actively contributing to their treatment, and this can have an ego-strengthening effect. The training includes the construction of the final image of themselves after recovery from the operation, which they rehearse during the preoperative period using their own ideas and the expert guidance of their therapist. It also involves explaining the principles involved in the images and fantasies. For example, if a blood vessel is tied sufficiently, there cannot be any bleeding; a tumour will shrink through lack of nourishment; or an important blood vessel is kept open just enough so that healthy tissues receive plenty of nutrients to speed up the healing process.

In the experience of one of the authors (KKA), there have been occasions when the anaesthetist and surgeon were amazed with the ease of the operation and the lack of any troublesome bleeding, and they could not wait to tell the patient, even when the patient had not disclosed the use of hypnosis. This enormously boosts the patient's confidence and demonstrates that it is not necessary for the hypnotist to accompany the patient at all, nor that the anaesthetist or surgeon need be the hypnotist.

Dentistry

Applications in this field are covered in Chapter 29.

Obstetrics and gynaecology

Chapter 28 discusses applications for these purposes (including childbirth).

Accident and Emergency

While there is plenty of scope for hypnosis in the Accident and Emergency Department, it seems that it is hardly used formally in this setting. (Patients at Accident and Emergency Departments are in a state of acute anxiety and confusion and may already be very receptive to the communications of the staff. Accordingly, it is not advisable for a nurse, doctor or policeman to say to the victim of a car accident, for example, 'You are lucky to come out of that crash alive', or 'Another inch and you would not be here'.)

Dabny Ewin, a surgeon and specialist in psychiatry in New Orleans, has worked in an emergency burns unit in which his favourite procedure is his version of the 'special place' technique, namely the 'laughing place'. Whilst the patient is thus engaged, suggestions of rapid healing of the burns are given. Ewin (1986) considers that an early intervention such as this does indeed promote a better clinical recovery, although evidence on this from controlled investigations is lacking.

Injuries

Here we are concerned with the long-term painful effects of injuries (i.e. beyond the immediate trauma and recovery period). Common are orthopaedic injuries owing to sports accidents, falls, road traffic accidents, spinal injuries, burns, and phantom limb pain following amputation (because of either injury or disease).

Within this category will be a range of disability and there are many patients who present with intractable pain and who require multidisciplinary teamwork (which may include hypnosis) and whose problems often attract the label 'chronic pain syndrome' (see below). The category also includes patients whose injuries are caused by the malevolence or inconsideration of others and who also may develop chronic pain syndrome. The latter patients may also be pursuing compensation claims, an extra factor to consider in treatment. They are often very angry and cannot accept that the world can be so unfair. For example, they may say, 'He walked away laughing. I've lost everything'. Maybe some will only be able to move forward once their claim is settled – it is often difficult to be sure.

Miscellaneous illnesses and complaints

Under this heading we include degenerative illnesses such as multiple sclerosis, arthritic conditions, conditions of the spine, low back pain (not directly caused by external injury), neuralgia, causalgia, temporomandibular joint pain, and burning mouth syndrome. Some of these patients' problems may come under the heading of chronic pain syndrome.

ACUTE PAIN VERSUS CHRONIC PAIN: TREATMENT ISSUES

There is no clear-cut distinction between acute and chronic pain, although some have suggested the latter to be anything up to 6 months, while others suggest as little as 6 weeks. Acute pain may be short-lived (e.g. during childbirth, following an injury or after surgery) or it may last several months (e.g. during the recovery period of a serious injury). It is of signal value – that is, it is telling the patient to be careful, take it easy and recuperate – and tends to perceptibly diminish over time. It is clearly related to some pathology or physical damage. Analgesics, and hypnotics for sleep disturbance (caused by pain and discomfort), may be helpful. In the treatment of acute pain, the focus of psychological treatment can be very much on pain relief, and hypnotic susceptibility appears to be a significant factor in determining the method chosen.

There are various ways of categorising chronic pain. Chronic periodic pain is acute but intermittent (e.g. headaches and menstrual pains). Chronic progressive pain is usually associated with malignancy, such as cancer. Some chronic pain, such as low back pain, can be classified as benign.

Of interest here is the syndrome of the chronic pain patient who presents as far more disabled and dependent than appears to be warranted by an examination of the existing pathology or injury. In these patients, the pain seems to dominate their lives unduly. They are often depressed (even clinically so) and almost always very angry. Their anger may be directed at their doctors or, in cases of injury, with any responsible party. They often use high doses of analgesics and may be dependent on them.

The treatment of such patients may be best undertaken in a multidisciplinary setting, say at a pain clinic, under the supervision of a consultant pain specialist. Unfortunately, not uncommonly the patient referred to the individual practitioner of hypnosis may have attended, or already be attending, such a clinic.

Treatment needs to address a wide range of aspects of their lives – physical and mental activities, general health and fitness, diet, weight, exercise, sleep, use of medication, relationships, self-esteem, anger, and so on.

Hypnosis may therefore be used to augment therapy in a variety of ways, not just at the level of pain management. Hypnotic susceptibility is probably not as significant a factor as in the case of the acute pain patient.

These patients often complain of multiple pains (e.g. low back pain, plus pain at the back of the neck, plus pain down the left arm, plus headaches) and it is a good idea to work on the problems one at a time, starting with what seems to be the easiest to treat.

Many of these patients feel so helpless and the future for them seems very bleak. Accordingly, therapy may be needed to assist them in developing a sense that, with improvement, good times lie ahead. Age progression and ego-strengthening are useful methods for this purpose. Although with pain patients one does not normally use psychodynamic approaches, such as regression methods, there may be some scope for using these in the case of chronic pain patients who may not be coping well because of what has gone before in their life. There may also be an argument that pain caused by an injury may be exacerbated by post-traumatic stress and this can be dealt with using procedures described in Chapter 30.

CONCLUSIONS

The use of hypnosis for pain management does not have to be a long drawn-out treatment. It is of proven efficacy and it is certainly safe. It reduces the patient's reliance on medication and its abuse, and it is not expensive relative to the cost of other treatments and the cost of painful conditions to the community generally. It provides the patient with a sense of mastery, independence and self-control. These are important for many patients who may feel a sense of total helplessness when the pain is with them all or most of the time.

REFERENCES

Benson V 1971 One hundred cases of post-anaesthetic suggestion in the recovery room. American Journal of Clinical Hypnosis 14: 9–15

Blankfield R P 1991 Suggestion, relaxation, and hypnosis as adjuncts to the care of surgery patients: A review of the literature. American Journal of Clinical Hypnosis 33: 172–186

Clarke J C, Jackson J A 1983 Hypnosis and behaviour therapy: The treatment of anxiety and phobias. Springer, New York

Crawford H J 1994 Brain dynamics and hypnosis: Attentional and disattentional processes. International Journal of Clinical and Experimental Hypnosis 42: 204–232

Eastwood J D, Gaskovski P, Bowers K 1998 The folly of effort: Ironic effects in the mental control of pain. International Journal of Clinical and Experimental Hypnosis 46: 77–91

Ewin D M 1986 Emergency room hypnosis for the burned patient. American Journal of Clinical Hypnosis 29: 7–12

Folkman S, Lazarus R S 1980 An analysis of coping in a middle-aged community sample. Journal of Health and Social Behavior 21: 219–239

Hart R R 1980 The influence of taped hypnotic induction treatment procedure on the recovery of surgery patients. International Journal of Clinical and Experimental Hypnosis 28: 324–332

Kessler R 1997 The consequences of individual differences in preparation for surgery and invasive medical procedures. Hypnos: Swedish Journal for Hypnosis in Psychotherapy and Psychosomatic Disorders 24: 181–192

Kessler R, Dane J 1996 Psychological and hypnotic preparation for anaesthesia and surgery: An individual differences perspective. International Journal of Clinical and Experimental Hypnosis 44: 189–207

Lester N, Keefe F J 1997 Coping with chronic pain. In: Baum A, Newman S, Weinman J, West R, McManus C (eds) Cambridge handbook of psychology, health and medicine. Cambridge University Press, Cambridge, p 87–90

Melzack R 1975 The McGill Pain Questionnaire: Major properties and scoring methods. Pain 1: 277–299

Melzack R, Wall P D 1965 Pain mechanisms: A new theory. Science 50: 971–979

Rainville P, Duncan G H, Price D D et al 1997 Pain affect encoded in human anterior cingulate but not somatosensory cortex. Science 277: 968–971

Rosenstiel A K, Keefe F J 1983 The use of coping strategies in chronic low back pain patients: Relationships to patient characteristics and current adjustment. Pain 17: 34–44

Wall P D 1978 The gate control theory of pain mechanisms: A re-examination and a restatement. Brain 101: 1–18

Wall P D 1999 Pain: The science of suffering. Weidenfeld and Nicolson, London

Weisenberg M 1998 Cognitive aspects of pain. International Journal of Clinical and Experimental Hypnosis 46: 44–61

27

Hypnosis and cancer

INTRODUCTION

In terms of physical health and illness, one diagnosis that people seem to dread most of all is being informed that they have cancer. No single person is exempt from the possibility that this will happen at some point in his or her life. In the UK, one in every three people will develop cancer and one in every four people will die with cancer (Department of Health 2000). This means that every year over 200 000 people are diagnosed with cancer and 120 000 will die with cancer in them. Not surprisingly then, cancer is the most researched of all illnesses.

PERSONALITY, STRESS AND CANCER

From ancient times, due acknowledgement has been given to the interaction of mind and body in the understanding and treatment of illness.

Hippocrates ($c.460-c.377$ BC), the father of medicine, said:

Whatever happens in the mind influences the body, and vice versa. In fact mind and body cannot be considered independently one from the other. He would rather know what sort of a person has a disease than what sort of a disease a person has.

Plato ($c.428-c.348$ BC) had similar advice for physicians:

Let no one persuade you to cure the head until he has first given you his soul to be cured, for this is the great error of our day in the treatment of the human body, that physicians first separate the soul from the body.

From the time of Galen ($c.130-c.201$ AD), it has been speculated that people of a certain personality type are more likely to develop cancer. In the last three decades, there has been an increasing awareness of the importance of emotion and stress in the management and prognosis of cancer sufferers. How much psychological factors play a part in aetiology remains speculative. Research has found some support for the so-called 'Type C', cancer-prone, personality (Eysenck 1994). Major characteristics are suppression of feelings such as anger, passivity in the face of stress and a need to conform. It is not possible for us to review the whole literature here but we can note, for example, that Cooper & Faragher (1993), in a study of 2163 women, showed that certain coping strategies and personality dispositions were associated with a reduced risk of developing breast cancer following a major life event such as bereavement or other loss. This was particularly so if individuals were unable to externalise their emotions and obtain appropriate help and counselling. Regular exposure to stressful situations appeared to reduce the risk of a malignancy. Pettingale (1983), in a controlled study of 160 women, found stress and suppression of anger were significant factors only in women aged under 50 years. Also, the same study showed no greater tendency for women who had experienced stressful life events to develop breast cancer than benign lumps in the breast.

Advances in our understanding of the genetic components of human behaviour and emotional expression, together with similar discoveries in the field of cancer, suggest there may be linked genes associated with the cancer-prone personality. However, in the experience of KKA, who has been running a cancer support group for the past 15 years, the intimation that the patient's personality and style of emotional expression may be linked to the development of cancer is very destructive for the patient's mood, anxiety, self-esteem and motivation.

Related to this are the communications that follow when a person has been diagnosed with cancer (see below). The fear of failure in handling stressful situations, which may jeopardise the patient's sense of control, will generate further guilt in addition to the guilt of failure in the first place that the patient has let everyone down by contracting the disease.

Nevertheless, attention to 'the mind' must remain an important factor in any conventional treatment. One could say that this is the 'cement' and the conventional methods are the 'bricks' in building the 'wall against cancer'. When there are no bricks, the cement plays the main part in its treatment.

PSYCHONEUROIMMUNOLOGY

In modern terms, what we have been talking about here is the field of psychoneuroimmunology, the interaction between psychological processes, the nervous system, the immune system and, in the clinical context, vulnerability to illness and recovery therefrom (Walker & Eremin 1995).

Spontaneous regression of malignant tumours and anecdotal miraculous cures have been known since ancient times. Since the initial use of vaccination for smallpox by Edward Jenner during the late 18th century, and a century later the discovery of antibodies by Emil von Bering and Shbasaburo Kitasato, ideas have been floated concerning the possibility of a vaccination against tumours. Around 1960, details of lymphocytes were revealed, resulting in great advances in immunology and our understanding of how the immune system attacks and destroys not only foreign antigens but also tumour cells. For detailed information on lymphocytes, their complex and intriguing genesis, maturity, immuno-specificity, chemodynamics and self-induced and self-regulated inter-functioning, the interested reader is referred to Janeway & Travers (1996).

The main players in tumour destruction are lymphocytes matured in the thymus gland (T cells) of which the large granular null cells, called natural killer (NK) cells, form the first line of defence. NK cells are spontaneous tumour killers (cytotoxic), while the involvement of macrophages and sensitisation by helper T cells releases cytokines (lymphokines) such as γ-interferon and interleukin 2 that help in the process of enhancing anti-tumour activity (Guillou 1988). This is exploited in immunotherapy by the in-vitro production of lymphokine-activated killer cells from lymphocytes taken from cancer patients.

One key factor that provides a rationale for psychoneuroimmunology is the distinction between the sympathetic adrenal medullary (SAM) system and the hypothalamic pituitary adrenal (HPA) system. Both systems are activated by what we loosely call 'stressors' and are intrinsic to survival by mobilising the organism to more effectively recognise and deal with challenge and danger.

In very simple terms, the SAM system is associated with the organism's response to an immediate challenge and involves the release of the hormones adrenalin and noradrenalin. The HPA system is thought to be associated with chronic stress, or stress that the organism is incapable of countering effectively, and involves the release of steroid hormones, notably cortisol. For present purposes, we need only state that activation of the SAM system appears to promote a temporary 'up-regulation' of certain immunological functions (this makes sense in survival terms) whereas activation of the HPA system may result in 'down-regulation' through the immunosuppressive effect of cortisol.

In the above, doubtlessly oversimplified terms, we are provided with a basis for predicting that chronic stress, particularly when associated with helplessness on the individual's part, may have a measurable adverse effect on immunological functioning and render the individual more vulnerable to illness and less able to recover. (In the latter case, 'stress' includes the effects and consequences of the illness itself, and the person's reaction to these.) However, we must not forget that there is a myriad of contributory factors relating to the individual's personality, lifestyle, environment, genetic predispositions, and so on. Readers are referred to Ader, Felton & Cohen (1991) and Fox & Newberry (1984) for a more detailed discussion of the subject.

It is not surprising, then, that researchers have endeavoured to discover if immunological functioning is affected by stress and by methods intended to alleviate it, such as relaxation and self-hypnosis. There are many such studies and it is not possible to review them here. Examples are Bartrop et al (1977) and Jemmot et al (1983) and, from the hypnosis literature, Bongarz et al (1987), Johnson et al (1996) and Ruzyla-Smith et al (1995).

Neither is it surprising that clinical investigations have been undertaken to determine if stressful life events (and, importantly, the individual's coping mechanisms) play any part in the aetiology of illnesses such as cancer (see earlier). Additionally, during the past three decades, great interest has been shown in the use of psychological methods, including hypnotic techniques, in the everyday management of cancer patients, and controlled studies have been conducted to evaluate such methods. Fawzy et al (1995) reviewed four major psychosocial interventions, namely education, behavioural training, individual psychotherapy and group interventions. These approaches have been found to benefit patients in terms of improved psychological well-being and quality of life, and extended survival period, as well as increased tolerance of treatments having unpleasant physical and psychological side effects. Accounts of this research are found in Fawzy et al (1990), Grossarth-Maticek et al (1984), Spiegel et al (1989), and Spiegel & Moore (1997). Active in this field have been Professor Leslie Walker (formerly of the University of Aberdeen, now at the University of Hull) and his colleagues and we summarise some of their findings below.

In the hypnosis literature, there has for many years been an interest in whether immunological activity may be directly influenced by suggestion and imagery. (For positive results see, for example, Black (1963) and Olness et al (1989), referred to in Ch. 25.) The clinical counterpart of this is often referred to simply as 'visualisation'. Simonton et al (1978) popularised the idea of healing by this means in their book *Getting Well Again*, which still provides a resource for many people who want to embark on helping cancer patients. Patients are instructed to visualise their host defences devouring and destroying malignant cells, either using prescribed images or, possibly better still, by creating their own metaphorical imagery.

Such techniques have formed a component of a therapeutic programme offered by Walker and his colleagues. They carried out a controlled clinical trial of relaxation plus guided imagery in 96 women with locally advanced breast cancer (Walker et al 1999). The intervention had beneficial effects on quality of life, mood and coping. In addition, the intervention brought about statistically significant changes in host defences, although this did not translate into prolonged survival 5 years after diagnosis (Walker et al 2000b). However, in a long-term study of 63 patients with lymphoma (with a mean follow-up period of 13 years 9 months), patients who had been randomised to relaxation, with or without hypnosis, as an adjunctive therapy for chemotherapy side effects, survived significantly longer than those receiving standard supportive care (Walker 1998, Walker et al 2000a).

THE IMPORTANCE OF COMMUNICATION IN THE MANAGEMENT AND TREATMENT OF THE CANCER PATIENT

All those who are involved with cancer patients should receive training in how to communicate with them in the best possible way. In the experience of KKA, a large proportion of the 'suffering' reported by patients and their families is due to what is said to them, the unwitting choice of the wrong words at the wrong time as well as the omission of what they really want to know. In particular, the communications at the time of the first encounter between the patient and the specialist can affect the patient's whole quality of life from then on. The anger and hurt that inevitably result from poor communication are largely the responsibility of the professionals.

Twenty-five centuries after Hippocrates' declaration (see above), the UK government has finally taken on board the importance of communication, as revealed in the NHS Plan (Department of Health 2000, p. 13):

We want patients and their family to be confident that they will receive the information, support and specialist care they need to help them with cancer, from the time that cancer is suspected throughout the subsequent stages of the disease. ... By 2002 it will be a pre-condition of qualification to deliver patient care in the NHS that staff are able to demonstrate competence in communication with patients. And for cancer we shall give staff additional training in communication skills, and in the provision of psychological support.

It is not the intention of this book to give details on how to break bad news to the patient, and the reader may refer to Buckman (1989) for guidance on this. The crucial points to remember when communicating with a newly diagnosed cancer patient can be summarised as follows:

- Patients will be unprepared, the news may well be the greatest shock that they have ever had, and they will remain in a state of disbelief and non-communication for some time – hours or even days.
- It is important to ensure that the interview is conducted in the best environment for the *patient*, one in which the patient can feel in control and supported, rather than vulnerable – for example, if possible seated, fully dressed and accompanied by relatives.
- The professional should endeavour to be calm and empathically receptive to anything that the patient would like to discuss, allowing plenty of time and, though an authority on the problem, never appearing *authoritarian*.
- The professional should carefully and gently attempt to find out all the things the patient and family wish to discuss at that very moment,

saying no more and no less than required, and helping the patient feel that he or she has overall control while the professional is there to give the best of advice, guidance and support.

• Information is shared with (not *told to*) the patient and others present, using language they will understand and with repetition, rephrasing and, where appropriate, the use of diagrams. This should be done patiently as many times as is required, and all details should be given. If necessary, this may be done in stages over several sessions, at the patient's own pace.

• Whatever is to be done (further investigations, treatment, etc.) should be precisely specified, and every opportunity given for instilling hope and the reassurance of effective management, continuous help and care, and the best possible quality of life.

So what happens when a person is told by the doctor, 'It is cancer'? These are some of the feelings commonly expressed by many cancer patients: 'All lights (of life) go out'; 'Complete darkness surrounds'; 'Everything worked for, everything being built, everything wished and wanted to have – meaning *everything* – is shattered into smithereens'; 'Everything in life stops dead. What now?'; 'Failed to escape from the dreaded. Now feel trapped and condemned to die without mercy'; 'Feels like inside the worst prison, while all the others are outside'; 'So different from all other people – a social outcast'; 'Ashamed'; 'Unworthy'; 'Guilty'.

They are confused and shocked. They feel guilty because they have failed in what everybody should try to win. They feel isolated, sad and hurt, and very angry about becoming such a loser. They drag up all their past failures and mishaps to make themselves out to be the worst person in the world. They are frightened about the inevitable suffering that they have to go through before they die, and that fear is beyond any description. They start grieving about their own death, and the mental pain is too much as they bring grief from the past, increasing their sense of abandonment. No amount of surgery, radiotherapy or chemotherapy can deal with all of this.

They need to know so many things because they are frantically searching for something, the tiniest straw, that will give them hope; *hope that will change how they feel, however small that change may be.* This is essential to any treatment. *Any statement however justified, that will destroy that hope has no place in the dealings with cancer patients. The same applies to anything that reminds them that they are dying.*

These patients have many questions that the doctors should try to answer truthfully, otherwise trust is destroyed. If there is no answer, one should say so. Worst of all is if the doctor gives a simple answer about the exact amount of time that patients have before they die, as it is the commonest question most patients would ask. Instead, the answer should be 'Nobody can be sure'. If the patient and the family wish to know the statistics, they can be told them, but the statistics are only probabilities: *there can and always will be exceptions.*

PSYCHOLOGICAL APPROACHES IN TREATMENT

All of this paves the way for introducing the patient to the psychological therapy. The metaphors used in the treatment of grief in this book (see Ch. 13) have been found (by KKA) to be extremely helpful in moving the patient away from the preoccupation with dying towards the idea of getting on with life and making it the best that it can be. The story of the villager who goes to hell and heaven (Ch. 13) is useful in demonstrating that, although the chief knew the exact day on which he was going to die, with the hope of cheating the angels he lived productively up to the last minute as if he were never going to die. Cancer patients need help to be aware that they are living *now*; they do not know the exact time of their death but they will know when they are 'there'. Therefore, they will want to concentrate on what they can do for the best the whole way along their journey.

Those patients who feel hopeless and helpless are ready to accept the philosophy that *they are not dead yet, nor dying, but they are living – yes, with a serious problem.* This is because they are looking for a ray of hope that will enable them to take control of the course of their life. This attitude helps them to get back into living their life again, emotionally, personally and socially.

At this point, the principles of psychoneuroimmunology are introduced in a language that patients will understand, likewise hypnosis and how it can help them. While all efforts are made to instil a positive attitude, it is essential to address any unresolved issues, including those from the past, as it is inevitable that these will take up a prominent place in the patients' emotional preoccupations. However, because they are shocked and confused, they are usually not immediately able to engage in such work.

Accordingly, the therapist (KKA) uses various metaphors to motivate the depressed patient. For example, a cartwheel is drawn with each segment representing different aspects of life – personal, social, sexual, relationships, professional, financial, etc. For the smooth and efficient running of the wheel, *all* of its segments should be given equal care and attention, rather than just one segment, namely cancer. When the wheel turns, as it has to do, non-stop, in life, it will break down when any unattended segment is on the ground bearing the weight. Another metaphor is that of filling a bucket with water; if there are holes in the bottom of it, all efforts to fill it will be wasted and so it is important to mend all the holes. The water represents all the positive measures taken, while the holes are the still unresolved negative influences. Patients are thus encouraged to open up and talk about anything that is bothering them – from the past, in the present, or anticipated in the future. Usually there is no holding back; indeed, the therapist (KKA) has never had a patient who rejected this suggestion. The therapist helps the patient resolve those issues using counselling and other psychotherapeutic methods including hypnotic techniques as described elsewhere in this book.

The applications of hypnosis with cancer patients

Hypnosis can be of value in the treatment of cancer in the following respects:

- General relaxation using self-hypnosis
- The control of anxiety and other negative emotions
- Ego-strengthening
- The creation of a sense of personal control over the disease by the use of imagery of self-healing, thus encouraging hope of containment of the tumour and combating the fear of failure of conventional treatment and of the return of the cancer
- The facilitation of radiotherapy and chemotherapy by the reduction of undesirable side effects
- The facilitation of anaesthesia, operative procedures (possibly by reducing bleeding), postoperative analgesia, and postoperative recovery
- Enhancing motivation by future rehearsal, thus helping replace the preoccupation with dying with ideas of a return to a productive lifestyle
- More general pain management.

Hypnotic procedures

One of us (KKA) has developed an approach which includes all of the above in one 15-minute self-hypnosis session that can be taught individually or in groups of any number. A tape recording of the initial session may be used with any patient who is physically too weak. Family members can be included, as they can substitute the suggested imagery of healing with that of staying strong to care for the patient. The therapy may also help them to cope better with their grief when their loved one dies.

Outline and preparation

The pre-induction discussion starts with establishing a clear understanding of the contents of the self-hypnosis exercise. Even with group therapy, this stage should still be undertaken on an individual basis. For ego-strengthening, it is necessary to explore those things that patients are or used to be good at, great or small. Patients are then shown how this material will be used during hypnosis by demonstrating how they can wholeheartedly celebrate all those good things. Patients may see themselves standing with their arms raised, waving their fists and shouting aloud, for example, 'I celebrate that I am good at loving everybody'.

The rest of the fantasy is carried out in an imaginary place. This is any place that they enjoy and value and find relaxing, and they must create it for themselves. It is not unusual to come across patients who have difficulties with imagination or fantasy, perhaps, for example, because they have been made to regard fantasy as being childish, and the exercise may therefore be embarrassing for them. These inhibitions can easily be overcome if the therapist describes what other patients have come up with, but it should be insisted that they use their own special imagery, the more fanciful the better, as long as it fulfils the above requirements. The same principle is used in constructing all further imagery.

The use of places or events from past experience is usually avoided for the following reasons. First, when patients bring to mind wonderful memories of their past, it is inevitable that they will feel sad as it is unlikely that they will have such a good time again. Second, *creative* fantasising may encourage a more profound trance experience (i.e. greater absorption) and it reinforces the idea that they are in charge; they are not to allow any other human being into the image because such intrusion will only restrict their freedom and mean potentially unhappy compromises. It is a good idea for patients to give a name to the place, such as 'magic place' or 'special place'. In cancer patients, words like 'peaceful', 'safe' and 'secure' may not be appropriate as these could imply the ultimate place, namely heaven.

To help with the removal of negative feelings, the idea of having a 'magic disposal unit' installed in the special place is suggested. For the construction of self-healing imagery, patients are first assisted in devising a metaphor for the cancer from their understanding of the disease. The therapist fills in any gaps for patients and helps them give the tumour an imaginary shape, size and colour, at the same time associating it with vulnerability. Once this is achieved, as in the 'symptom control imagery' we discussed in Chapter 25, patients use this image to create a therapeutic metaphor of how the disease can be effectively dealt with, using the best methods or agents, even special or magic things from their own special or magic place, as long as it is without the slightest doubt that success will be achieved. Patients may incorporate images of their natural defence systems – white cells, NK cells, etc. – as part of the metaphor, appearing in any shape and form that they fancy. Ideas derived from their understanding of how the surgery, chemotherapy or radiotherapy works also can be included, with the suggestion that these are all working together as a combined and united force, helping each other while at the same time each one is being sufficiently destructive by itself. This combination helps to remove any irrational anxiety on the patient's part as to whether psychological techniques may interfere with the patient's conventional treatment. Indeed, it may help patients feel that they are able to contribute to this by mobilising their own internal resources to the best possible advantage.

The next stage of the procedure may be directed towards the idea of neutralising the undesirable side effects of treatment, or facilitating surgery or other methods. This is done by rehearsal in imagination of the procedures in question, as described in the section on the use of hypnosis for labour and delivery in Chapter 28. That is, the patient imagines undergoing the full treatment from the initial preparation through to (where relevant) anaesthesia, surgery or other intervention, postoperative recovery (lack of pain, absence of side effects, etc.) and on to the final successful stage.

As always, the details of the imagery have to be individualised for each patient, illness and procedure and we leave that to the creative ability of readers and their patients. It is important that the therapist should have a full understanding of the clinical nature of the illness and the mode of action of the treatment in order to assist the patient in becoming well versed in them. Images and suggestions incorporated into the procedure may include the idea that every single ray of radiotherapy is targeted only at the tumour cells, likewise every molecule of the chemotherapy treatment; the installation of mechanisms to protect the healthy tissue; increased appetite (providing extra energy to help the healing and the rebuilding of health); the idea that the patient's own scavenger system is working overtime in efficiently removing debris and cleaning up the site, (so that the dead and decaying tumour is not left to rot in the body to make the patient feel sick); and disposal of all the waste in the urine and stool.

The therapist should be aware of the fact that not all patients are capable of visualising the images; they may use other modalities such as auditory or somatosensory or a mixture, but this does not make any difference and therefore one does not have to insist on visualisation only.

During age progression, patients may imagine their future selves engaged in routine activities as well as special events, while appearing contented and in good health. They may be reminded that the image that they create of their future self will be older than the person who is sitting in the chair, will be wearing different clothes, and so on, thus making them different from the patient doing the hypnosis, since depressed and demoralised patients may ask themselves, 'How can this poor specimen of a being ever become that person in the future?' The future may be immediate or extend into a ripe old age.

The hypnosis session

After the therapist has made sure that patients have a clear understanding of what is expected of them during the hypnotic session, they are invited to sit with both feet on the floor and to keep their eyes closed for the entire duration of hypnosis. Then they are asked to take a deep breath and to breathe out slowly and deliberately while listening to the sound of their breathing and thinking about something wonderful. In groups, it is emphasised that they should ignore the others and 'be selfish', focusing their attention on themselves only. When they have done this three or four times, their attention is drawn to the movements of their breathing, including the feel of their breath, while they breathe very slowly. Their attention is drawn to the experience of relaxation that is gradually spreading through their entire body. After the third breath, they are asked to *watch* their breath by imagining that the surrounding air is their favourite colour. While they are doing so, they can see it filling their lungs (if they cannot visualise this, they can certainly think of it happening) and spreading very quickly through their entire body, calming every part on the way, at the same time removing every bit of tension from their body and mind. (The therapist names all the important parts, including the brain and mind.) All the time, their attention is drawn to how well they are relaxing while they breathe in and out, as they can hear, feel and see all the tension being blown away, until they have the most wonderful experience that their body is feeling deeply relaxed, much more than they ever expected.

In the experience of KKA, this method of induction is well suited to this kind of therapy and has never failed to produce effective, if not always very deep, relaxation in all kinds of patients, especially cancer patients, who are often physically debilitated and have poor concentration, and even in groups of anything up to 40 people. With regular practice, deep relaxation is achieved after three breaths of listening, feeling and 'watching'.

Then patients are asked to 'float away' or simply be in their prearranged magic place. There, they are invited to explore and spend a short while enjoying that very private, exclusive relaxing place, where they can do whatever they like and be whatever they wish without any intrusions or restrictions from anything or anybody.

They are then guided towards the 'magic disposal unit' and encouraged to symbolically dispose of all the 'negative baggage' that they are carrying from the past or present. It is surprising that many of the patients achieve this goal so easily, unless the events associated with the negative emotion are too profound. If the latter is the case, then they may be invited to talk about such events so that the therapist can help them to resolve them.

Then is the time for ego-strengthening. Patients are invited to celebrate at least ten things that they are good at, while thinking of their resourcefulness behind each one, and to anchor those feelings using any standard techniques.

Being void of negative emotions, refilled with good ego-strength, and confidently motivated, patients are guided to the healing imagery and, if appropriate, future rehearsal of their medical or surgical treatment. For control of pain, ideas of isolating the tumour, for example by building steel or concrete walls around it, and cutting off the blood supply and all the nerves connected to it, may be more than enough to address the problem of pain. Additionally, however, any technique of pain control described in Chapter 26 may be included in the imagery.

Some patients create the images of healing and treatment in a symbolic body or object *outside* their own body, while others are comfortable imagining this going on inside them. It is important to let them have their own preferred way, but it is also necessary in the former approach, that they connect the imagery to themselves by experiencing the benefits and the results of what they are creating in their imagination.

Finally, the patient is age progressed to a successful outcome and reminded that the future person is indeed himself or herself. Thus patients can appreciate the result of all their hard work. They are then asked to reach out to their future self and to make the connection by feeling really pleased about that person while the latter is thanking them for all the good work they have done, without which that person would not be what he or she is now (i.e. in the future).

While anchoring that image, patients are asked to open their eyes and re-orientate to the immediate surroundings. The whole package is briefly explained once more and patients are asked to practise the procedure as many times as possible. It may be taped if the patient is too debilitated. Follow-up sessions are used to repeat the procedure, to fill in gaps or change inappropriately framed suggestions or imagery, and to introduce alterations that allow for progress or any new developments. Thus, the package functions as a versatile platform on which any variation of the play can be staged. Hence, it can be used for any organic disease.

Therapists working with cancer patients, especially when using these kinds of methods, run the risk of problems concerning emotional attachment or dependency and transference and counter-transference issues. Hence, it is a good idea that they have a supervisor who can help them handle these situations should they arise.

REFERENCES

Ader R, Felton D L, Cohen N 1991 Psychoneuroimmunology, 2nd edn. Academic Press, San Diego
Bartrop R, Lazarus L, Luckhurst E et al 1977 Depressed lymphocyte function after bereavement. Lancet 1: 834–836
Black S 1963 Inhibition of immediate-type hypersensitivity response by direct suggestion under hypnosis. British Medical Journal 1: 925–929
Bongarz W, Lyncker I, Kossman K T 1987 The influence of hypnosis on white blood cell count and urinary levels of catecholamines and vanillyl mandelic acid. Hypnos: Swedish Journal for Hypnosis in Psychotherapy and Psychosomatic Disorders 14: 52–61
Buckman R 1989 Communicating with cancer patients. The Practitioner 233: 1393–1396
Cooper C L, Faragher E B 1993 Psychosocial stress and breast cancer: The inter-relationship between stress events, coping strategies and personality. Psychological Medicine 23: 653–662

Department of Health 2000 NHS Cancer Plan: A plan for investment, a plan for reform. Department of Health, London

Eysenck H J 1994 Cancer, personality and stress. Advances in Behaviour Research and Therapy 16: 167–215

Fawzy F I, Kemeny M E, Fawzy N W et al 1990 A structured psychiatric intervention for cancer patients. II. Changes over time in immunological measures. Archives of General Psychiatry 47: 729–735

Fawzy F I, Fawzy N W, Arndt L A, Pasnau R O 1995 Critical review of psychosocial interventions in cancer care. Archives of General Psychiatry 52: 100–113

Fox B H, Newberry B H 1984 Impact of psychoendocrine systems in cancer and immunity. C J Hogrefe, New York

Grossarth-Maticek R, Schmidt P, Vetter H, Arndt S 1984 Psychotherapy research in oncology. In: Steptoe A, Matthews A (eds) Health care and human behaviour. Academic Press, London, p 325–341

Guillou P J 1988 Immunological approaches to the treatment of malignant diseases. Journal of the Royal College of Surgeons (Edinburgh) 33 (Feb.): 2–8

Janeway C A, Travers P (eds) 1996 Immunobiology, 2nd edn. Churchill Livingstone, London

Jemmot J B, Borysenko L Z, Borysenko M et al 1983 Academic stress, power motivation and decrease in secretion rate of salivary secretory immunoglobulin A. Lancet 2: 1400–1402

Johnson V C, Walker L G, Heys S D et al 1996 Can relaxation training and hypnotherapy modify the immune response to stress, and is hypnotisability relevant? Contemporary Hypnosis 13: 100–108

Olness K N, Culbert T, Uden D L 1989 Self-regulation of salivary immunoglobulin A by children. Pediatrics 83: 66–71

Pettingale K W 1983 Stress and cancer. Update July 1: 34

Ruzyla-Smith P, Barabasz A, Barabasz M, Warner D 1995 Effects of hypnosis on the immune response: B cells, T cells, helper and suppressor cells. American Journal of Clinical Hypnosis 38: 71–79

Simonton O C, Matthews-Simonton S, Creighton C 1978 Getting well again. J P Tarcher, Los Angeles

Spiegel D, Moore R 1997 Imagery and hypnosis in the treatment of cancer patients. Oncology 11: 1179–1189

Spiegel D, Bloom J R, Kraemer H C et al 1989 Effect of psychosocial treatment on survival of patients with metastatic breast cancer. Lancet 2: 888–891

Walker L G 1998 Hypnosis and cancer: Host defences, quality of life and survival. Contemporary Hypnosis 15: 34–39

Walker L G, Eremin O 1995 Psychoneuroimmunology: A new fad or the fifth cancer treatment modality? American Journal of Surgery 170: 2–4

Walker L G, Walker M B, Heys S D et al 1999 The psychological, clinical and pathological effects of relaxation training and imagery during primary chemotherapy. British Journal of Cancer 80: 262–268

Walker L G, Ratcliffe M A, Dawson A A 2000a Relaxation and hypnotherapy: Long term effects on the survival of patients with lymphoma. Psycho Oncology 9: 355–356

Walker M B, Walker L G, Simpson E et al 2000b Do relaxation and guided imagery improve survival in women with locally advanced breast cancer? Psycho Oncology 9: 355

FURTHER READING

The value of hypnosis in the treatment of cancer was acknowledged by the dedication of issues 2 and 3 of Volume 25 (1982–1983) of the American Journal of Clinical Hypnosis to 'Hypnosis and cancer'.

Hypnosis in obstetrics and gynaecology

PROLOGUE

Thy faith hath made thee whole: go in peace.

(St Luke, ch 8, vs 44–48)

Jesus thus spoke to a woman who came and fell down before him, trembling and declaring to him before all the people for what cause she had touched him and how she was healed immediately. Jesus was on his way to the house of Jairus, the ruler of the synagogue, to heal his daughter who lay dying. People thronged around him. The woman, who had had 'an issue of blood' for 12 years and had spent all her wealth on physicians with no betterment, touched his garment. Immediately, she stopped bleeding. Jesus asked who had touched him but nobody owned up, as a multitude of people was pressing around him. When he insisted that someone had touched him, as he felt that 'virtue' had gone out of him, the woman came forward, finding herself no longer hidden in the crowd.

In this chapter, we shall review the role of hypnosis in obstetrics and in the treatment of certain gynaecological problems. We shall first consider the range of applications in obstetric practice in chronological order, from the problems of conceiving through to labour and childbirth itself. Under problems of conceiving, we could include psychosexual difficulties but these are considered in Chapter 31 along with other psychological disorders.

INFERTILITY

Throughout history, beliefs and expectations, bolstered with faith, have shown great influence in the healing of 'women's complaints', no more so than in the search for remedies for infertility. Many writers consider that anxiety may sometimes contribute to either primary or secondary infertility, because of the interaction between stress and hormonal and immunological factors, and there is evidence to support this (Edelmann & Connolly 1986, Sanders & Bruce 1999). As long as a significant level of anxiety remains for whatever reason, there is the possibility of infertility. The anxiety may itself be related to the failure to conceive (Edelmann & Golombok 1989, Newton et al 1999, Pook et al 1999). Indeed, in the experience of one of us (KKA), it is not unusual for patients with fertility problems to conceive following the successful treatment of difficulties such as phobias, unresolved grief, panic attacks, depression and chronic constipation, using hypnosis for relaxation, ego-strengthening and psychodynamic exploration. Although these are only informal observations, they sometimes involve patients who have been unable to become pregnant after years of trying and when all investigations have failed. They request hypnosis for their other problems and assume that nothing more can be done for their infertility.

Some of the underlying psychological issues may be described by patients themselves, such as trauma associated with childbirth, either witnessed in the case of primary infertility, or self-experienced in the case of secondary infertility. Very occasionally, patients experience severe guilt for the traumatic labour that their mother experienced during their birth and the ill-health that followed, which their mother constantly reminds them of by blaming the birth. These patients often do not associate such trauma or guilt with infertility, though the associated emotion remains very strong. For some aspiring parents, there may be fears concerning the responsibilities of parenthood, the effects on their relationship of sharing a baby, and so on.

Patients may request hypnosis as a treatment for infertility by itself or as an adjunct to a trial of drugs or in-vitro fertilisation (IVF). Where psychosocial stress and anxiety are evident, then hypnotic procedures such as relaxation, ego-strengthening and self-hypnosis may be used. In addition, direct questioning during hypnosis concerning possible psychological contributions to the infertility may reveal issues such as those mentioned above. At other times, psychodynamic techniques such as ideomotor signalling may be used, as the cause may not be fully acknowledged at a conscious level.

In addition, the patient may be educated about ovulation and the process of conception. Such education is important in assisting with grief associated with miscarriage, in order to clear up any misunderstandings and inappropriate self-blame. Counselling programmes for infertile couples usually involve education in identifying the 3-day ovulation period by taking daily body temperature and having intercourse on those 3 days. The male partner is also advised on the optimal frequency and timing of intercourse in order to promote the greatest likelihood of conception.

To minimise anxiety during intercourse, posthypnotic suggestions may be given that pregnancy is a natural phenomenon and it will happen automatically; there is no need to *try to make it happen*. The most important thing the couple has to remember while making love is that it is done for pleasure, joy and, above all, the expression of their love for each other, 'sending the right signals to nature to do its part'.

The female partner, in particular, can be taught to imagine during hypnosis how to remain relaxed 'so the most natural thing that can happen to any woman – that is, to be pregnant – can happen spontaneously and naturally'. Guide the imagery as follows, adding and adapting it to the needs of the individual.

You are experiencing – by seeing, feeling and thinking – one of your ovaries. ... I don't know if it is the right or the left one, but *you* may know ... and it is releasing a healthy ovum (*or egg*). The ovum is caught by the hand-like end of the tube and is making its way to the womb. Its journey through the tube is taking 3 days, during which healthy sperm are meeting the ovum in the tube. You know that it is the best place for fertilisation to happen, this unique event of the start of your baby's life, by the entry of the healthiest sperm, so lovingly into your ovum ... the perfect union. You can see the fertilised ovum triumphantly entering the womb that is already well prepared to receive it with love and affection. The baby is now settling in very comfortably, but firmly attached to the top part to remain there for the full term. The baby is expecting ... and you, the mother, are giving ... all that is needed for him or her to grow into a beautiful and healthy baby, and also exchanging the best of love and affection and ... that most powerful feeling of being wanted.

During this imagery, the patient may reveal any problematic issues and the therapist must be observant for this and help the patient resolve them. Similar ideas may be applied, with suitable modifications, with patients undergoing an IVF programme.

We must not forget that the male partner may be under stress also, and it is important that this is addressed, since it is believed that stress in males may reduce fertility (see earlier references). He may also approach intercourse with anxieties because of worries about conceiving. Timing intercourse with the partner's ovulation cycle itself may be associated with 'pressure to perform'. He may himself have emotional concerns about being a father and sharing his partner with a child. As with his partner, these anxieties may relate to his relationship with his own parents.

The following are some examples from the caseload of one of the authors (KKA). We acknowledge that in none of these patients can it be *proved* that conception would not have occurred had it not been for hypnosis.

Case examples

Mia, a patient in her late 20s, approached the therapist with a problem of severe constipation. She was free of any physical abnormality but she was very anxious. Hartland's ego-strengthening and daily self-hypnosis to relax, increased her self-confidence. Later, she was able to ventilate her feelings about her relationship with her employer and her appalling working conditions, about which she was unable to assert herself. Within 3 weeks of self-hypnosis, aided by tape recordings of the three treatment sessions, a mood of calmness, assertiveness and confidence started to infiltrate all aspects of her life. As she began to feel more positive, she stood up to her boss and, to her surprise, things then turned around for the better. Her problem of constipation disappeared. Four months from the start of the therapy, she conceived for the first time; she then disclosed to the therapist that she and her husband had been trying for a family for the previous 8 years and had given up.

Natasha, a woman aged 31, was seen for panic attacks. Her explanation for the episodes was that she was having thoughts that earthquakes were going to happen where she lived and where she went on holiday. This fear prevented her from having any social life and she became more and more housebound and miserable. With the help of her therapist, she learned self-hypnosis with ease. Hartland's ego-strengthening routine was also incorporated. However, she did not show any progress with the panic attacks, even though she developed more positive attitudes in her everyday life. Accordingly, a psychodynamic approach was introduced; the 'jigsaw puzzle visualisation' technique was employed (see Ch. 19). She interpreted the result as indicating that the thoughts of earthquakes were symbolising the abused and unloved childhood she had experienced. Her husband was having a very stressful time at work and he was being unkind and aggressive towards her. At that stage of the therapy, she was able to talk about these problems and this helped her to resolve the anger, fear and hatred that she had been harbouring for many years. As in Mia's case, she became pregnant towards the end of the therapy and she told the therapist that it was a surprise because she and her husband had not been using any contraception during the 7 years since their marriage. After another 2 years, she had a second child.

Grief was the prevailing emotion in other cases of secondary infertility seen by the same therapist. A young woman, Julie, became depressed and lost her libido when her first-born son reached 18 months of age. Both she and her husband wanted another child and they started trying for one. Accordingly, she suppressed her negative feelings because she reasoned that all that was required to become pregnant was to have sexual intercourse. Nothing happened, and all the investigations indicated that there were no physical reasons why she should not conceive. After 2 years, the couple approached the therapist for help using hypnosis. Julie was still depressed. She was able to talk about her feelings for the first time, but only after she had had several sessions of deep relaxation and ego-strengthening. It was then suggested to her during hypnosis that from that time onwards, whenever she practised self-hypnosis, she might find that certain thoughts would repeatedly pass through her mind.

Julie later returned and disclosed that she had had recurring thoughts about her late mother. Her mother died when she was only 3 years of age, but she realised that she was still grieving for her and still feeling very sad. She commented that she was having irrational feelings that her own child was going to be motherless. She then became aware that grief had always been present in her feelings, but had become much stronger when her first child was born. She was afraid of dying, as her mother had done, when her child reached 3 years of age and then would have to go through all the heartache that she herself had experienced. Helping her with her grief (see Ch. 13) resulted in the lifting of her depression and soon she began to enjoy lovemaking. She became pregnant in the natural way.

Unresolved grief can be associated with a previous miscarriage and is often accompanied by anger towards the medical personnel for their insensitive handling of the tragedy. The stress may be inadvertently caused by words spoken, such as losing the 'fetus' instead of the 'baby'. Sometimes the message may be well meant but unhelpful, conveyed in a statement, such as, 'Don't feel bad, you still have time to have another one'; or it may be that nobody paid any attention to the mother's concerns. Also, patients can feel very guilty by making themselves believe that things went wrong because they were inadequate in some way and they indirectly 'caused the death of their baby'.

HYPNOSIS DURING PREGNANCY

When we examine the use of hypnosis during childbirth, we shall see that the mother-to-be will have been preparing for this by the regular practice of self-hypnosis during pregnancy. This practice may have advantages for mother and baby alike. Maternal stress during the prenatal period has been reported to affect fetal blood flow and increase fetal stress (Simkin 1986). Especially in the third trimester, it has also been reported to increase the incidence of obstetric complications such as pre-eclampsia, forceps delivery, prolonged labour, clinical fetal distress and primary postpartum haemorrhage (Crandon 1979).

Fuchs et al (1989) observed increased fetal movements (measured using ultrasound) in mothers who used hypnotic relaxation for their anxiety. The use of hypnosis during pregnancy has also been reported to result in fewer complications (Davenport-Slack 1975) and this may be due to reduced anxiety in the latter stages. Omer et al (1986) have shown, in a controlled study, that the practice of relaxation using hypnosis prolongs the pregnancy in cases of anticipated premature labour. Avoiding premature labour may result in an increase in the birthweight of otherwise low-weight premature babies.

Bonding with the baby

Bonding with the baby can start at any time during pregnancy. This is easily done by asking the expectant mother to converse with the baby inside her. During this, she takes the part of the baby in such a manner that the baby is conversing as an individual who is already in the outside world and is able to see, hear, touch and smell. The baby makes comments on what others are wearing, appreciating the colours of the flowers in the garden, the lovely fragrance of mum's perfume, and so on. The baby may even express disagreement with what mum, dad, siblings or relatives say and do. In the experience of one of us (KKA), this technique could have the potential to reduce anxiety, postnatal depression and sibling jealousy. For example, it is not uncommon for a child to show behavioural problems with the arrival of a new sibling. It may be that this problem can be anticipated and ameliorated by including the existing child as a partner in the pretend conversations. Most importantly, the expectant couple and any existing children will have ample opportunity to express their ideas and any concerns about how the new arrival will fit in with the present lifestyle of the couple or family. Thus, everyone involved will have some idea of how things are going to be well before the baby arrives.

Morning sickness (hyperemesis)

Vomiting is a very common symptom of pregnancy. However, it is possible that anxiety arising, say, from the 'horror stories of labour' may aggravate the symptom. In the experience of one of the authors (KKA), it may be more evident in unwanted or forced pregnancies and paradoxically also in the 'dream-come-true' pregnancies, as both groups of patients may experience a great deal of anxiety. It may also be that pregnancy occurring during a bad phase in the partners' relationship can precipitate severe vomiting, as in a case (seen by KKA) of a woman who was extremely dominated and badly treated by her husband and his family alike. She was seriously in fear of having no control or influence in the upbringing of her child. She could not keep these fears out of her mind, but, at the same time, she felt that she was not capable of doing anything about them.

Fuchs et al (1980) treated 138 women suffering from extremely severe vomiting in the first trimester of pregnancy. The authors used hypnosis with suggestions that the patients would experience calmness, composure and happiness, and that their pregnancy would progress well. A total of 87 of these patients were treated in groups and 51 were treated individually. In the former, no patients were hospitalised, and treatment was easier and more efficient. Altogether 61 patients were cured of vomiting and nausea, 24 were cured of vomiting but still experienced some nausea, and only two patients failed to improve at all.

Treatment involves achieving as profound a state of relaxation as possible and ego-strengthening suggestions are then given. The remaining suggestions are direct and aimed at relaxation and feelings of warmth in the abdomen in order to help the patient feel calm and comfortable. Further suggestions are given of how the baby is enjoying the experience and wanting to share this with the mother, and how much both the mother and baby are looking forward to further hypnosis training for 'the big day' to make everything pass easily and for them both to have a wonderful experience (see later). It is important to resolve any anxiety-provoking issues and to create a sense that the pregnancy is progressing normally. All of this can be rehearsed during self-hypnosis and if necessary put on a tape.

Hypertension during pregnancy

This can also be helped with training in deep relaxation and in the administration of suitable ego-strengthening suggestions. Direct suggestions may be given to imagine that the tension in the arteries is easing. The patient then practises this during self-hypnosis, which can be taped. Hypertension in pre-eclampsia should not be treated with hypnosis alone.

Anticipated premature labour and miscarriage

The principles of treatment are similar to those used for hyperemesis. Therapy consists of relaxation, ego-strengthening, education in the normal progression of pregnancy and labour, and resolution of any past, present and anticipated problems that may generate anxiety. Rehearsal of labour, as described below, with reference to the expected date of delivery, may also be undertaken.

In the case of repeated miscarriages, it is important to explore the possibility of unresolved grief or trauma. It is also of importance to work on the bonding of mother and baby as early as possible in pregnancy and to adhere to the principle that everything in pregnancy and labour is shared equally in a partnership between mother and baby.

PREPARATION FOR LABOUR AND DELIVERY

The use of hypnosis (or mesmerism) for analgesia in childbirth was recorded as early as 1831 (Chertok 1981), but the development of chemical anaesthesia in obstetrics pushed hypnosis into the background. More recently, in the 1970s, the introduction of childbirth education and parent classes, along with relaxation training during the antenatal period, further sidelined hypnosis in the practice of obstetrics.

Research

The search to demonstrate the superiority of hypnosis over the benefits of childbirth education and chemical analgesia began to appear in the 1970s (Harmon et al 1990). However, it may be argued that the inherent inclusion of education in most of the strategies that are used in obstetric hypnosis makes the debate rather futile.

Several recent clinical trials have nevertheless supported the efficacy of training in hypnotic procedures in preparation for childbirth. When hypnosis has been used for relaxation and purposes of analgesia, a significant shortening of the first stage of labour has been reported (Abramson & Heron 1950, Callan 1961, Davidson 1962, Harmon et al 1990). Other studies, however, have shown no difference in the duration of labour (Perchard

1960, Winkelstein 1958) while Freeman et al (1986) found that it was prolonged. However, while it may be true that shorter labour is desirable for the well-being of both mother and baby, measuring length of labour has inherent flaws and its validity as a positive indicator of labour is debatable. One thing is certain: the use of hypnosis reduces, if not removes, the need for medication and chemical analgesia, which are potentially distressing to the mother and baby. Harmon et al (1990) found fetal distress to be less on APGAR scores when hypnosis was used and it reduced the need for operative interventions such as the use of forceps and caesarean section.

Training for labour and delivery

In accordance with our guidelines for good ethical and professional practice, we emphasise that the therapist should be appropriately experienced and trained in obstetric practice.

The training of an expectant mother for the use of hypnosis during labour invariably takes place during pregnancy. Even though, with no prior training, hypnosis may be successfully used during labour or as a method of analgesia, say for episiotomy suturing, this is only so for highly hypnotisable patients. The earlier in pregnancy the training can start, the better prepared will be the expectant mother for the delivery. This also provides ample time for the essential process of education, and gives more opportunity to guide the progress of the pregnancy.

Educating the patient and her partner

It is not appropriate for us to outline the educational component that forms an essential part of the full hypnotherapeutic programme for the mother-to-be. We assume, instead, that readers who intend using hypnosis for these purposes are already trained in the knowledge that is to be imparted to the patient.

To maximise her confidence in the hypnotic approach, it is important to provide the expectant mother with sufficient understanding of the full process of labour, how it should proceed for the best, and how learning hypnotic techniques can make the whole experience as she would like it to be. This should describe exactly what will happen at the precise stages of the labour and delivery and the various roles that the mother, baby, father and obstetric team will take to make the whole delivery an enjoyable, safe and successful experience for all concerned. Therefore, these details will have to be reiterated to the mother-to-be many times so they become, as it were, second nature.

The language used should be appropriate to the level of knowledge of the patient. In most cases, it is better to avoid technical medical terms. For example, it is better to use the word 'baby' rather than 'fetus', as the latter does not connote affection, love, or human attributes; likewise, 'womb' rather than 'uterus', and 'afterbirth' rather than 'placenta'.

An exception to this is the case of a patient seen by one of the authors (KKA) who initially hated the word 'placenta', as her previous labour was premature and complicated owing to, so she was told, 'early separation of placenta'. When the details of the nature and the functions of the placenta were explained to her, and how hypnosis, in theory, might help the placenta to remain attached right up to the third stage, then she wanted to use this word. This was because she could be more precise in forming the imagery. Also, saying the word 'placenta' indicated to her that she was no longer anxious about a repetition of the previous problems.

Hence, the best way of knowing the words to choose is to ask the expectant mother, providing options and their meanings, and thus arriving at a list of terms with which she is comfortable. This will also assist with rapport by enhancing her sense of being in control of the proceedings.

The information provided should be such as to substantiate every instruction or suggestion (hypnotic and non-hypnotic) given. It should be emphasised that hypnosis will enable her to be in control without jeopardising the progress of labour or any other procedures used, while fully cooperating with the obstetric team. This makes it more likely that the instructions will be adhered to, and assists in removing any anxiety and mystique associated with childbirth by the patient and her partner. Any emotional problems may be addressed at the early stages.

Training in hypnosis: standard method

Training in hypnosis can be introduced at any stage of pregnancy, along with the educational component. Teaching self-hypnosis with progressive relaxation and ego-strengthening is the first step. The practice of relaxation on a daily basis may help a trouble-free antenatal period.

It will already have been explained in the educational part that the purpose of contractions during labour is to help the baby's journey by giving the baby that 'loving push'. Therefore, there is no need for any pain. The sensation of pain is merely an interpretation, at the cortical level, of the experience of contraction, as everybody is accustomed to describe contractions as 'pains', just as all such interpretations are learned and become habitual. Thus, the expectant mother will be able to learn to reinterpret the occurrences of contractions as 'squeezing of the womb', like a hand squeezing a rubber ball. From then on, she will experience contractions as only 'contractions' or 'squeezing' (in imagination and at delivery) and not as pain. The word 'pain' in fact will never be used in future rehearsals.

Also, in this particular approach, 'relaxation' is not emphasised; nor need it even be mentioned, as the mother, being in a jubilant mood, will stay confident, calm and composed. She will remain physically active and mentally alert (compare with active–alert hypnosis). This is to avoid any problem of her becoming too placid and deeply relaxed, and therefore unable to 'push' when this is most needed. She will not miss out on the thrill of helping the delivery of her baby. Also, there is thus no need to become deeply relaxed between contractions, and then have to reverse this when doing the pushing.

When the woman attains proficiency in self-hypnosis, a programme of the events of the entire process of labour is constructed, incorporating suggestions provided by the expectant mother. Here, we shall only outline the steps because every case needs to take into consideration the wishes, attitudes and ability of the mother-to-be, her partner, the obstetric team, and so on. It is very useful for her to visit the maternity unit and to meet the staff who might be in attendance. (The therapist or the community midwife need not accompany her.) This assures her that the imagined scene will correspond to the real one.

The delivery can be represented in imagination as a video, with the mother and baby as the main characters. In the video, the mother in labour, of course, looks different from the mother who is having the training; for example, she will be a few months older, she will be wearing different clothes, and her abdomen will be a great deal bigger. The mother may wish to identify the predicted date of delivery as 'the grand day', 'the big day', 'the victory day', or whatever.

This day starts in the imagined video or movie with the waking of the mother and her having breakfast. At the pre-discussed time in that day, the contractions start. That will be the sign from her baby, declaring that it is time for the baby to come out into the wide world, and the baby knows exactly what to do. Always emphasise that it is the baby who decides when to come out and the baby makes his or her own way, whether or not the mother wants this. So the mother's role is simply to lovingly help the baby to come out.

The 'movie' continues with the mother's informing her partner, calling the maternity unit, (or, in the case of home confinements, making the necessary preparations for the arrival of the midwife or doctor), travelling to the maternity unit, being admitted, being introduced to the staff, the setting-up of all the monitoring equipment, and so on. Also, the mother expresses her wishes concerning the way she wants to conduct the delivery.

The contractions progress as they should, the cervix opens and the waters break. The patient stays calm and composed but is full of energy, readily and actively helping the baby make his or her way out and being assisted by everybody. The baby gives out a big yell, announcing a triumphant arrival into the world. The mother herself celebrates the victory, and there are big smiles and congratulations all round. The process of bonding, encouraged during pregnancy, is completed when the baby is put on the mother's body and she holds him or her, likewise when the father also takes hold of the baby. This is followed by an image of her feeding the baby, and doing whatever has been arranged with the staff. Thus, the bonding that started in the antenatal period is reinforced.

Any other items that have been identified during the educational phase may be included, such as the amount of bleeding, the time for the second stage, the severance of the cord, the separation of the placenta, and the final contraction of the uterus. It is important to include every detail and these should remain fairly consistent from one rehearsal to another unless there are compelling reasons to alter the routine.

Once such a detailed fantasy movie is constructed, the patient undergoes hypnosis and imagines it as part of her self-hypnosis. In earlier sessions, the therapist may have to help her by relating the contents of the imagery as a running commentary until she is able to remember the details. Should this prove difficult, one of the sessions (the best one) may be taped and used for self-hypnosis. Whatever method is chosen, it is important to regularly practise self-hypnosis.

Nearer the time of the expected date of delivery, for example at 34 weeks, further imagery is added to the movie relating to the future care of the baby, such as breast feeding (with plenty of milk available) and suggestions of how much hypnosis is helping the child and the mother, how well the baby is accepted by her partner and the rest of the family and relatives, and how much happiness, love and care the baby is enjoying. This reinforces the part of the routine involving only the labour and delivery, as it helps with motivation. In cases of hyperemesis or any other problem during pregnancy, this second stage can be introduced in the strategy for such treatment. When the rehearsal of the first part is going well and there are no problems with the pregnancy itself, then it is only necessary to practise the second part on an occasional basis. The therapist may expand on the themes described if there is time and the patient is able to absorb this information.

The above 'self-hypnosis, imagery rehearsal strategy' helps the expectant mother to be self-sufficient in the use of hypnosis during labour and obviates the need for the therapist to be present during labour. However, it is a real bonus to have the therapist there.

One of us (KKA) has trained a number of women in this manner. Most of them did not involve their partner in the training. All of them did extremely well. One of the mothers, a consultant psychiatrist, commented, 'I was thrilled with the whole experience. When everything was finished I wanted to jump out of bed and run to the pub down the road for a pint'. A few of them even managed to correctly predict the actual timing of labour in the 'self-hypnosis, imagery rehearsal routine'.

Direct methods of hypnoanalgesia

If it is possible to have plenty of practice, then it is not necessary to use hypnoanalgesia as a separate technique, because all contractions will be perceived as such, and not as pains. Even if a little pain is experienced, the mother's pleasure and sense of achievement will over-ride this. Another advantage of this strategy is that even unfamiliar staff cannot disturb the routine. Even if they were to ask about 'labour pains' or otherwise introduce the idea of 'pain', the mother will spontaneously and instantly translate 'pain' into 'contractions' or 'squeezing'. (It is desirable to include posthypnotic suggestions to this effect in the routine.)

Some women, however, will require separate training in producing hypnoanalgesia when episiotomy or any other surgical procedure that might be undertaken during hypnosis is anticipated. Some patients may need such training as a standby, just in case the rehearsed programme is not effective, especially when there has not been much time for practice. In good hypnotic subjects, it may therefore be desirable to train them in pain control, but with the inclusion of essential precautions – for example, when and where they should use it and when they should not use it – by giving a clear explanation of the reasons for it. Even caesarean sections have been performed using hypnosis, but hypnosis will never be anywhere near routine practice. However, episiotomy suturing and the application of forceps are easily undertaken during hypnosis. Techniques of hypnoanalgesia or anaesthesia have been described elsewhere in this book (Ch. 26). Methods of choice are transferral of glove anaesthesia to the desired part, the use of imagery directly involving that part, or rendering the entire body painless by dissociation.

Risks and precautions

Once the patient has received training in the use of hypnosis, most likely she will take full control during labour of how and when it is used, rather than simply adhere to the therapist's instructions. The fact remains that everything owing to hypnosis is made to happen by the subject and not the hypnotist, who can only provide the training. The particular labour will only happen once and there is no guarantee that everything that is taught will be used, even though all seems to be working well during the rehearsals. This includes, in appropriate cases, the suggestion of profound analgesia, which can be tested for efficacy.

Even so, although the expectant mother may be a good subject and the therapist may have given the appropriate instructions, she may wrongly use them if those instructions were given in the mistaken belief that all hypnotic suggestions and posthypnotic suggestions *must* be acted upon.

The mother, at the time of labour, may suddenly lose trust in hypnosis, and decline to use it. Apart from the time that has been wasted, this presents no danger, unless she gives up in the middle of a surgical procedure that is being done solely using hypnoanalgesia.

Nobody should underestimate the function of pain for the protection of the person and the maintenance of alertness to potential danger. In a few individuals, it is easy to produce profound analgesia but if this is not used at the right time and in the right place, appropriate protection and effective performance will be compromised. It is only common sense that in all cases conventional methods should be ready at hand.

The risks are more serious when the patient overdoes the hypnotic relaxation, as a result of which she remains too placid and unhelpful when she should be actively working with the obstetric team. She may use hypnosis in such a manner that she appears to be so relaxed that vital signs of maternal and fetal distress, or the obvious indications of the progression of labour, may be masked and this may mislead the obstetric team. This is less of a problem in hospital, with all the electric monitoring, than in domiciliary deliveries, which are becoming more popular. The ideal situation is therefore for the hypnotist to be one of the obstetric team, and then is on hand to offer guidance as appropriate.

As it is usual for the mother's partner or another family member to be present, he or she should be aware of what the mother has been taught. This person may take an active role in the process by giving the mother carefully chosen reminders to signal the use of hypnosis at the appropriate stages. This role depends on the ability of the person to remain calm and composed. People fulfilling this role will have their own perceptions of what the mother is going through during labour based on their own emotional make-up. The mother will be the better judge as she will be concentrating on the labour itself and what is best for her and the baby, and she is likely to put other emotions into the background until after the delivery.

Case example

Roxanne, an expectant mother (seen by KKA) who was well trained in the procedures, was enjoying the experience of labour, but her partner assumed that she was in distress as he observed her having strong contractions. He pleaded with her and the obstetrician that she should be given an epidural. She resisted this for a while as she was more excited about how well her hypnosis training was proceeding and how she was not in any form of distress. However, she finally gave way to her husband's repeated appeals and accepted the epidural because she felt so pressured and distracted by his behaviour and she wanted some peace so she could proceed with the delivery. Roxanne later regretted this decision because it deprived her of the special experience she was hoping to have. She resented her husband for what had happened and would not have him present at the birth of their second child.

Postnatal progress

It is the impression of one of the authors (KKA) that the benefits of hypnosis during pregnancy and at the delivery may extend to the postnatal period in relation to such matters as bonding, the incidence of postnatal depression, how calm and relaxed the babies are and how well they sleep, and stimulation of lactation by suggestion. It remains for research studies to demonstrate whether these impressions are valid.

SOME GYNAECOLOGICAL CONDITIONS

Painful conditions, such as dysmenorrhoea, endometriosis, vulvodynia and idiopathic chronic pelvic pains, may benefit to some degree from straightforward techniques of hypnotic pain management. Anxiety is usually a part of these conditions, either from the suffering related to the problem itself or from co-existing life stresses. This itself may aggravate the suffering and thus may create a vicious cycle of anxiety and pain. Teaching relaxation in the form of self-hypnosis and encouraging its regular practice can stop this cycle.

Sometimes there may be unresolved emotional problems and some gynaecological conditions may be caused by emotional traumas. The patient may never associate these with her physical condition, in which case the use of hypnosis in a psychodynamic framework may be productive. Psychodynamic methods of exploration and resolution, as described in Chapter 19, may be used in such cases.

A working model for using hypnosis with painful gynaecological conditions

The following working model is used by one of us (KKA) as an explanation for patients of how and why they suffer from many of the above conditions when the doctors tell them that they cannot find anything physically wrong that may account for the pain or the severity of pain experienced. Like all working models (see Ch. 15), its main strength will lie in its acceptability to the patient and its effectiveness as a basis for a therapeutic intervention; the literal validity of the model is a matter for controlled research.

The patients in question commonly experience mistrust and frustration, and more stress and guilt as it seems that their problem is all of their making or they are malingering, even though they know that they do really experience the pain and are not making it up. Offering a simple working model will help these patients immensely. For example, in the case of vulvodynia, it may be stated that the sensory experience of pain, burning, soreness, and so on is created in the brain (or the cortex) in response to information in the form of electrical impulses that originate in the tissues of the vulva. The experience is not created by the vulva at all. In fact, all kinds of electrical impulses are transmitted to the brain from every part of the body, rather like a telephone network. These sensory impulses are analysed by the brain by reference to data available in the memory banks which are located all over the cortex. Billions of brain cells and the interconnecting junctions, the synapses, are involved with this analysis in order to provide meaning for those incoming impulses and the most appropriate name, such as 'pain', 'soreness' and 'burning'. However, impulses are arriving all the time and the meaning and the label will normally be 'it is normal and it is all right to ignore it'. For example, the patient's 'conscious brain' is usually ignoring impulses arriving from the wrist about the presence of a watch being worn.

Once those impulses are identified by the brain as 'a sensation of pain', that 'sensation of pain' is referred back to the part where the impulses came from, in this case the vulva. The person then consciously experiences 'pain in the vulva' or whatever sensation the brain has given to those impulses. Sometimes naming may be non-specific and the patient experiences 'a strange but very uncomfortable sensation' which she cannot describe more precisely.

Once the patient has understood the above mechanism of normal sensory experience, one can then progress with the working model to explore how such normal functioning can appear as 'an illness'. Many of the patients may have originally had some sort of vulval infection or minor injury in that part. At that time, the brain appropriately created the sensation of pain to make the patient pay attention to this area. Simultaneously, she experienced anxiety associated with the pain and illness, especially when under stress from any source. The brain records both 'anxiety/stress' and 'pain' and may create an association between the two. When the patient is faced with anxiety or stress at a future date, the brain now also experiences pain and projects that pain to the site of the previous illness, even though there is now no physical problem in the vulval area. The patient will then naturally think that the infection or illness has returned and go to the doctor for treatment. However, the specialists genuinely fail to find any illness and declare that there is 'nothing wrong' with the vulva. This will only provoke further anxiety.

In the experience of one of the authors (KKA), it is a very common finding that when one is faced with stress and anxiety at any time, negative feelings or anxiety that were associated with previous events but have been 'forgotten' or 'suppressed' tend to surface and even take up a prominent place in the person's everyday thoughts and feelings. The patient almost always provides such evidence. One may then assume that those negative feelings (guilt, anger, anxiety, hurt, etc.) become attached to the existing anxiety of having 'vulvodynia with no clinical evidence' and these negative feelings gradually take up a prominent place in the patient's life.

Because vulvodynia presents as constant and prolonged suffering, it is difficult for therapy to be directed on the previous traumatic events and their effects or on the current anxiety (which is usually the vulvodynia itself) and the best option will be to focus on both. Once again, from the experience of KKA, working with the effects of previous trauma provides substantial lasting benefits. Therefore, it is worthwhile considering a psychodynamic approach in treating vulvodynia of unknown origin. The therapist can introduce the 'unconscious–conscious' model as a prelude to the psychodynamic work. It is not uncommon, however, that the patient may identify possible relevant traumatic experiences without any exploratory work. Some patients may find that they can alleviate the pain simply by using this new understanding, while seeking resolution of the emotional issues by their own means.

If patients can understand these explanations (which may be simplified accordingly), they usually have no hesitation in accepting them, as they are seeking a way forward while the clinicians are 'failing'. This working model also opens up the possibility of various metaphors to ease or block the pain or to experience normal sensation. For example, using hypnotic imagery, they may 'isolate' the imagined part of the brain where the memory of 'pain in the vulva' is located, thus symbolically preventing the normal impulses entering that part; instead they project to the part of the brain where they are processed as 'normal'. Relaxation and ego-strengthening may be sufficient to deal with the effects of the previous traumas. However, in practice the majority of patients require exploration and resolution of the identified trauma.

REFERENCES

Abramson M, Heron W 1950 Objective evaluation of hypnosis in obstetrics: A preliminary report. American Journal of Obstetrics and Gynecology 59: 1069
Callan T D 1961 Can hypnosis be used routinely in obstetrics? Rocky Mountain Medical Journal 58: 28–30
Chertok L 1981 Sense and nonsense in psychotherapy: The challenge of hypnosis. Pergamon Press, New York
Crandon A 1979 Maternal anxiety and obstetric complications. Journal of Psychosomatic Research 23: 109–111
Davenport-Slack B 1975 A comparative evaluation of obstetrical hypnosis and antenatal, childbirth training. International Journal of Clinical and Experimental Hypnosis 12: 266–281
Davidson J A 1962 An assessment of the value of hypnosis in pregnancy and labour. British Medical Journal ii: 951–953
Edelmann R J, Connolly K J 1986 Psychological aspects of infertility. British Journal of Medical Psychology 59: 209–219
Edelmann R J, Golombok S 1989 Stress and reproductive failure. Journal of Reproductive and Infant Psychology 7: 79–86
Freeman R M, Macaulay A J, Eve L et al 1986 Randomised trial of self hypnosis for analgesia in labour. British Medical Journal (Clinical Research) 292: 657–658
Fuchs K, Paldi E, Abramovici H et al 1980 Treatment of hyperemesis gravidarum by hypnosis. International Journal of Clinical and Experimental Hypnosis 28: 313–323
Fuchs K, Zimmer E Z, Eyal A et al 1989 Is there any influence of maternal hypnosis on foetal well-being in utero? In: Waxman D, Pedersen D, Wilkie I, Mellett P (eds) Hypnosis: The Fourth European Congress at Oxford. Whurr, London, ch 7, p 196

Harmon T M, Hynan M T, Tyre T E 1990 Improved obstetric outcomes using hypnotic analgesia and skill mastery combined with childbirth education. Journal of Consulting and Clinical Psychology 58: 525–530

Newton C R, Sherrard W, Glavac I 1999 The Fertility Problem Inventory: Measuring perceived infertility-related stress. Fertility and Sterility 72: 54–62

Omer H, Freidlander D, Plati Z 1986 Hypnotic relaxation in the treatment of premature labour. Psychosomatic Medicine 48: 351–361

Perchard S D 1960 Hypnosis in obstetrics. Proceedings of the Royal Society of Medicine 53: 458–460

Pook M, Krause W, Rohrle B 1999 Coping with infertility: Distress and changes in sperm quality. Human Reproduction 14: 1487–1492

Sanders K A, Bruce N W 1999 Psychosocial stress and treatment outcome following assisted reproductive technology. Human Reproduction 14: 1656–1662

Simkin P 1986 Stress, pain, and catecholamines in labour, Part 1: A review. Birth 13: 227–233

Winkelstein L B 1958 Routine hypnosis for obstetrical delivery: An evaluation of hypnosuggestion in 200 cases. American Journal of Obstetrics and Gynecology 76: 153–159

Hypnosis in dentistry

INTRODUCTION

A famous person once commented that the greatest blessing of techno-logical progress in the 20th century was the improvement in routine dental treatments. Indeed, it is only relatively recently that a visit to the dentist (or whoever took on that role) was inevitably associated with agony and dread. Not surprisingly, therefore, there is a tradition of using mesmer-ism and hypnosis to ameliorate the ordeal. John Elliotson himself (see Ch. 1) in the 19th century included dental extractions amongst many other surgical procedures that he carried out solely using mesmeric passes to effect analgesia.

Even today, despite all the advances, anxiety about going to the dentist is still very prevalent, and sympathy is automatically offered to anyone who is due for an appointment. Historical and cultural influences play their part: in the country where one of the authors (KKA) grew up, it was an exciting adventure to go to a dentist.

Dental anxiety results in a restless or rigid patient in the dental chair and this makes the patient feel helpless and often the dentist also. A handful of such cases in a day is enough to cause more exhaustion and stress than any dentist would wish for.

One adult in three has moderate-to-severe fear of dental procedures (British Dental Association 1995) and this problem is very prevalent amongst children. Genuine dentally phobic people often do not see the den-tist at all. In extreme cases, the result is that the entire mandible sequestrates owing to osteomyelitis, separating in a single piece.

Other problems include gagging. Constant gagging while the dentist is trying to take an impression means that an unsatisfactory outcome is inevitable. Indeed, the gagging patient may not be able to wear dentures at all, however perfectly they have been made, and may keep returning to the surgery to complain. Also, the treatment of temporomandibular joint (TMJ) dysfunction can be daunting for the patient as well as the dentist. Bruxism (habitual grinding of the teeth) is another problem whose consequences are evident to the dentist.

The use of hypnosis in adults and children can provide some answers to these problems. As most dentists who use hypnosis acknowledge, it can make routine dentistry less stressful for the practitioner and can be extremely rewarding. Equally, hypnosis has a place in emergency treatment, such as with the patient who presents with an acute dental abscess.

LEGAL AND ETHICAL ISSUES

The matter of whether it should be made explicit when hypnotic procedures are being used has been discussed in Chapter 8. Relaxation, imagery and distraction techniques are commonly used by dentists as and when they deem them appropriate, and the business of introducing them as 'hypnosis' interrupts the session and takes up time that dentists may not have allowed for. We suggested in Chapter 8 that unless techniques such as eye fixation and arm levitation are used (procedures that are more characteristic of the second approach to hypnosis), the practitioner is justified in referring to 'relaxation' or 'imagination'. We are not sure what the position is in countries such as the USA, where the use of hypnosis may have legal implications.

As always, dental practitioners must only use hypnosis for problems that are of concern to dental care. It is not unheard of for patients, knowing that their dentist uses hypnosis, to ask for help with their non-dental problems. The dentist should resist these requests and encourage these patients to seek more appropriate help, or refer them to their general medical practitioner, who will advise them of the most appropriate professional person to see.

GENERAL CONSIDERATIONS IN TREATMENT

Crucial to easing the patient's anxiety is the creation of an ambience that is friendly and reassuring. Efforts to achieve this should start with the reception staff, by their conveying warmth and friendliness when they take appointments by the telephone, and greeting the patient at the reception desk in a pleasant manner. This attitude should also be adopted by the nurse and the dentist. The waiting area can be made less clinical and more homely. Appropriate pictures, including pictures on the ceiling above the dental chair, will help calm patients, especially children. Soft music is another good idea.

Rapport and trust are enhanced when the patient is given a full explanation, in non-threatening language, of what is going to happen; undue surprise or shock is thus avoided. Parents should be allowed to stay with their children. The instruments which may appear most threatening to very anxious patients should be kept out of sight if possible.

Putting all those ideas in place will take away the sting of any painful procedures. They are also important for success in any hypnotic interventions.

The most essential ingredient of any dental procedure, and one that is most important when hypnosis is used, is some form of signal that the patient can make to stop the treatment immediately and to discuss any problems. Without this, patients are likely to hold on to the fear of losing control. A common misconception of hypnosis is that 'trance takes away personal control' and patients therefore fear that they are going to be hurt and can do nothing about it. Losing control is the most significant feature of dental anxiety or phobia.

Let us now review the common applications of hypnosis in dental practice. We shall leave the most common application, namely assisting the anxious patient, until the end.

THE AMELIORATION OF DISCOMFORT AND PAIN

As we stated earlier, dental treatment is all too often still associated in the public mind with anxiety, discomfort and pain. Yet dentists assert that nowadays patients overestimate the amount of real pain that is experienced during routine dental procedures. It seems that the main problem is that patients anticipate pain. For example, they may think, 'What if the drill slips and catches a nerve?' On the other hand, some pain is not uncommonly experienced and it cannot be said that dental treatment can be anything better than 'uncomfortable'; as patients, we have to lie back with our mouths wide open, and are therefore unable to communicate with our 'assailant' (the dentist) in the usual way. We are thus rendered passive and are unable to see where all the action is taking place – namely, in our mouth. This adds to the sense of uncertainty and apprehension. Many patients also have more general anxieties relating to medical settings, injections, the sight of blood, and so on.

Consequently, dentists trained in hypnosis find that simple suggestions and imagery conducive to calmness and comfort can help ameliorate the unpleasantness and discomfiture that patients experience to varying degrees, even when chemical analgesia and anaesthetics are administered (in which case these techniques may be a prelude to the injection). Some dentists, in fact, use hypnosis as an adjunct to relative analgesia. With less anxious patients, suggestions, imagery and distraction techniques may be administered informally, without a hypnotic induction. With more anxious patients, and where pain is likely to be significant, formal methods are required.

For young children, distraction may be the most appropriate ploy. If one is using guided imagery, one can suggest that patients go to a safe place where they will enjoy doing something interesting; meanwhile, the dentist can do all that has to be done and give the reassurance 'nothing will bother you at all'. (Note the avoidance of the word 'pain' or 'hurt'.)

The popular method of directly suggesting hypnoanalgesia is transference of glove anaesthesia (see Ch. 25). It is important to test the effectiveness of the suggestion before transferring the analgesia to the desired area. Producing glove anaesthesia has the added advantage of demonstrating to the patient that 'hypnosis works'. When indicated, it is in order to suggest that the analgesia will continue to give adequate comfort during the post-operative period, provided that necessary safeguards are also suggested, such as seeking advice when complications arise.

At the end of the session, always congratulate the patient for the successful use of hypnosis; this is in itself ego-strengthening and will facilitate future sessions. If appropriate, teach the patient the whole of the procedure for self-hypnosis, including the suggestions relating to pain control, but without the testing of analgesia. If the patient practises this regularly, this will enable the practitioner to omit the induction, deepening and administration of analgesia suggestions, and this will speed up future treatment. A well-practised patient does not even have to go to a practitioner who is adept at hypnosis.

Patients presenting with any form of dental pain may have similar kinds of hypnotic interventions to provide instant analgesia, or at least to render the pain more tolerable for as long as is necessary. It should of course be ensured that the patient will have proper treatment in due course. On the other hand, one may proceed with treatment where this is warranted and if the patient responds well to the suggestion of analgesia. Medical and dental practitioners report that in their experience, someone who is in agonising pain and therefore highly anxious, usually proves to be well motivated and responsive to hypnotic suggestions to help them cope. Hypnoanalgesia and hypnoanaesthesia also have the benefit of producing no side effects.

CONTROL OF BLEEDING

The literature on hypnosis and the control of bleeding reports mixed results (Enqvist et al 1995, Hopkins et al 1991). There are also reports of the successful use of hypnosis in the management of haemophilia (Dubin & Shapiro 1974, LeBaron & Zeltzer 1984, Lucas 1975, Swirsky-Sacchetti & Margolis 1986), although not all have obtained positive results

(Lichstein & Eakin 1985). Dentists who use hypnosis often aver that bleeding control is easily achieved by direct suggestions of 'no bleeding', 'less bleeding' or 'no need to bleed'. When images of cold and ice are used to create analgesia, they may also be allied to the suggestion that the blood vessels are constricting and therefore the loss of blood is reduced. Posthypnotic suggestion of minimal bleeding during the healing period may be given, but it is important to include the suggestion of having sufficient bleeding to form a clot to occupy the socket, thus preventing the possibility of dry-socket bone infection.

BRUXISM

Jaw clenching and teeth grinding at night are invariably out of a patient's control. One theory is that bruxism is an expression of pent-up anger and helplessness (Pierce et al 1995). Whatever the case, as bruxism is an expression of tension, training the patient in general relaxation using hypnotic techniques is the first step. This may be followed with suggestions focused on relaxation around the muscles that move the jaw. Once this feeling of relaxation is well established there, anchor it with a clenched fist or fists and give posthypnotic suggestions that whenever the patients clench a fist or fists, the jaw muscles will become profoundly relaxed. Rehearse the anchoring method and teach patients, by covert practice, how to use it as a means of releasing anger and frustration in everyday life (see Ch. 12). Also give ego-strengthening suggestions relating to self-control. Cognitive rehearsal is next carried out with the suggestion that the patient is in bed and tension is building up in the jaw muscles and this automatically makes the patient want to clench the fist(s). As soon as the patient clenches the fist(s), the previously anchored relaxation returns to the jaw muscles, displacing the tension there.

When the patient has repeated the procedure a number of times and shows confidence in the method, further posthypnotic suggestions are given that the patient will practise all of this at home before bedtime. A tape recording may be prepared for this purpose. Being able to control unwanted negative thoughts and feelings will help the patient fall into a natural, relaxing sleep.

GAGGING

Reflex gagging may present as anything from a mild form of choking to violent retching when the palate is simply touched or, for example, during the taking of impressions. The fauces, base of tongue, palate, uvula and posterior pharyngeal wall have maximum sensitivity and so form trigger zones. Certain conditions such as chronic nasal obstruction or sinusitis may increase the predisposition to gag (Bartlett 1971). Psychological contributions are represented by conditioned protective reflexes from earlier experiences or existing stresses and anxieties. Simply the sight, sound and even the thought that something out of the ordinary is going to enter the mouth may precipitate gagging.

Helping the patient understand the nature of gagging removes some of the embarrassment and possibly even some of the anticipatory anxiety. Hence, hypnosis for eliminating gagging starts with an explanation of its nature. The reflex action begins with the sensation of touch, either real or imaginary, in the mouth, especially at the trigger zones. Therefore, in theory, if those areas are made to feel numb, this should eliminate the reflex cycle of gagging.

After hypnotic induction and deepening, introduce appropriate ego-strengthening suggestions that create a positive expectation of success. These are followed by suggestions of relaxation of the throat muscles. Encourage the patient to breathe slowly and steadily through the nose. This instruction is useful for patients whose gagging is associated with a fear of asphyxiation. Now introduce the image of how well the patient will be in the future when all the treatment has been carried out and, if relevant, when the patient is able to tolerate the new dentures. Anchor the positive feelings and the images by the clenched fist method, or with an imagined word, etc. Rehearse the anchoring and create the positive experience several times. In the same session or, if time is not available, in the following session, proceed to produce glove anaesthesia and then transfer this to the trigger points to make them as numb as required in order to stop the gagging reflex. The numbness can be created by directly suggesting that these areas are gradually becoming numb, or that they are experiencing tingling that leads to numbness. These suggestions may be augmented by suitable imagery.

Once this is achieved, start with the gradual, step-by-step desensitisation process in imagination. At every level, and whenever there is any sign that the reflex is being activated, instruct the patient to use the anchor to reinforce the feelings of calmness, self-control and confidence in success, and remind the patient to breathe slowly through the nose. Success at each stage is fed back to the patient to reinforce continued confidence.

Once the patient is able to go through the procedures confidently in imagination, progress to the use of real materials, using if necessary instruments of the smallest size and then gradually increase to normal size. For example, in the case of intolerance of dentures, one can start with a small-sized plate or a toothbrush, beginning on the front parts of the tongue and progressing to the back of the mouth. Instead of instruments, one could use cotton buds, tongue spatulas or even spoons.

It may not be possible to achieve full competence in one or two sessions, and therefore it is highly beneficial to bring all these ideas together into a self-hypnosis routine for the patient to practise several times at home.

Case example

With some patients, all the efforts at desensitisation may fail in spite of achieving a good response to hypnosis itself, and this may indicate some underlying psychological gain or unacknowledged problems. In such situations, a psychodynamic approach using hypnosis may reveal unexpected reasons for the difficulty. A middle-aged woman, Nita, was referred for treatment to one of us (KKA) for severe gagging and failure to have impressions made. She had the same experience with a toothbrush if it accidentally touched the back of her mouth. She failed to make progress with the already described methods of desensitisation. The affect bridge technique (Ch. 19) elicited the memory of her being sexually abused in the form of forced oral sex by her father. It was then that she herself began to interpret her smoking as a defence: 'He can't put it in when there is something burning near my mouth'. The trauma was effectively resolved and so also the gagging. To the patient's own surprise, she never wanted to smoke again.

Nita's case is an unusual example of what may happen when hypnosis is used psychodynamically, but it also highlights the limitations of the dental practitioner who will not be trained in dealing with such matters. However, where there is a conditioning experience, it is most likely to be having something stuck in the throat that causes choking and fear of asphyxiation or being forced, while feeling sick, to finish up one's food by parents.

TEMPOROMANDIBULAR JOINT DYSFUNCTION

The nature of TMJ dysfunction is very complex. Structural malfunctions and diseases are the commonest contributors, but the problem may be more psychosomatic in nature. The pain or discomfort may be confined to the joint or joints, but it may spread to anywhere in the facial region, sometimes resulting in an inability to tolerate dentures. When the usual treatment has failed, hypnotic techniques, in the form of pain control and relaxation, may prove effective, or they may be used as an adjunct to traditional treatment. It is not unusual to find a tender spot on the temporalis muscle, ipsilateral to the TMJ pain. Relaxation of the muscles of mastication, and pain control methods described in Chapter 25, especially focused on the 'tender spot', may be all that is required in many cases.

TMJ dysfunction may have emotional concomitants that require the assistance of professionals trained in psychological therapies and counselling, but hypnosis can be an extremely useful adjunctive procedure, especially when symptom-oriented methods have failed, when it can then be used psychodynamically to help the patient acknowledge and resolve any underlying problems.

Case example

Agnes, a patient of one of the authors (KKA), was a widow in her late 50s, who had reached the state of being unable to wear dentures without experiencing severe pain and a very uncomfortable tingling sensation in her face and temporomandibular region. The problem started as 'discomforting' sensations on the left side of her face when she was wearing her dentures. Her dentist made some new dentures for her but after several unsuccessful attempts at wearing them, she was referred to a dental hospital. Despite further treatment, the discomforting sensations turned to pain and tingling that spread to the inside of her mouth, the TMJ area and the opposite side of her face. Eventually, she was having pain at times when she was not even wearing the dentures. She was referred to neurologists for investigative tests but she herself finally came to the conclusion that there were psychological aspects to her problem, and hypnosis was offered.

During hypnosis, the affect bridge procedure triggered her expression of grief as she described the scene of her husband's sudden death. He was lying on the floor when she walked into the room and his dentures were out of his mouth and 'staring at her'. She expressed guilt at 'not doing anything to prevent his death'. This was resolved by counselling. The pain lessened for a while but came back as before, even though she was expressing more of the grief. She was unable to reveal any more reasons for the continuation of her grief and of the pain.

A modified form of the dream suggestion technique (Ch. 19) was then introduced in the hypnosis session. She could accept a working model describing how the normal sensory input into the brain from the affected parts could be distorted on its way to the cortical 'cognition centre' by the actions of 'messengers' from some parts of her memory store, especially memories relating to certain emotional trauma or guilt (see Ch. 28). Such distortions could change a normal feeling to a feeling of pain.

Once Agnes had accepted this model, it was suggested during hypnosis that an imaginary agent had been planted in the pathway of the sensory input and this would recognise the 'messengers'. This agent would identify the nature of their mission and this would be revealed to her in a dream.

Sure enough, the patient reported a dream about her son, who was showing extreme anger and throwing things at her. She then broke down with feelings of extreme guilt because, soon after her husband died, she left the house where they had lived their entire married life. Now she felt that she had thus abandoned the love that they had for each other. She was left asking herself how she could have done such an injustice to her beloved husband.

The solution was at hand, as the therapist, during hypnosis, reassured her that 'Love is always carried in your heart and it goes with you all the time wherever you go. It does not live in the bricks and mortar of the house'. This was illustrated to her by the therapist's own experience of the love for his father that he carries in his heart even though he now lives thousands of miles away; this love is no less than when he was in his father's house. Her grief then eased, she completely recovered from the pains, and she was able to wear her dentures with no problem.

DENTAL ANXIETY AND DENTAL PHOBIA

As we noted at the beginning of this chapter, one in three patients attending any dental surgery suffers some degree of anxiety to the level of panic. Hypnosis is an effective tool in helping such patients to undergo dental procedures with confidence and enabling a dental visit to be a regular experience for them.

Depending on the severity of the anxiety, the dentist's use of hypnotic procedures may be informal (blending in with the dentist's usual patter, say to distract the patient or to encourage the patient to engage in some pleasant imagery) to a formal course of therapy, beginning with history-taking and followed by a programme of desensitisation (see below). Although hypnosis is often cited as being time-consuming, dentists who use hypnosis find that patients with moderate degrees of anxiety often respond well to relatively brief formal induction methods. Severe cases, notably those who have avoided dental treatment (the true dental phobics), do, however, require a more structured programme.

If the anxiety is not too severe, the dentist will find that the procedures we have outlined in earlier chapters – hypnotic induction and deepening (e.g. the 'safe place' method), suggestions of continuing calmness and relaxation, ego-strengthening, an anxiety management method such as the clenched fist procedure, posthypnotic suggestions, and self-hypnosis to rehearse dental appointments – collectively lend themselves well to the task of helping the dentally anxious patient. For more severe problems, the following programme of treatment may be undertaken.

Therapy starts with history-taking and assessment, and this includes establishing a hierarchy of the anxiety-provoking situations and stimuli (see Ch. 20). These may be the smell of anaesthetic, the feel of the probe in the mouth, the sound of the drill as it is turned on, and so on. Standardised dental anxiety scales may be used (Humphries et al 1995). Special attention is given to the kinds of physical symptoms associated with anxiety, as these are targeted in the desensitisation procedure.

When the patient is ready, one can go through the preparation and preliminaries outlined in Chapters 5 and 6 (the first approach to hypnosis). Then, take the patient through a sequence of induction and deepening procedures to establish a state of deep relaxation. We suggest including the 'safe place' method as this is good for distraction purposes and for calming patients if their anxiety level becomes too high. Suggestions of total body relaxation are repeated along with ego-strengthening suggestions appropriate to the patient's goals. Relaxation and resourcefulness (drawn from previous achievements) are then anchored, for example using the clenched fist procedure, or using an image or a word chosen by the patient. Age progression may also be used to create images of having a better life, when the patient is cured of the fear and is the proud owner of a good set of teeth. The patient is instructed to practise regularly the whole routine in self-hypnosis.

When patients reach proficiency in creating a sense of calmness and relaxation using their anchors, they may be taken through the desensitisation programme (as above) step-by-step in imagination. Patients are asked to dwell on each fear-provoking situation, to experience the fear, and then to follow with the anchoring method for reinstating a sense of relaxation, calmness and self-control. Once they are able to remain calm with that image, with their permission one proceeds to the next stage in the hierarchy, and so on. It is important to be aware that even though all of this is done in imagination, the physical and emotional stress to the patient can be extreme. Therefore, patients should be able to signal when they wish to stop the image and, for example, switch to their safe place. Hand or finger signals to indicate 'Yes' or 'No' or 'Stop immediately' are the most efficient way of communicating during hypnosis.

Once the patient has gained confidence in the imaginary rehearsal of the full treatment session, one can begin the actual dental treatment, proceeding step-by-step with plenty of reassurance and feedback for every sign of success (a good form of ego-strengthening) and with encouragement and reassurance that all is going well. This also means that the next stage or the next treatment session will be easier.

Unfortunately, some patients' dental anxiety may be so severe that they never go to see a dentist, and therefore dentists may not see many dental phobics at all. Such patients may 'break into a cold sweat' when anything about dentistry is mentioned in their presence, and may even be afraid of cleaning their teeth, or they do so under great sufferance. Hence, this causes their teeth to deteriorate to an appalling condition and this often contributes to poor self-esteem, distancing from relationships, a failure to achieve certain goals in life, and a host of physical and emotional problems, including social phobia and agoraphobia. Therefore, clinical psychologists, psychiatrists and general medical practitioners are often the first point of contact with these patients (whom they may be seeing for other reasons). Even though dental practitioners trained in the treatment of the dentally phobic patient are often the best people to treat them, they may have to provide a special room that bears no resemblance to the dental surgery and has a separate entrance. This may be obligatory if the dentist is to persuade such patients to seek treatment in the first place. The therapy can, however, start with a non-dental therapist and be carried on by a dentist trained in hypnosis, once the patient reaches the point of being able to see a dentist (though not to go through any dental procedure). In the final stage of the therapy, the patient obviously has to be exposed to the actual dental surgery and treatment.

Case examples

Patients resistant to the above programme may, as we have seen earlier, benefit from a psychodynamic approach. A patient, Jenny, in her late 30s approached the therapist (KKA), who was also her GP, with a problem of panic attacks. She normally worked at a supermarket check-out but she had become unable to go to work because of panic attacks that started to happen when there were people around. Her marital relationship began to suffer as she was becoming more and more housebound, could not go on holiday, and could not accompany her husband motorcycle racing, something that she normally loved to do. She also felt that she was being ridiculed by her children.

(continued)

Case examples (*continued*)

After several sessions of ego-strengthening and counselling, she had the courage to tell the therapist that it was dental phobia that was the root cause of her problems. She did not dare to open her mouth in front of anybody because her teeth were in such bad condition. She had not seen a dentist since she was 10 or 11 (after which age she could refuse her parents' instructions to do so), but could not understand the reason.

During hypnosis, she was asked, as her 'adult self', to imagine travelling back through her life looking for the earliest memory of her being troubled and frightened. (This is a variation of the affect bridge method, the patient being an 'observer' or 'disso-ciated'.) She then reported seeing herself at the age of 6 suffering from toothache and being on the way to the dentist. Her father was quite cruelly telling her that if she did not behave, the dentist would cut her head off; he would then have to sew it back on again, and there would be a large scar on her neck. The little girl firmly believed that she would come back without her head. The adult self was then instructed to help and reassure the 7-year-old child (see Ch. 19).

The care of this patient was then transferred to a dentist trained in hypnosis, who carried out the desensitisation programme with no problems and all her teeth were restored. Jenny then experienced a new lease of life.

Naomi, who was 17 years old, ran 3 miles non-stop to her home, raced upstairs, and sat on her bed, panting with fear. Her grandmother, who had just been with her in the local hospital dental department, then arrived back by bus. All that had happened was that the junior dental surgeon approached Naomi with a needle and syringe to take some blood prior to a dental operation. She had been referred to the hospital because she refused to see her family dentist as she had a phobia of needles and dentists.

She failed to respond to a desensitisation programme. A psychodynamic approach was then pursued using Wolberg's theatre visualisation technique (Ch. 19). She began describing a set of bright lights and a man appearing in a white coat. With undue eager-ness, the therapist (KKA) intervened by asking, 'Is that man a doctor?' She then alerted herself, very distressed. The session continued with the reinstatement of hypnosis and relaxation. Naomi was then asked to watch her 'dissociated ego' at an easel painting pictures concerning her problem. She then spontaneously regressed to the age of 7. She was alone in the dentist's chair, frozen with fear, and unable to talk or cry, as her mouth was held wide open. The dentist was 'poking around with a needle' prior to extracting one of the teeth. Naomi began to whimper and when allowed to cry, she 'let it all out'. All she (the child) wanted at that time was to have her mummy hold her hand and then the dentist could do whatever was needed.

Naomi's grandmother, who was chaperoning her during the hypnosis session, was recruited in the role of her mother and held her hand and comforted '7-year-old Naomi'. Little more was needed. On alerting, Naomi showed no signs of anxiety as she took a needle and syringe in her hand and then allowed the therapist to take a blood sample.

Most often, dental phobia is linked to a bad experience in the dental surgery (Öst 1985). We also sometimes hear horror stories as young children. These expectations may then be confirmed at the dentist's by what otherwise might have been only minor pain, but which is now perceived as 'terrible hurt'. Treatment may be focused on unravelling such memories, which are understandable but based on distorted information, and encouraging the 'younger self' to have a more realistic perception and understanding with the help of the 'adult self' in conjunction with a trusted therapist. Hypnosis can be the best medium to achieve this.

REFERENCES

Bartlett K A 1971 Gagging. A case report. American Journal of Clinical Hypnosis 14: 54–56
British Dental Association 1995 Dental phobia. Fact file, June. British Dental Association, 64 Wimpole Street, London WIM 8AL
Dubin L L, Shapiro S S 1974 Use of hypnosis to facilitate dental extraction hemostasis in a classic hemophiliac with a high antibody titer to Factor VIII. American Journal of Clinical Hypnosis 17: 79–83
Enqvist B, von Konow L, Bystedt H 1995 Pre- and perioperative suggestion in maxillofacial surgery: Effects on blood loss and recovery. International Journal of Clinical and Experimental Hypnosis 43: 284–294
Hopkins B, Jordan J M, Lundy R M 1991 The effects of hypnosis and of imagery on bleeding time: A brief communication. International Journal of Clinical and Experimental Hypnosis 139: 34–139
Humphries G, Morrison T, Lindsay S 1995 The modified Dental Anxiety Scale: Validation and United Kingdom norms. Community Dentistry and Oral Epidemiology 12: 143–150
LeBaron S, Zeltzer L K 1984 Research on hypnosis in hemophilia – preliminary success and problems: A brief communication. International Journal of Clinical and Experimental Hypnosis 32: 290–295
Lichstein K L, Eakin T L 1985 Progressive versus self-control relaxation to reduce spontaneous bleeding in hemophiliacs. Journal of Behavioral Medicine 8: 149–162
Lucas O N 1975 Use of hypnosis in hemophilia dental care. Annals of the New York Academy of Sciences 240: 263–266
Öst L G 1985 Mode of acquisition of phobias. Acta Universitatis Uppsaliensis (Abstracts of Uppsala Dissertations from the Faculty of Medicine) 529: 1–45
Pierce C J, Christman K, Bennett M E et al 1995 Stress, anticipatory stress, and psychological measures related to sleep bruxism. Journal of Orofacial Pain 9: 5–16
Swirsky-Sacchetti T, Margolis C G 1986 The effects of a comprehensive self-hypnosis training program on the use of factor VIII in severe hemophilia. International Journal of Clinical and Experimental Hypnosis 34: 71–83

FURTHER READING

We thoroughly recommend the following monograph that is devoted to hypnosis in dental practice and contains chapters on history; the hypnotic treatment of dental anxiety and phobia in adults and children, gagging and denture intolerance, bruxism, TMJ dysfunction; and pain management.

Mehrstedt M, Wikström P-O (eds) 1997 Hypnosis in dentistry. Hypnosis International Monographs, number 3. MEF-Stiftung, Konradstrasse 16, 80801 Munich, Germany

Below is a selection of individual papers on topics that we have covered in this chapter.

Barsby M J 1994 The use of hypnosis in the management of 'gagging'. British Dental Journal 176: 97–102
Clarke J H, Persichetti S J 1988 Hypnosis and concurrent denture construction for a patient with a hypersensitive gag reflex. American Journal of Clinical Hypnosis 30: 285–288
Clarke J H, Reynolds P J 1991 Suggestive hypnotherapy for nocturnal bruxism: A pilot study. American Journal of Clinical Hypnosis 33: 248–253
Eli I, Kleinhauz M 1985 Hypnosis: A tool for the integrative approach to the treatment of the gagging reflex. International Journal of Clinical and Experimental Hypnosis 33: 99–108
Forgione A G 1988 Hypnosis in the treatment of dental fear and phobia. Dental Clinics of North America 32: 745–761
Golan H P 1989 Temporomandibular joint disease treated with hypnosis. American Journal of Clinical Hypnosis 31: 269–274

Kelly M, McKinty H, Carr R 1988 Utilisation of hypnosis to promote compliance with routine dental flossing. American Journal of Clinical Hypnosis 31: 57–60

Rodolfa E R, Kraft W, Reilley R R 1990 Etiology and treatment of dental anxiety and phobia. American Journal of Clinical Hypnosis 33: 22–28

Thompson S A 1994 The use of hypnosis as an adjunct to nitrous oxide sedation in the treatment of dental anxiety. Contemporary Hypnosis 11: 77–83

Hypnosis for anxiety disorders

INTRODUCTION

This chapter covers the application of hypnosis to those problems that are designated as 'anxiety disorders' according to the Diagnostic and Statistical Manual of Mental Disorders (DSM-IV; American Psychiatric Association 1994). We are also concerned with anxiety that is problematical but not of the scale of a clinical disorder ('exam nerves', lack of confidence in social situations, driving test anxiety, interview anxiety, etc.).

In fact, we have already covered, in previous chapters, much of the material that is relevant to this subject. We shall therefore draw together what we have previously covered and present some modern theoretical ideas that can inform a psychological approach, augmented by hypnosis, to assist people with anxiety problems. We shall adhere mainly to a cognitive-behavioural understanding, but one that allows the therapist to adopt a psychodynamic model when this seems appropriate.

THE MANIFESTATIONS OF ANXIETY

Anxiety is an everyday feeling, yet it is universally experienced as aversive. Why then do we become anxious? Why do we *suffer* from it? Would not life be so much better without it? The answer must be that it is adaptive in some way and necessary for survival. One obvious advantage is that it is associated with the 'adrenalin' response that energises the body for an effective 'fight-or-flight' reaction. Yet, we also have an adrenalin response when we are excited and enjoying ourselves. So why is anxiety experienced as so unpleasant and why does it seem to be associated with so many problems?

In recent years, there has been an increase in experimental and theoretical interest in the relationship between emotion (particularly anxiety) and how our being emotional affects the way the mind and brain process (interpret, register, encode and recall) information and vice versa.

This work has examined the three major manifestations of anxiety, namely the everyday emotion of anxiety (state anxiety); the characteristics of people whom we describe as anxious (trait anxiety); and clinical anxiety (anxiety disorders) – and the relationships between all three.

State anxiety

The experience of anxiety is complex and multiply determined. Initially, we have an infinite range of possible sources for the anxiety that may be located externally (e.g. a large dog or an impending job interview) or internally (e.g. a pain of unknown origin). In the spirit of cognitive therapy, we say that it is not the situation or the event itself that causes anxiety but our interpretation or appraisal of it (although some occurrences are better explained by conditioning).

It is customary to consider how a person's anxiety is expressed at different levels, namely:

1. *Physiological* (increase in heart rate, respiration, sweating, etc.)
2. *Cognitive* (how the situation is interpreted and appraised; this includes thoughts such as 'What if … ?', 'I will not cope' etc., which are worries influenced by long-term memories)
3. *Behavioural* (how we respond behaviourally to the situation, say by escape, avoidance, dependency, protective actions, posture, gestures, and vocalisations).

An important finding about these three levels is that there is only a low correlation between them. That is, if we measure objectively the physiological, subjective and behavioural responses, we find that their relationship is much lower than we would suppose and this has important theoretical consequences. What determines the level of *experienced* anxiety (i.e. how anxious the person actually feels) is the person's *perceived* rather than actual intensity of response on each of these three levels. So, for example, patients might perceive that they are in a high state of physiological arousal but objective measures may not bear this out.

With increasing levels of perceived threat, the way the above information and that coming from the external environment are processed are subject, in most people, to certain biases that favour the early detection and recognition of danger. There are two main cognitive biases associated with high levels of anxiety: the first is a selective attentional bias to possible sources of threat and the second is an interpretational bias. The latter refers to a tendency to interpret events in a threatening way, even when realistically there is little threat present.

It follows that if two people are put in the same situation, whilst they may differ in their *objectively* rated anxiety, their *subjective* experience of anxiety may be even more different in terms of both quality and intensity. The differences are determined by a number of factors, notably constitutional ones (e.g. whether the two people differ in their trait anxiety or neuroticism – see below) and previous experiences which are encoded in long-term memory (which may be remote or more recent).

There is also some evidence that as anxiety increases, this facilitates access to anxious memories. (It was previously held that this kind of bias was only a feature of depression.)

The adaptive function of these biases is obviously to facilitate the early detection and recognition of danger in potentially threatening environments ('hypervigilance' theory).

Trait anxiety

How many core dimensions of personality are there on which one can usefully and efficiently represent all human beings? The late Raymond Cattell (Cattell et al 1970) considered there are 16 main ones; according to the late Hans Eysenck (1967), there are three. Many now consider that the answer is five (Digman 1990). Whatever classification is used, all include trait anxiety or neuroticism (or 'negative affectivity').

Trait anxiety is usually measured by questionnaire, and studies on twins now suggest that 31% of the variation in trait anxiety in the population is due to heredity (Pedersen et al 1988). Contrary to intuition, physiological measurements of people both in low- and high-stress situations do not discriminate low- and high-trait anxious individuals. There are a number of reasons for this. As we have seen, anxiety is multi-dimensional in nature; also people differ in what makes them anxious and in experiments on anxiety the stressors used may not be relevant to the anxieties of all participants.

Most interestingly, people who score low in measured trait anxiety are not an homogeneous group. They consist of genuinely low anxious individuals and 'repressors' (Eysenck 1997, Myers 2000). Repressors report (usually genuinely) that they do not feel very anxious, yet they have very high levels of physiological activity even in moderately stressful situations. Repressors manifest the opposite cognitive biases to high anxious individuals. Under conditions of increasing stress, they disattend to threat and have defensive styles of denial and intellectualisation in the presence of danger (usually social rather than physical threat). They tend not to acknowledge high levels of physiological, cognitive or behavioural manifestations of anxiety. This avoidance defence interferes with their ability to cope effectively with stress.

Repressors also score highly on measures of 'social desirability', for example on the Marlowe–Crowne Social Desirability Scale (Crowne & Marlowe 1964). They tend to be conformist and are motivated to avoid disapproval (and perhaps to seek approval). They show a childhood history involving indifference and antipathy from one or both parents.

Repressors show a significant tendency to develop somatic symptoms under stress (see Wickramasekera 1993). Hence, they are less likely to describe 'anxiety' as their reason for seeking treatment. In women with breast cancer, repressors show more rapid progress of the disease (Jenson 1987).

It is important to bear in mind that we are here talking about tendencies; in reality, human nature is far too complex to allow us to divide people into two different groups like this without the risk of gross oversimplification. Also, we must avoid making value judgements; no doubt many successful and otherwise fulfilled people have a repressive style of coping.

Clinical anxiety

Anxiety is maladaptive when the person is overattentive to possible sources of threat, makes unrealistic appraisals and interpretations about the potential danger of external and internal events, and is unduly influenced by memories that evoke anxiety. M. W. Eysenck (1997) has suggested that there is continuity between state anxiety, trait anxiety and clinical anxiety. However, anxious patients are more likely than anxious non-patients to interpret feelings of anxiety as implying danger and 'catastrophe'. They are therefore more susceptible to a 'positive feedback loop' involving experienced anxiety on the one hand and, on the other, perceived physiological, cognitive and behavioural anxiety and the influence of anxiety-provoking long-term memories.

The above author also proposes that the various anxiety disorders are associated with cognitive biases for different components of anxiety. Thus, panic disorder (without agoraphobia) is associated with biases primarily with respect to physiological activity and bodily sensations; social phobia with behavioural anxiety ('action tendencies'); obsessive–compulsive disorder with cognitive anxiety, notably an inflated sense of responsibility; and specific phobia is most associated with cognitive appraisal of environmental stimuli. General anxiety disorder patients are similar to high trait anxiety patients and tend to have selective attentional and interpretive biases on several of these sources of information.

TREATMENT APPROACHES

Treatment approaches, with and without the use of hypnosis, can be targeted at different levels – physiological, cognitive and behavioural – although changes at any one of these levels will effect changes at the other levels. Specifically in cognitive therapy we have procedures, the aim of which is to:

- Reduce excessive attentional bias to stimuli that are interpreted as threatening
- Encourage a more realistic interpretation of stimuli and events that are misinterpreted as threatening or whose threat is exaggerated
- Reconstruct and reinterpret salient memories or schemas associated with the feared situations.

In addition, at the physiological level, we have behavioural procedures, such as relaxation techniques, that are aimed at directly reducing the level of autonomic arousal associated with anxiety.

In preparation for this work, a useful (and indeed, not infrequently therapeutic) exercise is to ask the patient to relive in imagination an example of the specific problem situation and then explore the physiological responses, the attentional and interpretive biases, the behavioural responses adopted, and possible underlying schemas and salient long-term memories.

Physiological anxiety

Attention to this level is particularly important in the treatment of panic disorder, generalised anxiety disorder and hypochondria, but it is a good starting point for the treatment of most anxiety disorders. This is because first, we can provide the patient with a more rational understanding of the physical changes associated with anxiety and panic; second, when patients are able to control the physical changes, they have a greater sense of empowerment; and, third, the relaxation techniques assist in building a good rapport between patient and therapist.

1. Direct symptom control

We have presented relaxation and self-control methods in previous chapters. The main effects of these are a reduction in arousal, and the anxious feelings are thereby less noticeable. If the patient hyperventilates, then one of the breathing techniques described in Chapter 12 will eliminate the adverse effects of this.

Exposure therapy in the case of specific fears, such as phobias for creatures (spiders, birds, moths, etc.) and height phobia, is presumed to reduce physiological arousal by extinction, habituation or reciprocal inhibition. It is probably better if one can use in vivo exposure for these rather than imaginal exposure, in which case it is likely that hypnosis will be redundant, although some practitioners augment the treatment with an anxiety management technique.

2. Correcting attentional biases

Reduction in arousal by relaxation and self-control techniques means less attention is paid to the symptoms of anxiety. An attention-switching strategy may be used; in fact, all self-control techniques have this effect anyway (e.g. breathing, self-talk and safe place imagery). Some attention-switching strategies – e.g. for blushing fears, self-consciousness owing to anxiety, and hypochondriacal fears – were described in Chapter 20. These may be rehearsed in imagination during hypnosis and self-hypnosis, posthypnotic suggestions may be given, and so on.

3. Correcting interpretative biases

Simply teaching a patient an effective self-control method leads to the modification of more general beliefs; for example, the patient may be able to move away from the belief that 'These feelings control me' to 'I can control these feelings', a very significant step.

One may wish to provide the patient with some relevant facts concerning physical arousal and panic. For example, the patient can learn to reframe the experiences thus: 'My body is only doing what it does when I am very active or very excited'. If the patient hyperventilates, then this will result in a wide spectrum of symptoms that, if the patient does not understand them, can be misinterpreted in a catastrophic manner, which then leads to more anxiety, more hyperventilation, and so on.

Wilkinson (1988) gives a good account of hyperventilation and its treatment, incorporating hypnosis. We can in fact distinguish acute and chronic hyperventilation. During acute hyperventilation, the person is in an obvious state of panic; breathing is rapid and often shallow (but occasionally may be profound and slow) with overuse of the chest muscles as opposed to the diaphragm. The patient may be informed that this type of breathing is appropriate for strenuous exercise or excitement. Chronic hyperventilation is more persistent in the person's everyday life but is often unnoticeable.

The relevant effect of hyperventilation is depletion of carbon dioxide in the bloodstream and nervous tissue, which leads to autonomic arousal in favour of the sympathetic component. Carbon dioxide depletion in the bloodstream leads to increase in alkalinity ('alkalosis'), vasoconstriction and therefore a decrease in uptake of oxygen by the nervous tissue. This may lead to feelings of dizziness and faintness, and even depersonalisation. However, in a healthy person it will not cause fainting, the blood pressure being raised (in contrast to fainting owing to the sight of blood or injury, which is associated with low blood pressure).

Depletion of carbon dioxide in the nervous tissue leads to increased neuronal activity and excitability, increased motor activity, sensory aberrations such as visual and auditory disturbances and paraesthesiae (tingling) in the extremities, and increased sympathetic dominance. Overuse of the thoracic muscles may lead to chest pains.

Acute hyperventilation is obvious (in vivo or from the patient's description). Not uncommonly, the patient will complain, 'I can't breathe properly'. Panic symptoms, 'tinglings', feelings of unreality, faintness and heaviness in the limbs are also commonly reported.

Chronic hyperventilation is associated with frequent sighing or yawning, breathlessness and feeling the need to breathe more, tiredness, aching of chest muscles, globus, wind, bloating (possibly caused by swallowing of air), anxiety and the sudden occurrence of panics. The causes may be 'stress' (particularly in people who lead a sedentary life). Chronic carbon dioxide depletion leads to a compensatory excretion from the bloodstream (via the kidneys) of bicarbonate ions to restore the resting pH value of the blood. Therefore, the person has to continue to overbreathe and breathing may then be effortful and accompanied by a feeling of respiratory insufficiency.

Acute hyperventilation and panic may be triggered by momentary increases in arousal – sudden shock, excitement, yawning, exertion, fleeting anxious thoughts, and so on. This is more likely to happen in people who suffer from chronic hyperventilation, thus explaining why some patients complain, 'My panics can just came out of the blue'.

The main points to get across to patients are that hyperventilation is not dangerous and there are no catastrophic outcomes, even fainting. Patients can be encouraged to test reality with you; both of you hyperventilate and discover that for as long as you are willing to go on with this, nothing terrible happens. Only do this with a healthy patient (e.g. not with someone with a heart problem, asthma or epilepsy or with an expectant mother).

Again hypnosis may be used to assist cognitive rehearsal of the reinterpretation of the symptoms in the ways already described.

The external situation

This is particularly important for situational phobic anxiety.

1. Correcting attentional biases

Attentional biases to the environment are not necessarily just through the senses; for example, an anxious car passenger may be constantly anticipating being hit from behind, yet not actually be always looking in that direction.

Attentional biases may be selective, as in the case of the agoraphobic or claustrophobic person who may be constantly checking to see if an exit from the room is accessible. On the other hand, hypervigilant patients, say those with travel phobia or fear of the dark, describe how they are on the alert for anything happening. Finally, some patients may avoid attending to particular aspects of the environment; for example, socially phobic individuals may avoid looking at other people by keeping their eyes and head down.

Working cognitively entails (i) the identification of the nature of attentional biases to the external environment and (ii) the *normalisation* of attention. In the case of some patients, this may actually entail their *avoiding* attending to aspects of their environment. For example, hypervigilant travel phobic patients may be asked to look down at their lap for periods of time. In behavioural terms, this may be construed as avoidance behaviour but, in cognitive terms, it is 'reality testing' and challenging the belief that 'I am in constant danger and must be alert and ready to act'.

The changes in distribution of attention may be rehearsed in imagination and specific posthypnotic suggestions given.

2. Correcting interpretative biases (cognitive restructuring)

This is a large part of cognitive therapy and involves helping the patient gain a more rational and realistic appraisal of the situation, thus reducing the perceived threat. This may be done directly by instruction – for example, educating the thunderstorm phobic person on the relative dangers of other phenomena and activities. However, as we said in Chapter 21, it is better to elicit the reinterpretations from patients themselves.

Again, hypnosis and self-hypnosis, using imaginal rehearsal and posthypnotic suggestion, may be used to augment these procedures.

Behavioural anxiety

In Chapter 21, we outlined the rationale for identifying and eliminating behavioural responses to unrealistic cognitions and beliefs. Behavioural anxiety does not appear to lend itself too well to the analysis of attentional and interpretative biases, although M. W. Eysenck (1997) summarises evidence from social psychology laboratories that socially anxious individuals overattend to their anxious behaviour (body posture, fidgeting, speech dysfluency, etc.) and are inclined to overestimate how much other people are noticing it and judging them by it. Consequently, rehearsal of a relaxed body posture will eliminate the cues that inform such people that they are anxious, likewise a more external focus of attention (see the section on attention switching in Ch. 20).

Common manifestations of behavioural anxiety are avoidance, escape, dependency, checking, obsessions, holding onto things, bracing oneself, avoidance of eye contact, and overapologising. Elimination of these and the substitution of more appropriate behaviour may be rehearsed in imagination using past, present and future situations.

Cognitive anxiety

Here we are concerned with cognitive activity that goes beyond the immediate automatic thoughts and interpretational biases that we have discussed up until now. According to M. W. Eysenck (1997), it is patients with obsessive–compulsive disorder who accelerate their anxiety by attentional and interpretative biases to cognitive anxiety. We shall shortly discuss this particular disorder.

Typical of the kind of cognitive anxiety we are discussing is what is commonly called 'worrying'. Worrying may occur in response to past events ('What would have happened if … ?'; 'I wonder if I caused any offence?'; and so on). As such, it may involve a reappraisal of memories. People who have had 'narrow escapes' often worry in this way, and this can be one route to the acquisition of a phobia.

Case example

Mrs M. (seen by MH) was flying home from holiday with her husband and another couple, when the plane hit some turbulence. The other lady panicked dramatically, but Mrs M. remained calm and was able to reassure and comfort her friend. In the months afterwards, she ruminated on the idea 'What if it was me who had panicked?' and imagined that she would make a complete fool of herself in front of the other passengers. When the time approached for Mr and Mrs M. to start thinking of a holiday again, she found that she was terrified by the thought of flying.

Thus we see a second type of worrying, one with a future orientation: 'What if X happens?' Characteristic of this is anticipatory anxiety, which nearly everyone experiences.

Both types of worrying can be adaptive in the sense that they are about being prepared for coping with danger. (People who worry that they could have been killed in an accident may be construed as endeavouring to ensure that they are well prepared next time.) In fact, Janis (1971) wrote of 'the work of worrying' by patients waiting for surgical operations; those who worried to a moderate degree felt better after their operations than those who claimed not to be worried at all.

Worrying about the future is very difficult to control. Hypnotic relaxation and self-control procedures are not particularly effective in helping people dispose of this type of worrying. One could reframe the worrying by informing patients, with some justification, that worrying is preparing them for the event in question and therefore a good thing. It is not uncommon to discover that the worst part of facing an anxiety-provoking situation is the lead-up period. Perhaps the function of worrying is to encourage the anxiety to peak *before* the event. Hence, one could suggest the 'worrying chair' technique described in Chapter 20. It is important, however, that patients who are worrying about some out-of-the-ordinary occurrence, such as a dental appointment or an aeroplane journey, should be encouraged not to cancel the event because of their worrying.

Worries are often expressions of deep-seated or core beliefs and these may be challenged. For example, a rational emotive therapist may challenge Mrs M. (above) about her apparent need to always be seen as calm and composed. Surely there are worse things to worry about than being seen to panic? Some paradoxical methods also address such worries. For example, people who worry that they might draw attention to themselves in public (say by having to go to the toilet at the cinema and causing the people in the same row to have to stand up) may be instructed to do just that.

We have discussed formal 'thought-stopping' and 'decentring' methods in Chapter 20. In the next chapter, we shall describe another distraction technique that may be useful for obsessional worrying by depressed people.

Schemas and significant memories

As we described in Chapter 21, there are times in cognitive-behavioural therapy when it may be useful to depart from the here and now and review earlier experiences that may be related to the development of longstanding dysfunctional assumptions or schemas. We have described ways of accessing these, the affect bridge being an especially useful procedure. In Chapter 19, we also described the use of ego-state therapy combined with regression. This can be a very effective manoeuvre from a cognitive therapy perspective because the patient takes responsibility for reappraising the event or situation, and the high level of emotion that often accompanies this procedure seems to have a kind of binding effect on the new cognitions and attitudes generated.

OBSESSIVE–COMPULSIVE DISORDER

The above methods may be used in a treatment programme for anxiety disorders such as generalised anxiety disorder, panic disorder, agoraphobia, social anxiety, and specific phobias, although in all of these the therapist should be mindful of the importance of in vivo exposure, especially when working with specific phobias, in which case hypnosis may not be particularly useful.

A similar caveat applies to the treatment of obsessive–compulsive disorder (OCD). The term OCD covers a range of problems characterised by the occurrence of excessive maladaptive thoughts and the overwhelming compulsion to perform some action contingent on these thoughts.

The treatment of choice for OCD is usually response prevention on exposure to anxiety-provoking situations. The mode of action of this may be construed both in behavioural terms (elimination of escape and avoidance) and in cognitive terms. In the latter case, the major cognitions around OCD are to do with the avoidance of some dreadful consequence (usually involving others) if the obsessional thoughts or compulsive actions are not carried out. Hence, response prevention may be construed as reality testing.

There is very little work reported on the use of hypnosis with OCD and it is known that patients with OCD, even when they have been successfully treated, tend to be low in hypnotisability (Hoogduin 1988), although there are bound to be individual exceptions. We do not recommend that readers attempt to use hypnosis with OCD patients unless they are experienced in cognitive-behavioural treatment, otherwise much time may be wasted.

OCD patients are of course anxious, but their anxiety need not be manifest at the physiological level to the same extent as those patients with other anxiety disorders who report high levels of autonomic arousal, with or without panic. M. W. Eysenck (1997) regards the main focus of attention and interpretational biases of OCD patients to be on their cognitive activity. Readers may understand the difference by imagining what it is like when one is, say, at the cinema worrying about whether one locked the door on leaving home. Compare this to the anxiety experienced when confronted with physical danger. Consequently, physical relaxation methods may play only a limited role in the treatment of OCD.

One of the features of OCD thinking is 'thought-action fusion' whereby the patient considers that thinking of doing something unacceptable is as bad as actually doing it, or that thinking about some disturbing event makes it more likely to be true or to happen in reality. Another characteristic of the thinking in OCD has been described as an 'inflated sense of responsibility' for the possible occurrence of untoward events. That is, OCD patients appear, for example, to believe that were they *not* to carry out their cognitive or behavioural rituals, then something terrible would befall other people.

Cognitive therapy methods have been increasingly used with OCD to challenge the patient's irrational thinking. Hence, hypnosis may be used to rehearse cognitive restructuring (as well as abstaining from compulsive behaviour) in various key situations imagined by the patient. Imaginal techniques (such as imagining *not* acting on the obsessional thoughts) could also be used to clarify the nature of the supposed dreadful consequences that the patient so fears. For an illustration of the hypnotic augmentation of flooding and response prevention for compulsive hand-washing, readers may consult Scrignar (1981).

It should be noted, however, that the theoretical rationale underpinning cognitive-behavioural treatment contraindicates the use of thought-stopping, decentring or distraction methods. Indeed, OCD patients invest much energy on strategies aimed at controlling, suppressing or neutralising their obsessional thoughts and this seems to be counterproductive. Instead, the patient must fully confront and challenge the maladaptive thoughts.

Although Freud and his followers enunciated theories about OCD that, stripped of references to psychoanalytic concepts, are not dissimilar to the cognitive model, it does not appear that psychoanalysis or psychodynamically oriented therapy has a good track record in the treatment of OCD. Nevertheless, it may be important to consider where in OCD the 'inflated sense of responsibility' comes from. The developmental model of cognitive therapy for anxiety disorders was presented in Figure 21.1; a very similar model for OCD has been presented by Salkovskis (1989), the key component being that the relevant formative experiences in the person's life concern the inculcation of a sense of responsibility for others, a need to take great care, and so on.

Now, children can certainly come to feel unduly responsible for events that happen (or could happen) in their family life. This may arise from punitive attitudes on the part of parents, who may explicitly blame their children quite unrealistically for upsetting events ('You've made your mother very ill', 'This is all your fault', etc.); or children may come to believe (or even hope) that they have some ability to forestall some dreadful happening such as the break-up of their parents' marriage. Although there is little evidence currently to support the use of regression methods in therapy for OCD, it may be worthwhile researching the possibility of augmenting a cognitive-behavioural approach with schema-based methods using hypnosis.

POST-TRAUMATIC STRESS DISORDER

Post-traumatic stress disorder (PTSD) is classified as an anxiety disorder under DSM-IV. It is however a complex disorder in that the patient complains of a considerable range of symptoms that are manifestations of extreme arousal and anxiety and some depressive tendencies.

As we also stated for OCD, hypnotic procedures in therapy for PTSD should be undertaken adjunctively by those therapists already experienced in the treatment of patients with this disorder. Here we shall present a number of ways in which hypnosis may augment a course of therapy.

General considerations

Largely, we suspect, for the expediencies of legal practice, to fulfil a diagnosis of PTSD a minimum number of criterion symptoms must be present. However, for clinical purposes those therapists who work with traumatised patients will see many who do not fulfil the necessary criteria, yet are clearly suffering. Treatment is not necessarily different for patients who fall below the threshold for a full diagnosis of PTSD.

Patients vary considerably in severity. Also, in our experience, those patients involved in compensation proceedings are beyond the acute stage of the disorder when they present for therapy. This may be a consequence of protracted litigation, whereby treatment awaits either the final settlement or some interim payment, or if the client is referred to a health service specialist or clinic with a long waiting list for treatment. This is also usually the case at the time of the client's assessment, which may be over a year since the accident. For example, in 205 road traffic accident cases (interestingly, one-third male and two-thirds female) seen by one of us (MH), only 10% were considered to fulfil full criteria for a DSM-IV diagnosis of PTSD by the time they were assessed for medicolegal purposes. The remainder had residual symptoms, travel anxiety being very common (classifiable as a phobia in around one-third of all cases).

In such cases, where the patient is still reacting with anxiety to thoughts and images of the incident, some form of image desensitisation and reprocessing procedure (see below) may be undertaken in the early stages of therapy. In more serious cases, it may be wise initially to work on anxiety management, symptom control and ego-strengthening before embarking on confrontation and reprocessing of the traumatic imagery.

Those patients who have sustained physical injuries may require help in, for example, pain management. Some patients may also be quite markedly depressed. Major depression may occur alongside PTSD or may be a consequence of the restrictions imposed on the patient by the disorder itself or any physical injuries sustained. The most catastrophic consequence for a patient is loss of employment, which in our experience puts the patient at great risk of major depression. Patients describe how their lives have been 'turned upside down' and they feel helpless and hopeless.

Where the trauma resulted from the negligence or malevolence of another person, patients often feel great anger and a sense of unfairness. There is often guilt too, as a result of irrational self-questioning of the type 'Was I (partly) to blame?' but also shame that, for example, 'After all this time I should have been able to pull myself together'. In Britain at least, anything short of displaying 'a stiff upper lip' (an expression, incidentally, of American origin) is equated with mental weakness and cowardice, and it is customary nowadays for any media announcement that 'survivors and witnesses of the tragedy are being offered counselling' to be greeted with a chorus of groaning and sneering and claims that the country is facing something tantamount to national decline.

All of this serves to emphasise the importance of carefully assessing the patient's symptoms and problems and planning the course of therapy.

There is some evidence that patients with PTSD are higher than average in hypnotisability (Cardeña 2000). This may mean that high hypnotisability predisposes a person to develop PTSD, or that PTSD renders people more hypnotisable. Spiegel & Cardeña (1990) draw a parallel between PTSD and hypnosis. For them, the three major components of hypnosis are absorption, dissociation and suggestibility. They compare these components to (respectively) the intrusive reliving of traumatic events, 'psychic numbing', and hypervigilance and heightened sensitivity to environmental events, all of them symptoms that are observed in PTSD. For the purposes of considering the various ways hypnosis may augment therapy, we shall use the DSM-IV classification of symptoms.

Intrusive memories and images

Under this heading, we include the distress caused by recalling the trauma, frightening flashback images, nightmares and the avoidance of thoughts of the incident. There is a range of behavioural and cognitive techniques for addressing these problems. These are based on theories and working models of PTSD that postulate that in some way the details of the traumatic experience fail to be processed or encoded in long-term memory in the normal way. There are indeed theories, and some evidence, that neural activity associated with traumatic memories is in a different part of the brain to normal memories (van der Kolk 1996). Thus, the memories remain vivid and intrusive, with all the attendant emotion. This is obviously maladaptive and not conducive to survival. Consider that until only recently in the evolution of humankind, daily life was full of threat and exposure to danger. Survival would be impossible if, after each fearful encounter, the memory of the event and the fear evoked remained in their raw state. Individuals would be condemned to react with extreme anxiety, escape and avoidance to every situation in which they had experienced fear. Clearly, this would be disastrous for the carrying out of activities that are essential to survival, such as hunting and defending one's own self and one's territory. Some mechanism is needed to enable the individual to remember and learn from the experiences, yet not be forever incapacitated by them. It seems that with PTSD this process is, for some reason, stalled.

A simple behavioural explanation may be analogous to a phobia. The experience of terror is so overwhelming that the person continually attempts to avoid thoughts, images, memories and reminders of it. The person cannot easily do this in the case of the internal experiences and they persistently intrude, despite his or her efforts to prevent them. This 'battle' persists and it is difficult for the anxiety associated with the trauma to dissipate by the natural processes of habituation and desensitisation.

The concept of dissociation or some pre-attentive inhibitory mechanism may be incorporated into the above model, particularly where there appear to be blanks in the person's memory of the trauma that cannot be accounted for by inattention, forgetting, organic amnesia, and so on.

Another way of understanding what is happening is to recall that we endeavour to interpret and make sense of what happens to us in terms of our existing ways of mentally structuring and understanding our world, or our cognitive schemas. When something happens that cannot be accommodated into our existing ways of understanding our world (in Ch. 21 we use the analogy of a map), then we need to adjust the latter to 'take on board' what we have experienced. Occasionally, however, we experience or witness something that is so overwhelmingly terrifying, or so alien to what we have come to understand about our world and expect from it, that we simply cannot come to terms with what has happened. When something happens to dramatically challenge one's core beliefs, one is left struggling with a world that seems completely different to what one has hitherto implicitly accepted. How often do we hear comments such as 'You read about these things but you never expect them to happen to you'?

One implicit and very important assumption that people commonly have is 'I am safe' (Hodgkinson & Stewart 1991). Following a trauma, the person's core belief system now includes the important assumption 'The world is very dangerous'. Hypervigilance and avoidance behaviours are the consequence of this. Of course, this is neither a rational nor an adaptive response. For example, a person may have driven, and been driven, tens and even hundreds of thousands of miles before having a road traffic accident. Afterwards, the person feels and behaves as if an accident is certainly going to happen again at any moment. Of course, an accident *may* happen again, but as a general (and adaptive) rule, we do not experience anxiety and avoid situations when the probability of injury or death is very low, otherwise we would not do anything!

As well as the belief 'I am now always vulnerable', PTSD may also be associated with drastic changes in self-perception and self-esteem. From 'I am a competent person', the individual's core self-beliefs may now be 'I am incompetent'; 'I am guilty'; 'I am weak'; and so on. Such beliefs may arise from self-recrimination associated with what individuals perceive to be their failure to act appropriately at the time of the trauma – 'I should have realised what was going to happen'; 'I should have prevented it'; 'I should have fought back' (in the case of an assault); and so on. Negative self-regard is also associated with patients' disappointment with themselves in not 'getting over' the incident – viz. 'I used to think of myself as a strong person who coped. Now I'm just a bag of nerves'.

Therapeutic strategies for intrusive thoughts, memories and images

Therapeutic strategies that focus on the thoughts, memories and images of the trauma have a common component, namely they encourage exposure to internal events. Such procedures are consistent with the theoretical ideas discussed above and with the working model of unconscious–conscious activity presented in Chapter 18.

The simplest method, therefore, is to encourage the patient to keep talking about what happened. Some patients avoid doing this in their everyday life, but others may protest that they have talked about it enough. However, a plausible hypothesis is that while *seeming* to talk exhaustively about the incident, they may be adopting avoidant or 'blunting' defence strategies, so that they do not fully confront the memories. Accordingly, a more structured approach may be called for.

Image habituation

A behavioural strategy of proven value is 'image habituation'. This is similar to desensitisation for a phobia. A number of key images associated with the trauma are chosen and the patient is required to focus vividly on each one in turn, repeating the sequence many times. This is also done as a daily homework assignment using a tape recording that cues in each image. (One of us – MH – uses a written list instead.) The reader should consult Vaughan & Tarrier (1992) for a full exposition of this procedure.

The aim of the procedure is to reduce the patient's anxiety and distress on exposure to each image. A key instruction in this method is that patients must imagine each scene as vividly as they can, and must not employ any ameliorating strategies such as relaxation, blurring of the image or cognitive reconstruction.

These techniques for confronting traumatic memories may, in themselves, lead to adaptive reappraisal and reconstruction of the incident, the patient's role in it, and the patient's maladaptive cognitions regarding himself or herself and the world in general. Apart from desensitisation, one working model is that the processes of reconstruction and reappraisal are free to occur naturally once patients have fully assimilated the trauma into their normal long-term memory.

In contrast, explicit cognitive reappraisal and restructuring may be required in addition to image desensitisation. A full description of this work is beyond the scope of this chapter, but we shall refer to how image exposure methods may be augmented by cognitive reappraisal techniques as we go along. In fact, we have already encountered one such technique, namely ego-state therapy. For example, a survivor of an accident may be asked to imagine going back to the original scene and providing the necessary comfort and reassurance to the 'self' in the accident, important messages being 'You survived' and 'You did the best you could'.

Two methods from the hypnosis literature

From the hypnosis literature, there are several variations on the theme of confronting the memory of the trauma. Two of these will now be described. They both involve gradual exposure, with the patient initially in the role of onlooker, rather than flooding, and so the likelihood of extreme abreaction is reduced. For this reason, they are particularly useful in severe cases of PTSD.

Both methods require that patients have some ability to maintain and manipulate realistic imagery, and some dissociative capacity is advantageous. The induction and deepening methods used for these procedures are those presented for the first approach in Chapter 6 and include the safe place technique. It is initially explained to patients that they are going to be asked to review the traumatic experience, but this will be done in such a way as to minimise any distress. Initially they will observe the scene from a detached standpoint. It is emphasised throughout that patients are in full control and can immediately 'switch off' any image if this proves too distressing. It is also explained during hypnosis that if at any time patients wish, they may return in imagination to their safe place. Both procedures may be augmented by ideomotor signals although this does not usually confer any significant advantage.

The first technique is the screen method. We encountered this approach in Chapter 19 when we presented procedures for age regression, and there are many ways in which the method may be varied. It is suggested to patients that they are sitting in a comfortable chair and are looking at a television screen which is at present turned off. They have hold of the remote control and are therefore able to alter the focus, brightness, volume, etc.; they may stop and start the video playback whenever they wish, may switch channels to something more pleasant, and may turn off the television at any point.

Initially, patients are asked to select a programme which they find pleasant and amusing, such as a favourite film. In imagination, they can also practise controlling the screen, flipping channels, changing the programme, and so on. One can also ask them to practise going to their safe place, or one may have set up a positive anchor such as the clenched fist or, say, the pressure of the therapist's hand on the patient's shoulder. Another 'safety device' is asking them to imagine 'floating out of themselves' to a place where they can watch themselves watching the screen.

Patients are to run through the memory from start to finish. If it proves too emotional, then they are to switch off for a while, or freeze the video, or adjust the brightness so that it becomes much dimmer, and so on. However, it is essential that the video is watched in full. One can ascertain patients' affect and cognitions by, for example, asking them to freeze the video and eliciting these. Eventually, patients can be encouraged to 'play with the image'. The video can be run backwards and forwards, the colour may be changed, the brightness, the sound, and so on. The purpose is for patients to be able to tolerate the images without the associated affect.

One ego-state method that can be used is to ask patients to imagine that the screen is divided (as described in Ch. 24 for insomnia) and to imagine their 'healthy', 'resourceful' part in one half, ready to intervene in the replay of the event, which is in the other half of the screen, to comfort the 'self' that was traumatised, and so on. The therapist helps patients to reappraise the trauma both during the procedure and afterwards, when they are alerted.

The second technique is similar but uses the image of a protective bubble. It has been described by Alden (1995) with acknowledgements to Daniel Brown (unpublished work, 1992). The preliminary instructions are very similar to those for the screen method. The technique may actually be used as an induction and deepening routine.

Patients imagine that they are enclosed in a safe, protective bubble. This is just the right size to give them a sense of space and yet also a sense of containment and protection. The walls of the bubble are, of course, transparent, but they are sufficiently thick to give them full protection, though not so thick that they are unable to have any contact with the world outside.

Patients can then describe the bubble, how the walls feel, the colours, and so on. To help patients absorb themselves in this image, the therapist simply reflects back the comments patients make. The therapist then asks patients to imagine floating around inside the bubble and enjoy the sense of comfort and protection. It is suggested that they are floating in a carefree way, enjoying the security, and breathing naturally and easily, relaxing with every breath. These suggestions of deepening comfort, relaxation and safety are repeated a number of times in a manner similar to the hypnotic induction procedures described in Chapter 6. The suggestion may also be given that 'Although only a short time in reality may pass, you have all the time you need to go as deep as you need'. When patients are as deeply relaxed and absorbed as they wish, they may then give a signal that they are ready to proceed.

The next stage is to ask patients to imagine that the bubble is actually floating around, taking them to anywhere that they wish. This can be a safe place, and when they are there they give a signal. Patients can then describe where they are, and further suggestions may be given of feeling comfortable and secure. Alternatively, one can suggest a specific place to patients, for example, a comfortable beach or a garden.

Patients can then be instructed to imagine coming out of the bubble, walking around the special place, and finding a spot in which to rest, just as described in the deepening method given in Chapter 6. You may also establish a positive anchor for the feelings of being in this safe place.

Once patients are familiar with this method, it can then be used to broach the memories of the traumatic incident in a manner similar to the screen technique. Patients are encouraged to review the memories from the safety of the protective bubble until the original affect dissipates. Cognitive restructuring may be undertaken and patients may be encouraged to leave the bubble, knowing that at any time they may return. For example, ego-state work may be undertaken, as described above.

Eye movement desensitisation and reprocessing (EMDR)

This is an image exposure method in which the therapist introduces cognitive restructuring techniques as and when they are required. Otherwise, the therapist relies on the patient to reappraise the trauma as the memory and images are confronted. This kind of reprocessing is assumed to be facilitated by the patient's making rapid lateral movements of the eyes while keeping the traumatic image in mind. To aid this, the therapist moves a finger from side to side, or the patient may follow a row of lamps that light up in sequence. One theory is that these eye movements are related to rapid eye movements in dream sleep, or involve some kind of inter-hemispheric processing and integration. Thus, there may be a neurological mechanism that facilitates the reprocessing and assimilation of the traumatic memories.

EMDR has grown in popularity since its beginnings in the 1980s. It is *not* another fad like neurolinguistic programming (see Heap 1988a, 1988b for accounts of the latter). Its proponents are hard-nosed, clinical psychologists and psychiatrists, drilled in the tenets and disciplines of cognitive-behavioural psychology. There are many clinical trials and meta-analyses in respected peer-review journals that attest to its clinical effectiveness. Yet many authoritative commentators seem unable to bring themselves to give this treatment approach their full stamp of approval. Some therapists even consider that EMDR is hypnosis in another guise.

There appear to be at least two aspects of EMDR that worry many people. The first one is the way in which the eye-movement procedure was discovered. This was not the accumulation of careful laboratory investigations, but the casual subjective observation of EMDR's founder, Francine Shapiro, whilst strolling through a park in 1987 (Shapiro 1995). The second concern is the lack of any good theoretical justification for the eye movements. This worry is compounded by the recommendation in EMDR manuals (e.g. Shapiro 1995) that if the patient does not respond (or does not like) lateral eye movements, then one can use diagonal or vertical movements, or alternating finger-snapping in the left and right ears, or even alternately tapping the patient's knees.

In Chapter 15, we pointed out that a treatment may be effective for reasons not predicted by the theoretical model on which it is based. The fact that lateral eye movements are not essential to treatment outcome should lead us to conclude that a model that designates the eye movements with some special role in reprocessing traumatic memories is erroneous. Nevertheless, this does not in itself mean that we should abandon EMDR. Perhaps one explanation is that the eye movements, finger-snapping and knee-tapping facilitate reprocessing because they act as distracters which disrupt the habitual defensive ploys that patients engage in whenever the traumatic incident is brought to mind.

Since its inception, EMDR has become more elaborate and more cognitive in orientation (hence the 'reprocessing': it was originally known as EMD). EMDR practitioners interweave cognitive restructuring within the basic procedure. Cognitive restructuring may relate specifically to the trauma itself (e.g. 'I did the best I could') but preferably to here-and-now self-appraisal (e.g. 'I am a worthy person'; 'I am capable of being loved'; and 'I am safe').

Other imagery techniques

There are other imagery techniques and some of these directly attempt to change the raw images in some way so that they no longer exert an overwhelmingly destructive influence on the patient's state of mind. We shall not discuss these but the reader may recall our description of the technique of 'telescoping trauma with too late comfort' in Chapter 19 in which the most traumatic image is repeatedly paired with the image of rescue, safety, relief, and so on.

Techniques for nightmares

Some patients have recurring nightmares associated with the trauma. Often the kind of work we have described above will result in an easing of nightmares, but sometimes it is necessary to address these directly. One can use image habituation methods (and EMDR) but successful outcomes have also been reported (Kingsbury 1993) that ask the patient to change the dream in some way. A popular method is to ask the patient (if this is not too frightening) to relive the nightmare, and as the most fearful point of the nightmare is approaching, to change the outcome to one more positive. For example, if the patient is about to be attacked, the change could be, say, the assailant explodes or falls through the floor. (It may be that the more dramatic and absurd the new outcome of the dream, and the more appealing to the patient, the more effective will be the intervention.) Other ploys are imagining 'switching channels to a better programme' – that is, a more pleasant dream – which may be done using the imaginary television procedure, and sending the distressing image 'the wrong way' down a telescope so it vanishes in the distance. Using hypnosis, one can give a posthypnotic suggestion about the new outcome of the dream and ask the patient to rehearse this new outcome during self-hypnosis.

It is not clear if these techniques actually change the content of the dream so much as reduce its impact and frequency. This indicates that the underlying mechanism is probably more akin to desensitisation.

Finally, night terrors (which occur in stage 4 of non-REM sleep) appear to respond well to direct posthypnotic suggestion and stress reduction (Hoogduin & Hagenaars 2000, Koe 1989, Kramer 1989) as well as resolution of an earlier traumatic experience (Kraft 1986).

Hypervigilance, hypersensitivity, distress on exposure to reminders, and avoidance of these

Again, if one is able initially to reduce the impact of the traumatic images and memories, then some easing of general anxiety and anxiety on exposure to reminders may be achieved. However, phobic anxiety may persist in many cases (e.g. fear and avoidance of the original scene of the trauma, the dark, fire, car travel, dogs and heights, and even agoraphobia, depending on the nature of the trauma). This is because the phobic anxiety is continually reinforced by the patient's behavioural and cognitive coping strategies. This may be by avoidance of or escape from the feared situation, which, as we have seen, maintains and even exacerbates the degree of anxiety experienced. However, even when the person confronts the situation, the overwhelming impulse is to interpret every little incident as highly threatening. This, and the tendency to act accordingly (e.g. in the case of car travel, adopting bracing or holding postures, being overvigilant, and warning the driver unnecessarily) again maintain and exacerbate the anxiety and it is difficult for the person to become desensitised.

Therefore, therapy with a PTSD patient may well include cognitive-behavioural methods for reducing general anxiety and phobic anxiety and, as we have seen, hypnotic procedure may augment these.

Anger and hostility

Patients with PTSD are often very angry about what has happened to them. Their psychological (and sometimes physical) suffering also affects their tolerance level, and very commonly they are irritable and prone to angry, and occasionally violent, outbursts. All too often it is their family who is on the receiving end of their temper, and this compounds their sense of guilt and shame. Anger-management training may therefore be expedient, and the self-control methods described in Chapter 12 may augment this component of treatment.

Sleep

Sleep impairment is common in PTSD, even in the absence of nightmares. Sleep may improve on its own as the patient responds to treatment of the intrusive thoughts and memories, but if the impaired sleep pattern has become habitual, then the procedures outlined in Chapter 24 may be applied.

The depressive symptoms of PTSD

Criterion C of DSM-IV includes a number of symptoms that may be construed as depressive in nature – emotional numbing, loss of interest, social withdrawal, a foreshortened sense of future, and so on. Also, as we have said, the person may suffer a profound loss of self-esteem. Indeed, severe cases may also be diagnosed with major depression. These problems will be compounded if there are physical injuries, disability, loss of amenity (owing to physical and psychological problems and financial losses) and loss of employment.

Therapy for PTSD may need to address the 'cognitive triad', namely the patient's outlook on his or her world, self and future, and hypnotic procedures may play a role, as described in previous chapters.

Conclusions concerning hypnosis and PTSD

Psychological procedures for post-traumatic stress can be very effective for the milder, less chronic cases and the main focus of therapy may be on the intrusive thoughts, memories and images. With more severe and chronic cases, the therapy is much more involved and complex and the therapist needs to prioritise which problems to address first. One requirement is to counsel patients about the nature of PTSD, as often they are bewildered by their symptoms and problems, and not infrequently ashamed of themselves. It may be expedient initially to help patients cope with their general symptoms of anxiety and mood swings and to counsel the family. Given the known higher hypnotic susceptibility of these patients, it is well worth considering the adjunctive use of hypnotic procedures.

The question is occasionally raised about the use of hypnosis with PTSD patients who may have to appear in court. This may arise in personal injury litigation or in criminal cases that have yet to be tried. As we have stated elsewhere, there is a risk of memory distortion when using hypnosis, but it is possible that this is also a risk with other imagery methods (Brown et al 1998). Where distortions arise using these methods, they are likely to involve specific details of the incident rather than extensive confabulation, and these may not affect issues of liability and guilt. In fact, in the UK, the vast majority of personal injury cases are settled out of court and often liability is not contested when the case is heard. Nevertheless, there may be occasions when it is possible for a sharp defence lawyer to pick up on the fact that a claimant has been the subject of hypnotic procedures and then challenge the authenticity of the claimant's testimony. This is probably more likely to happen in the USA than in Britain.

We suggest that where a trial may be pending in which liability or guilt is to be determined, the therapist should confer with the patient's legal advisors concerning the use of hypnosis and similar procedures prior to the trial. The forensic use of hypnosis is further discussed in Chapter 33.

REFERENCES

Alden P 1995 Back to the past: Introducing the 'bubble'. Contemporary Hypnosis 12: 59–68
American Psychiatric Association 1994 Diagnostic and statistical manual of mental disorders, 4th edn. American Psychiatric Association, Washington DC
Brown D P, Scheflin A W, Hammond D C 1998 Memory, trauma, treatment, and the law. Norton, New York

Cardeña E 2000 Hypnosis in the treatment of trauma: A promising but not fully supported, efficacious treatment. International Journal of Clinical and Experimental Hypnosis 48: 225–238

Cattell R B, Ebeer H W, Tatsouka M W 1970 Handbook for the Sixteen Personality Factor Questionnaire (16PF). Institute for Personality and Ability Testing, Champaign

Crowne D P, Marlowe D 1964 The approval motive. Wiley, New York

Digman J M 1990 Personality structure: Emergence of the five-factor model. Annual Review of Psychology 41: 417–440

Eysenck H J 1967 The biological basis of personality. Charles C Thomas, Springfield

Eysenck M W 1997 Anxiety and cognition: A unified theory. Psychology Press, Hove

Heap M 1988a Neurolinguistic programming: A British perspective. Hypnos: Swedish Journal of Hypnosis in Psychotherapy and Psychosomatic Medicine 15: 4–13

Heap M 1988b Born-again mesmerism? The Psychologist 1: 262–263

Hodgkinson P E, Stewart M 1991 A handbook of disaster management. Routledge, London

Hoogduin K 1988 Hypnotisability in obsessive–compulsives. Hypnos: Swedish Journal for Hypnosis in Psychotherapy and Psychosomatic Disorders 15: 15–19

Hoogduin K, Hagenaars M 2000 Hypnosis in sleep terror disorders. Hypnos: Swedish Journal for Hypnosis in Psychotherapy and Psychosomatic Disorders 27: 180–190

Janis I L 1971 Stress and frustration. Harcourt Brace Jovanovich, New York

Jensen M R 1987 Psychobiological factors predicting the course of breast cancer. Journal of Personality 55: 317–342

Kingsbury S 1993 Brief hypnotic treatment of repetitive nightmares. American Journal of Clinical Hypnosis 35: 161–169

Koe G G 1989 Hypnotic treatment of sleep-terror disorder. American Journal of Clinical Hypnosis 32: 36–40

Kraft T 1986 The successful treatment of a case of night terrors (parvor nocturnu). British Journal of Experimental and Clinical Hypnosis 3: 113–119

Kramer R L 1989 The treatment of childhood night terrors through the use of hypnosis: A case study. International Journal of Clinical and Experimental Hypnosis 37: 283–284

Myers L B 2000 Deceiving others or deceiving themselves? The Psychologist 13: 400–403

Pedersen N L, Plomin R, McClearn G E et al 1988 Neuroticism, extraversion, and related traits in adult twins reared apart and reared together. Journal of Personality and Social Psychology 55: 950–957

Salkovskis P 1989 Obsessions and compulsions. In: Scott J, Williams G, Beck A A (eds) Cognitive therapy in clinical practice: An illustrative casebook. Routledge, London

Scrignar C B 1981 Rapid treatment of contamination phobia with hand-washing compulsion by flooding in hypnosis. American Journal of Clinical Hypnosis 23: 252–257

Shapiro F 1995 Eye movement desensitisation and reprocessing: Basic principles, protocols, and procedures. Guilford Press, New York

Spiegel D, Cardeña E 1990 New uses of hypnosis in the treatment of posttraumatic stress disorder. Journal of Clinical Psychiatry 51: 39–43

van der Kolk B A 1996 Trauma and memory. In: van der Kolk B A, McFarlane A C, Weisaeth L (eds) Traumatic stress: The effect of overwhelming experience on mind body and society. Guilford Press, New York

Vaughan K, Tarrier N 1992 The use of image habituation training with post-traumatic stress disorder. British Journal of Psychiatry 161: 659–664

Wickramasekera I 1993 Assessment and treatment of somatisation disorders: The high risk model of threat perception. In: Rhue J W, Lynn S J, Kirsch I (eds) Handbook of clinical hypnosis. American Psychological Association, Washington DC, ch 27, p 587

Wilkinson J B 1988 Hyperventilation control techniques in combination with self-hypnosis for anxiety management. In: Heap M (ed) Hypnosis: Current clinical, experimental and forensic practices. Croom Helm, London, ch 11, p 115

Hypnosis in the treatment of miscellaneous psychological problems and disorders

INTRODUCTION

In this chapter, we consider the application of hypnosis to some of the main psychological problems that one encounters in psychotherapeutic practice. The scope of this book does not allow us to cover *all* problems and disorders; nor are we providing a comprehensive account of how to treat the problems that we are discussing. Even if we were to do this, it would be no substitute for proper professional training in the understanding and treatment of these problems. Therefore, the kind of readers we have in mind at this point are professionally qualified persons who are experienced in treating one or more of the problems and disorders that we are covering, who are training or have trained in clinical hypnosis, and who wish to have some ideas for incorporating hypnotic procedures into existing treatment strategies.

In addition, another kind of reader may be the professional whose practice does not include the problems covered here, but who is interested in how hypnosis can be used in their treatment. Such readers may even pick up from this chapter some useful ideas for treating those problems that do fall within their professional remit. Finally, although not strictly in the area of psychological problems and disorders, we have briefly included some ideas about the use of hypnosis in human performance, such as sport.

As we shall restate later, the plan for the eclectic application of hypnosis in therapy, presented in Chapter 22, should serve practitioners in good stead as they contemplate the application of hypnotic procedures to the problems and disorders discussed here.

HYPNOSIS IN DEPRESSION

Psychotherapy with the depressed patient should be undertaken with great caution since, as a psychiatric disorder, depression is life-threatening. As always, we stress that if you are considering using hypnosis for this disorder you should already be well experienced in treating these patients. Any therapy for depression has to take place over a period of time (i.e. there are no one-session cures) and there will be times when the patient's mood will worsen for reasons that are both related and unrelated to therapy. At such times, the risk of suicidal action on the part of the patient should not be far from the therapist's mind. Two possible reasons related to therapy are as follows.

First, there are times in therapy when progress appears to have come to a halt or even reversed. This can be especially difficult for depressed patients, who typically feel pessimistic and many have already decided that nothing is going to make any difference to how they feel. We saw in Chapter 11 how complete insensitivity on a therapist's part to the patient's lack of progress precipitated the latter's serious suicide attempt.

Second, material often arises in a session that is distressing for patients. They may then leave the appointment with these unhappy thoughts, only to return to an unsympathetic environment or to resume responsibilities that do not make any allowances for their feelings at the time. For this reason, one must always be careful about, say, asking the patient to bring to mind unhappy memories, as in an age-regression technique. That is, while the scheme presented in Chapter 22 can be used to plan a course of therapy augmented by hypnosis, we recommend that the revisiting of difficult memories be undertaken very selectively and only when therapists are as sure as they can be that this is going to be productive for the patient.

It is worth mentioning here that, until relatively recently, hypnosis was said to be contraindicated for clinically depressed patients on the grounds that any elevation in mood that may result from a session of hypnosis may be just sufficient to mobilise patients to decide to end their life. Our belief is that there is no evidence that hypnosis poses a risk in this regard.

Psychotherapy for depression

Traditionally, psychotherapy in the form of psychoanalysis or non-directive therapy is viewed as ineffective for depression. For one thing, depressed people tend to be very passive and find it difficult to engage in a therapy in which therapists themselves assume a passive role.

In the last 30 years, a system of therapy for depression has evolved using both behavioural and cognitive procedures. This is now very highly structured and can be presented in 'manualised' form with instructions to the therapist on how to conduct the sessions. It is based on a well-developed theory, supported by research investigations, on the determinants of mood states and depressed mood in particular. The philosophy of this approach can be summarised by the statement 'Consider depression as something that you *do* and *think* rather than something that you *feel'*. Accordingly, the focus of the therapy is in the here and now; what happened in the past that might have predisposed the patient to behave and think in these ways is relevant (Fig. 21.1 may be adapted as a model for depression), but it is not something that is considered to be a fruitful area of exploration. Instead, therapy is very much concerned with helping patients to understand what it is that they habitually do, and the ways in which they habitually think about themselves, their world and their future, that result in their experiencing such debilitating disturbances of mood. The aim is then to change these ways of behaving and thinking so that patients can still think and respond to the world in a realistic manner, yet not be overwhelmed by depression. Readers unfamiliar with this information are referred back to the discussion of cognitive therapy in Chapter 21, and most notably the recommended reading, if they wish to explore the subject in greater detail.

Cognitive-behavioural therapy for depression has stood up well to evidence-based research. Accordingly, we recommend that if readers wish to offer hypnosis-augmented psychotherapy to depressed patients, then it makes sense that this is within a cognitive-behavioural framework. There are now rigorous training courses for professionals, some of them accredited and even organised internally by universities.

Psychotherapy for depression augmented by hypnotic procedures

In this section, we describe a number of procedures that in themselves do not collectively provide a course of treatment for depression but which may be incorporated into a programme of cognitive-behavioural therapy.

Alladin's cognitive hypnotherapy of depression

As it happens, a systematic attempt to harness hypnotherapeutic procedures to the formal cognitive-behavioural treatment of depression has been undertaken by the clinical psychologist Assen ('Sam') Alladin. Summaries of this are given in Alladin & Heap (1991) and Alladin (1989, 1992).

A working model for this approach is Alladin's dissociative theory of depression. This uses the idea of 'negative self-hypnosis' developed by Araoz (1981). Depressive thinking is considered to be automatic, dissociated, subconscious and 'syncretic' – that is, holistic and not just verbal or 'in the left hemisphere'. Alladin asserts that this is more typical of right hemisphere cognitive activity and is out of conscious control. (Alladin cites evidence of a right hemisphere disturbance in depression and greater right hemisphere activity during hypnosis.) Thus, this thinking exerts a powerful influence on mood, affect, self-image, and so on, and in this respect is akin to self-suggestion. This accounts for Araoz's use of the term 'negative self-hypnosis' to describe this kind of thinking.

One does not have to lend one's unconditional support to this working model in order to apply the therapeutic procedures thus generated.

In Alladin's cognitive hypnotherapy of depression, there are initially four sessions of routine cognitive therapy. Hypnosis is introduced at session five; this includes Hartland's ego-strengthening routine, taped for daily use. (Readers may wish to heed our recommendations in Chapter 11 concerning ego-strengthening before choosing a routine for the patient.) In subsequent sessions, cognitive restructuring is practised using imagined scenes, past memories and future situations, and posthypnotic suggestions for countering irrational depressive thinking are given in the usual way. Use of these procedures is based on the theoretical assumption that hypnosis allows better access to maladaptive cognitions and beliefs and the means of changing them – that is, it is tapping into the patient's negative self-hypnosis.

Other procedures include planning realistic goals, the use of activity schedules, anxiety management training (e.g. the Calvert Stein clenched fist technique) and assertiveness training. Two others are of special interest.

The first of these is termed 'first aid for depression'. The therapist takes patients through a sequence of images and ideas that are designed to bring about some elevation of mood, however marginal, during the therapy session. It is useful on those occasions, especially the first appointment, when patients come to the session in the depths of depression. The therapist has the simple aim of ensuring that when patients walk out of the clinic they feel better than at the start of the session. Even if this elevation in mood is only temporary, it conveys to patients the message that something can be done to lift their mood. The routine incorporates a humorous image that patients can bring to mind at any time, the suggestion having been given that, during the moment that they are thinking that thought, their mood will be better.

This routine is useful for an early session of treatment but abbreviated forms may be useful at any point in therapy. It was originated by Dan Overlade, and readers should consult the original reference for the full instructions (Overlade 1986).

The second procedure is an attention-switching method for eliminating depressive ruminations ('negative self-hypnosis'). Patients make a written list of 15 objects, people, situations, events, etc., that are pleasant or at least neutral, and that they are able to imagine. With the list in their lap, instruct patients to close their eyes and take them through a brief relaxation procedure (e.g. a breathing technique).

Then give them the instruction, 'Open your eyes and read item 1 to yourself' and after 5 seconds say, 'Close your eyes and think of that item'. After

15 seconds say, 'Open your eyes and read item 2 to yourself', and after 5 seconds, 'Close your eyes and think of that item'.

Go through all the items in this way. This takes around 5 minutes. Time each opening of the eyes with the patient's inward breath and the closing of the eyes with breathing out. Interpose suggestions such as 'That's fine' and 'Just continue to relax'. At the end of the procedure, encourage the patient to keep the eyes closed for a while and continue to relax.

Alladin instructs his patients to do this several times a day, particularly when they have started on a destructive, mood-depressing chain of thinking. A method similar to this is to rehearse with the patient during hypnosis several pleasant scenes and these are to be immediately substituted for any depressive images that arise during the patient's daily life.

Alladin (see Alladin & Heap 1991) reports that his own experience of using his 'cognitive hypnotherapy' programme with 20 patients does not suggest that it gives a better final outcome for clinical depression but patients seem to improve more quickly and to have less anxiety and greater confidence as a result.

Hypnotic induction

Alladin uses a traditional relaxation induction. However, depressed patients typically tend to be inactive and spend much of their time ruminating on their life. It has been suggested that relaxation and meditative procedures that involve relaxation and a sustained inner focus of attention may not be useful for people who are depressed (Carrington 1993). One might therefore consider using the second of the two approaches to hypnosis (Ch. 7), which emphasises suggestibility rather than relaxation and inner absorption.

Alternatively, why not experiment with an active–alert method using a form of repetitive exercise such as pedalling an exercise bicycle? These methods were described in Chapter 10 and they are also summarised in Bányai et al (1993). There is some sense in using such methods with depressed people, both for the reasons given above and because exercise can have a mood-enhancing effect. Ego-strengthening instructions may be used with such methods, as was described in the section on weight loss in Chapter 24.

Use of a cue word to identify depressive patterns of thinking and behaving

When a posthypnotic suggestion has been given, say, specifying the cognitive reappraisal of a given problem situation, then the type of distortion that the patient habitually uses can be employed as a cue or anchor.

> **Case example**
>
> Joe (seen by MH) had the usual depressive habit of filtering out all the positive aspects of his daily circumstances. After exploring this habit in detail with Joe, and helping him understand what he was doing, his therapist gave him the posthypnotic suggestion that whenever he was thinking in this way in his daily life, he would immediately recall the word 'filter' and then bring some realistic positive thoughts about his life to mind.

Planning future activities

There are several variations of this procedure, which may be incorporated into cognitive-behavioural therapy. Using age progression, patients are asked to imagine, say, that they are relaxing at the end of the day, ready to go to bed, looking back on the day and feeling *a little* better in mood than at present. Then allow patients plenty of time to come up with a realistic answer to the question 'What is it that you have done between now and then that is helping you feel better?' For example, one patient said that she had visited her neighbour that evening. Ask patients to imagine engaging in the most rewarding part of that activity (or, if the activity is a chore, then this could be the moment it has been completed) and direct patients to anchor the good feeling, say with a clenched fist. Now, bring patients back to the present and ask them to agree to engage in that activity later in the day. Tell patients that as soon as they think of engaging in that activity they are to re-establish the anchor, and this will remind them immediately of the good feelings they will experience when they are engaging in or have completed that activity. The exercise may be repeated for longer periods, say up to 6 months. Major activities, such as applying for a job, may be broken down into smaller steps; for instance, the first step may be buying the local newspaper to look in the jobs column.

The usefulness of this procedure is due to the fact that depressed people find it difficult to mobilise themselves to engage in any activities, even those that could lift their mood somewhat.

> **Case example**
>
> Ivan, a very depressed patient (seen by MH), spent almost the whole of one session of therapy describing what a terrible week he had had. Only when it was time to close the session did he mention that, for the first time in a long while, he had been swimming. He said that he ached a great deal afterwards, but while he was in the water he did feel better. The final words of the therapist, therefore, were that he should now commit himself to going swimming at least once a week. However, when he attended his next appointment, he confessed that he had not returned to the swimming pool. He had thought about it, but thinking about the effort of finding his swimming trunks and towel and walking in the rain to the bus stop put him right off the idea!

Such is depression; but we all know the feeling when we have to do some simple task such as fill in a form or do the ironing, and somehow we manage to put a big obstacle in our way by thinking of the activity in the most negative manner. The solution, then, is to age progress to the most satisfying part of the task (which may be its completion), to anchor that feeling, then to give yourself the suggestion that as soon as you think of performing that activity, you will make your anchor and bring the satisfying image and feelings to mind (thus distracting you from any negative, immobilising thoughts).

Metaphors

There is no harm done in introducing an apt metaphorical allusion to depression during therapy. For example, Hawkins (1991) used the story of a monk who was feeling depressed. The theme of the story was that in winter, even though the trees may appear to be dead, their roots are still very much alive, and when spring comes the trees will be stronger than ever. Another metaphor for depression was used by one of us (MH) with a depressed woman whose hobby was painting but who had abandoned this since becoming ill. Her therapist described how someone who liked painting woke up one morning and decided to paint a picture. However, she could only find the black and white paints. She felt upset and desperate as she believed that she had lost her coloured paints for ever. However, it was only the case that the paints had been mislaid and gradually as the day continued she found more and more of her paints and was then able to enjoy once again painting an exciting and colourful picture.

PSYCHOSEXUAL PROBLEMS AND DISORDERS

In this section, we consider how hypnotic procedures may be used to augment a course of therapy for sexual dysfunctions and disorders that are primarily psychological in origin. Common problems are low or impaired sexual drive; impaired sexual arousal (including erectile dysfunction in males and lack of vaginal lubrication in females); dyspareunia and vaginismus associated with penetration in females; and problems in the orgasmic phase, including, in males, premature and retarded ejaculation.

General considerations

There are a range of organic factors (including illnesses and general health, medication, and alcohol and drug usage) that affect sexual experience and functioning, and it is important that patients are given a thorough medical examination prior to embarking on a course of psychological treatment. Psychosexual problems may be part of a more general psychological reaction or disorder – for example, worry, depression, and post-traumatic stress – and it may be that therapy should address these broader problems, at least in the initial stages.

Increasingly, medicine and medical procedures are providing possible solutions to psychosexual problems, the most prominent example of this most recently being the drug sildenafil (Viagra) for male impotence. Therefore, the therapist and the patient's medical doctor or specialist (with the involvement of the patient or patient couple) should give consideration to the adjunctive use of medication should this possibility arise.

Readers may also be aware of a clinic in their locality that specialises in psychosexual problems and perhaps marital difficulties generally. In Britain, these come under the National Health Service and are staffed by a multidisciplinary team whose members have a mental health background. In most localities, there are also relationship counsellors who may also have been trained in sexual counselling.

Programmes of therapy for psychosexual problems have been developed, perhaps the most influential being those of Masters & Johnson (1970). These usually have a behavioural emphasis. Whenever possible, both partners attend the sessions, although therapy may include individual sessions for each partner. Many believe that it is important to have two therapists, one male and one female.

There are several components of treatment. These include: assessment; education; a programme of desensitisation that often begins with a prohibition on intercourse and intimate contact; miscellaneous therapeutic procedures according to the nature of the problem; advice on sexual techniques; more general relationship counselling; and individual counselling or psychotherapy when required by one or both partners, say, as a result of emotional problems concerning past experiences.

Hypnosis in psychosexual therapy

Hypnotic procedures may be incorporated into the above kind of programme (Beigel & Johnson 1980, Degun & Degun 1991). Often these will be only appropriate for sessions with one partner, but some may be adapted for joint sessions.

Hypnotic induction and deepening

As always, the practitioner should give thought to the purpose of the induction and decide what the emphasis should be – trance (absorption) or suggestibility. For example, if the problem is dyspareunia caused by anxiety and tension, then the former approach (Ch. 6) is preferable. If loss of self-confidence, say associated with erectile dysfunction, is prominent, the induction and deepening routines in Chapter 7, which endeavour to maximise the patient's expectation of a good response to suggestion and treatment, may be better. Indeed, for the aforementioned problem, some practitioners incorporate the arm levitation procedure, and directly or indirectly allude to how penile erection may occur in response to an image.

Relaxation and desensitisation

Because excessive anxiety is at the root of many sexual problems, relaxation and self-hypnosis are almost always an important part of therapy. Each partner (or the partner who cannot relax) is taught to relax and encouraged, for example, to imagine enjoying lovemaking with all the time that is needed. Similarly, hypnosis may be incorporated into a desensitisation programme for dyspareunia or vaginismus that involves the insertion of dilators of gradually increasing calibre. Misra (1985) also uses, in a desensitisation format, a graded series of slides that depict sexual scenes.

Posthypnotic suggestion

In many of these procedures, posthypnotic suggestions may be given in the usual manner to enhance the patient's expectation of a successful outcome, likewise the use of self-hypnosis. Some practitioners use direct suggestions and posthypnotic suggestions of increasing sensitivity of the erogenous parts.

Ego-strengthening

Ego-strengthening suggestions may relate specifically to pertinent sexual matters, but many patients have a more general problem of low self-esteem and lack of assertiveness, and ego-strengthening may address these.

Fantasising and metaphor

Particularly for problems of low sexual drive and arousal, patients may be encouraged to develop their own sexual fantasies (which may include memories of previous fulfilling sexual experiences). This may be facilitated by the provision of erotic literature. Some practitioners have used metaphorical imagery. For example, Hammond (1990) provides a script describing how preferences for enjoyable things such as foods or television programmes change with age. Another script asks the patient to imagine being in a 'control room' in the brain (the hypothalamus) and being able to operate a dial or lever that can increase or decrease sexual arousal.

Psychodynamic methods

Underlying any psychosexual problem may be emotional difficulties and conflicts that are associated with previous relationships. Interconnected with these, or in their absence, may be problems concerning the existing relationship and these may be acknowledged in varying degrees, or denied altogether, by one or both partners.

The source of the problem may be sexual in nature, as when a patient has experienced a trauma such as rape or sexual abuse as a child. Or the person's first licit sexual experience (with a previous partner or the present partner) may have been an unpleasant one. However, the underlying problem may involve early relationships but not those of an explicit sexual nature – say, a strict upbringing, religious indoctrination that instilled a sense of shame and guilt, or overprotective parenting. There may be some covert resentment or hostility in the present relationship that interferes with the expression of intimacy; or the partners may be replaying a relationship from earlier in one or both of their lives – say, a mother and son arrangement – in which sexuality would be taboo.

Some anxieties and conflicts may relate to feared consequences of intercourse, such as pregnancy or parenthood (entailing, say, loss of independence). When the problem is in the orgasmic phase, fear of overwhelming emotion or loss of control may be an underlying problem. One may speculate that this may relate to the blocking of emotional expression during a previous trauma (Oystragh 1980, Wijesinghe 1977).

For the purposes of exploring and resolving these kinds of problems, the psychodynamically based hypnotic procedures described in Chapter 19 may be of value. For example, the IMR signalling method may provide a safe means whereby to communicate information that is very difficult for the patient to broach in the normal way. The affect bridge regression method and 'part' or ego-state therapy are also commonly used.

Conclusions concerning psychosexual problems

The above represents a summary of hypnotic procedures that may be used in a structured programme of psychosexual therapy, and some additional papers are given in the reference list at the end of this chapter. These methods require a high degree of rapport and trust between therapist and patients. It is very important that sufficient time is allowed for the development of a good therapeutic relationship. The therapist must at all times fully inform patients of what each procedure entails and obtain their unequivocal permission to proceed at each stage. For example, we know of a patient with dyspareunia whose doctor used hypnosis to relax her while he conducted an intimate examination. At one point, he gave the suggestion that she would soon enjoy making love with her husband again. While this of course was her hope, she was shocked by what the doctor had said. He had not discussed with her beforehand whether she specifically wanted this aspect of her problem addressed during the examination and she assumed at that stage that her dyspareunia had a physical cause.

Needless to say, therapists must at all times behave with the correct degree of professional detachment and not place themselves in any compromising position. This may mean that for some procedures the patient's partner should be present or a member of staff such as a nurse. If this is not possible, it may be appropriate to make a recording of the session.

EATING DISORDERS

Aside from obesity that is not necessarily classified as a psychological disorder (though nonetheless interferes with one's daily life and is a health hazard), the general practitioner, clinical psychologist and psychotherapist will have as part of a normal caseload individuals for whom weight and weight control are a major preoccupation whether or not they are of normal size. These patients vary in the degree and type of psychological dysfunction or psychopathology; some may present with psychological concerns that are not unusual in the general population, while others may be emotionally very vulnerable, have significant personality problems (and even a personality disorder), and may engage in self-harming behaviours such as drug and alcohol abuse and self-mutilation. The upbringing and family background of people with eating disorders display an equal degree of variability. The majority are young women, but in recent times more male patients have been reported as well as younger patients.

When the subject of eating disorders is raised, one immediately thinks in terms of two major diagnostic categories, anorexia and bulimia nervosa. However, there are many patients who do not clearly fall under one of these two headings and may at different times have fallen into both categories.

Let us therefore look at these disorders from the point of view of symptomatology. Patients with eating disorders will have some of the following problems. They will be overly preoccupied, and usually dissatisfied, with their weight, size and shape. They have a morbid fear of being overweight. They may be underweight, and often clinically so, but many patients with an eating disorder are of normal weight or are not technically obese. However, except for some 'successful' anorexics, they believe that they are too fat. Indeed, they may genuinely misperceive their size. To control their weight, they adopt drastic and inadvisable methods, notably severe dietary restraint, excessive exercise, vomiting after eating, and the use of laxatives and diuretics. Some engage in uncontrolled episodes of excessive eating (binges) and these are usually followed by drastic attempts to 'compensate' by the aforesaid means.

Restricting anorexics tend to be lower than average in hypnotic susceptibility possibly because of the need to maintain control, whereas bulimics tend to be higher in susceptibility (Pettanati et al 1990). Moreover, although there will be many exceptions to this rule, those patients with bulimia tend to show a greater degree of psychopathology. They may also disclose dissociative types of experiences, particularly with regard to their bingeing, vomiting and other self-harming behaviours.

These differences have implications for therapy, but two of the most obvious contrasts between anorexic and non-anorexic patients are that, first, the former patients will be displaying symptoms associated with emaciation (such as depressed mood, lassitude and absence of menstrual cycle) and second, these patients value their underweight state (Fairburn 1985). Hence, therapy, which can only be deemed a success if the patient's weight increases, is immediately threatening. (Of 43 patients with eating disorders referred to one of us (MH) in 1 year, seven failed to attend at all, *all* of these patients being anorexic.)

Conversely, non-anorexic patients do not usually value their bingeing, vomiting and other related activities. They irrationally fear *weight gain* should they resume a normal eating routine, but a cognitive-behavioural programme can still make this a priority (Fairburn 1985). The patient of normal weight will discover that fears of weight gain are unfounded, and the overweight patient may even lose some weight. Also, these patients tend to be easier to engage in psychotherapy because of the aforementioned tendency for psychological disturbances to be more apparent than with anorexic patients. Indeed, for many anorexics the main reason for their problems may be regarded as 'dieting taken too far'.

Therapy for eating disorders

Patients with eating disorders, notably those with chronic anorexia nervosa, are difficult to treat successfully, and therapy should be targeted at a wide range of issues, eating-related and otherwise. Fairburn (1985) has presented a 20-session programme of cognitive-behavioural therapy for bulimia nervosa, claiming that 85% received significant benefit and 25% were symptom-free at the end of treatment. Fairburn asserts that cognitive-behavioural therapy is the treatment of choice for bulimia nervosa, but it obviously does not suit all patients. Serfaty et al (1999) evaluated a similar programme of cognitive-behavioural therapy for patients with anorexia nervosa, with promising results, but less successful than Fairburn (1985) for bulimics (see also Fairburn 1997, Garner & Bemis 1985). Other treatments are group therapy (which may be undertaken on a residential basis) and family therapy. Some treatment programmes may involve all of these approaches.

The adjunctive use of hypnosis with eating disorders

Hypnotic procedures have been used to augment a programme of psychotherapy with patients of both the anorexic and bulimic types and those with a mixed presentation. For these purposes, the scheme outlined in Chapter 22 for a course of eclectic psychotherapy may prove a useful guide.

Which of the two approaches to hypnosis is used (Ch. 6 or Ch. 7) depends on a consideration of the aim of hypnosis.

Ego-strengthening

Many patients have a problem of self-esteem, and anorexic patients will often invest with a misplaced sense of achievement their ability to maintain their weight at an unhealthily low level. For some, this 'achievement' may also signify independence by offering evidence that they are in control of their own bodies and their own eating in ways unauthorised by authority figures such as their parents. The therapist therefore needs to ascertain what issues are associated with low self-esteem, and these may be targeted by ego-strengthening. Vanderlinden & Vandereycken (1990a, 1990b) have used ego-strengthening coupled with age progression to the stage of separation from the family.

Rehearsal in imagination of cognitive and behavioural strategies

As with other problems, hypnotic procedures such as cognitive rehearsal and posthypnotic suggestion may be used to augment a course of cognitive-behavioural therapy. For example, Vanderlinden & Vandereycken (1990a, 1990b) have used imaginative rehearsal of appropriate eating. They also ask the patient to imagine life without the problem (plus the positive consequences) and life with the problem (plus the negative consequences). Hawkins (1991), in a single-case presentation, used the Spiegels' affirmations for weight control (see Ch. 24), namely:

For my body nourishment is essential.
I need my body to live.
I owe my body this respect and attention.

The patient rehearsed these ten times daily for a week. Hawkins also used the fantasy in which patients meet a friendly animal with whom they can share their problems and who can give them advice. (The idea that the person – adult or child – has an imaginary wise counsellor is a useful technique in cognitive therapy.)

Gross (1982, 1984) used suggestions of greater interoceptive awareness (hunger and fullness) and rehearsal of being in control 5 and 10 years from the present time.

We have discussed in Chapter 24 how, in a treatment programme of weight reduction, patients can be encouraged to think of satisfying activities that they can engage in instead of overeating. This ploy is also used in the treatment of eating disorders (Fairburn 1985) to eliminate bingeing and purging. 'Parts' or ego-state therapy may be used to this effect and this is described later.

Changing the body image

For this purpose, Hawkins (1991) used what may be called the 'double mirror technique'. Patients are asked to close their eyes and imagine that they are standing between two full-length mirrors. They are asked to look at themselves in the mirror behind them and see a reflection of themselves as they are now, and then to allow the reflection to fade and become colourless. Then the following instructions are given (p 114):

Now walk away from that mirror and look at the mirror in front of you. Imagine yourself as you would like to be, feeling good and happy about that. See this reflection brighter, clearer and more colourful and walk towards it, and become that person. You know that this is already happening, even though you may not fully appreciate it yet.

Gross (1982, 1984) used suggestions of having a healthier body image. He also used the image of a photograph of the person now, and an image of a future photograph modelled on a favourite person of healthy size.

Barabasz (1989) describes the treatment of five patients over a six-session course of therapy, including assessment. Two behavioural sessions (40 minutes each) were undertaken in front of a full-length mirror; the therapist gave positive feedback for accurate comments made by patients about their body shape and size, while patients touched their body from head to foot. Three 'behavioural hypnosis' sessions then ensued in which patients imagined the areas acknowledged as emaciated 'filling out to a normal, pleasing, attractive form'. Also, with eyes closed, patients imagined themselves again 'filled out to a normal attractive form'. These procedures were successful for all five patients, but two had relapsed at follow-up.

Ego-state therapy

Ego-state therapy is especially useful for bulimic patients when they describe their bingeing and purging 'dissociatively'. For example, they may say, 'It's as though I am standing watching myself doing it', 'I don't know why I do it, it's not like me', or 'Whenever food is put in front of me, I get really scared – I don't know what it is'.

When using ego-state therapy, it is useful (as in the reframing method) to acknowledge the 'bulimic part' as an 'ally' rather than as an 'enemy'. One can ask patients to imagine the last time they wanted to binge (or vomit). Then they are to concentrate on the 'bulimic part' or the 'part that wants to vomit'. The question that can then be asked is 'Can I communicate with the bulimic (vomiting) part?' One may use IMR signals if preferred.

The therapist then explores with patients the 'intention' of the part in question. If, for example, it is to protect patients in some way, further analysis may reveal conflicts and feelings that may be explored using the affect bridge method. One may also encourage a 'dialogue between parts'. For example, patients can be 'the part that wants to binge' and address 'the part that doesn't want to binge'. Ultimately, one goal of this approach can, figuratively speaking, be to secure the cooperation of the 'part that wants to binge', and thus to explore other, more satisfactory, means of achieving the same ends as bingeing.

Another way of introducing this technique is to ask patients to imagine being in a situation in which they would normally binge (or vomit) and then to suggest that this has not occurred. The question is then posed, 'Is there any part of you that is feeling bad in some way right now?'

A somewhat rarefied version of the above approach is the IMR reframing method. This has been used by Torem (1987) and the procedure may consist entirely of IMR signals to questions posed by the therapist. These responses are elicited at each of the following stages:

1. State the intention to communicate with the 'bingeing', 'purging' or 'starving state'.
2. Seek permission to communicate with this part.
3. Elicit the purpose of the behaviour. This may be done by a verbal response or, if this is not forthcoming, that idea that there is a purpose may be acknowledged by an IMR signal.
4. Ask that part to consider more adult (or adaptive) ways of achieving the same purpose.
5. Check that these new ways are acceptable (again using IMR signals).

It is always important to bear in mind that the above ways of communicating between patient and therapist are based on a metaphor or working model with a range of useful applications that is limited by the therapeutic context and the patient's ability to make sense of it.

Additional reading on hypnosis for eating disorders

There is quite a sizeable literature on hypnosis for eating disorders and some additional papers and chapters are given in the reference list below.

HYPNOSIS IN SPEECH AND LANGUAGE THERAPY

There is comparatively little, good, clinical research on the application of hypnotic procedures in speech therapy, and only a few anecdotal reports. In Britain, in the 1980s, some speech therapists formed the Scottish Society for the Practice of Hypnosis in Speech Therapy and this later became the British Society. At the time of writing, this society appears to have become dormant. Two of its members have presented a review of applications of hypnosis in speech and language problems (Dunnet & Williams 1988).

Stuttering

Lees (1990) has presented a thoughtful review of ways in which hypnosis may be used to help stutterers. As anxiety and tension are part of this problem, then relaxation and self-control techniques are obvious procedures to incorporate into therapy. Lockhart & Robertson (1977) used the clenched fist procedure and self-hypnosis for tension control in 30 stutterers with good results. Ego-strengthening may also be useful, as self-esteem is likely to be an issue.

Although psychodynamic therapy should not be seen as the preferred approach to this problem, regression to early memories of stuttering and their resolution may be included in conventional treatment by those therapists experienced in psychodynamic methods. For example, Gibson & Heap (1991, p 87–88) describe the successful use of regression and ego-state therapy with a woman who had a mild stutter. The memory elicited was her first day at a new school, aged 7, and stammering when asked her name. The 'adult part' was asked to go back in time and comfort the 'child part' in the usual way, and this seemed to have a profoundly beneficial effect.

Doughty (1990) and Kraft (1994) each provide an account of the successful treatment of a single case of stuttering. The former used hypnosis to facilitate systematic desensitisation and the latter used hypnosis for relaxation in conjunction with non-directive psychotherapy. Moss & Oakley (1997) present an experimental single-case study of a stutterer who was successfully treated by anxiety management using an anchoring procedure and ego-strengthening.

Psychogenic dysphonia

A number of therapists have published accounts of the use of hypnotic procedures in the treatment of psychogenic dysphonia (Giacalone 1981, Hill 1990, Horsley 1982, Little 1990, Opris 1973). These therapists have used standard methods of relaxation, self-control, suggestions and imagery of symptom alleviation, imaginal rehearsal, self-hypnosis and posthypnotic suggestion. Morris (1991) also used a metaphorical image that acknowledged the possibility of primary or secondary gain; the patient imagined a bath full of water and the therapist suggested that only when we make a decision to remove the plug is the water granted freedom to escape.

Speech and language therapist Alison Pennington completed a research dissertation at the University of Sheffield on psychogenic dysphonia in 1997. This compared standard speech and language techniques with the addition of physical relaxation or hypnotic techniques. The latter included a traditional induction and deepening routine (eye-fixation with progressive relaxation, followed by imagery of walking down ten steps to a 'special place'); a suggestion that any problem that was affecting the voice would reveal itself;

ego-strengthening; posthypnotic suggestions of general improvement; and the practice of self-hypnosis. The group undergoing the standard therapy and relaxation also received non-directive counselling. There were 15 patients in each group; they were seen for one assessment session and four treatment sessions. Follow-up was at 2 months. Overall, the standard treatment group showed no improvement on measures of vocal characteristics and quality of life whereas significant improvements were obtained with the hypnosis group.

Clearly hypnotic procedures should be more widely applied to these problems.

COMMON NERVOUS HABITS

Nail-biting, thumb-sucking and similar nervous habits may be treated with the usual stress-release training and appropriate positive and ego-strengthening suggestions. Covert positive reinforcement during hypnosis is one choice of therapy. This is done by eliciting, either from the history or during hypnosis, memories of events associated with positive feelings and self-esteem. Such events are relived during hypnosis and the good feelings are repeatedly anchored, for example, by making a fist. In the case of children, one can ask them to imagine (perhaps with age progression) how good and clever they will be when they grow up with the best of habits. The anchoring process is rehearsed several times and then the client is asked to perform overtly the habit to be removed, e.g. the thumb-sucking act. As the hand is rising towards the mouth, and just before it touches the lips, the client is to bring it down and instantly enact the previously established positive anchor. This is repeated several times so that the positive feelings will reward the act of stopping the habitual response, thus eventually extinguishing it. (The procedure also contains elements of habit reversal.) Finally, the client rehearses how just the very thought of sucking the thumb is being dismissed by making a fist.

Wagstaff & Royce (1994) investigated a single-session hypnotic treatment for nail-biting using direct suggestions that emphasised the benefits of stopping the habit, and the daily rehearsal of self-suggestion. This intervention was successful at 5-week follow-up for seven of 11 subjects (a 12th subject did not return). Only one of the control group stopped the habit.

HUMAN PERFORMANCE

Under this heading, we have in mind people who are required to hone their skills to a high standard, failing which they, and sometimes others, will suffer adverse consequences. In the hypnosis literature, the most common client group is sports people, notably those who are performing at championship level. Others are people who perform on stage, people whose work involves extreme precision under stress (e.g. surgeons) and anyone taking an examination.

A detailed exposition of this work is beyond the scope of this book and readers are referred to more specialised sources, a sample of which is given after the reference list at the end of this chapter. However, the self-control and cognitive-behavioural techniques that have been described in previous chapters may all be applied in this particular area. The following are special considerations.

General tension and relaxation

It appears to be universally accepted that in order to perform efficiently and effectively, one's level of arousal needs to be at an optimum. Arousal focuses attention on the relevant range of stimuli and energises the body for action. Hence, under-arousal means that our concentration is apt to wander and we are not primed to give of our best. Over-arousal (which may be associated with anxiety or anger) leads to mistakes, inefficiency in the use of the body's energy, and distraction by the symptoms of arousal itself (racing heart, shaking limbs, sweating, etc.). Hence, a careful assessment of the client's performance is required to determine if there is a problem of undue tension, in which case relaxation and tension control methods are indicated, or under-aroused, when motivating imagery and 'psyching up' routines are more appropriate. To this end, the alert–active methods described in Chapter 10 may be particularly appropriate.

Some performers become over-tense when they are being observed or judged, whereas at other times, (e.g. during practice) they are fine. We shall explore this problem in due course.

Honing of skills

This kind of work is particularly appropriate for those clients whose performance requires a high degree of perceptual-motor skill and precision and is already at a very advanced standard. Consequently, the therapist will probably be someone with expertise in coaching such individuals. Normal coaching procedures are augmented by rehearsing in imagination the skills to be practised (e.g. the swing of a golf club or racquet, or the drawing and release of the bow in archery). A particular pattern of tension in the relevant muscle groups is required, and performance may be marred, say, by an over-tense muscle or muscle group. Hence, the 'feel' of the correct response may be an important focus of practice. One ploy is for clients to imagine observing themselves in practice and playing the role of the coach.

Adverse reactions to spectators, audience and examiners

The presence of spectators or an examiner may cause anxiety and self-consciousness and can be distracting for the person. It is not uncommon, say, for someone who is undertaking a driving test to perform less well than during a lesson. Unless there are more deep-rooted problems of self-esteem, there are at least two different approaches. The first is to help the person ignore the spectators, say by transferring the feelings, thoughts and mental set that prevail during a successful rehearsal into the observed or examined performance. Covert rehearsal and anchoring methods may be used here.

A second approach entails exploring with clients their attitudes and feelings towards the crowd, the audience, or the examiner (present, as in a driving test, or remote, as in a written examination). Do performers perceive them as hostile, critical and not on their side, and imagine that they are just waiting for them to fail? We cannot be sure that this is not an accurate perception, and for some performers and examinees this may be a mind-set that can bring out the best in them. However, if you are a performer, then it may be better to imagine that observers and examiners are on your side and want you to do well. In the case of a written examination, say one that involves essay writing, one can imagine that one is communicating directly to the examiner, who is interested and keen to hear what one has to say. In the case of a driving test, one might even make the point of greeting the examiner in a friendly but polite manner and exchanging pleasantries before the test. All of this may help to relax overly tense and self-conscious performers and provide some positive motivation so that they can do their best.

Miscellaneous

Top performers often have to cope with publicity and media intrusion, that even extend into their private lives. They may have to balance the time and effort they have to dedicate to the pursuit of their careers with demands in their private life, such as their families or close relationships. Failure to achieve their ultimate goal may be interpreted by them as failure to achieve anything worthwhile at all. In team sports, disagreements and rivalries (tension between team members and with managers and coaches, etc.) may have an adverse effect on their performance. Consequently, counselling in handling all of these sources of stress may be beneficial for the performer and hypnosis may play a role in this.

REFERENCES

DEPRESSION
Alladin A 1989 Cognitive hypnotherapy for depression. In: Waxman D, Pedersen D, Wilkie I, Mellett P (eds) Hypnosis: The Fourth European Congress at Oxford. Whurr, London, ch 6, p 175
Alladin A 1992 Depression as a dissociative state. Hypnos: Swedish Journal of Hypnosis in Psychotherapy and Psychosomatic Medicine 9: 243–253

Alladin A, Heap M 1991 Hypnosis and depression. In: Heap M, Dryden W (eds) Handbook of hypnotherapy. Open University Press, Milton Keynes, ch 4, p 49
Araoz D L 1981 Negative self-hypnosis. Journal of Contemporary Psychotherapy 12: 45–52
Bányai E I, Zseni A, Forenc T 1993 Active–alert hypnosis in psychotherapy. In: Rhue J W, Lynn S J, Kirsch I (eds) Handbook of clinical hypnosis. American Psychological Association, Washington DC, ch 13, p 271
Carrington P 1993 Modern forms of meditation. In: Lehrer P M, Woolfolk R L (eds) Principles and practice of stress management, 2nd edn. Guilford Press, London, ch 5, p 139
Hawkins P 1991 The use of hypnosis in the treatment of bulimia. In: Heap M (ed) Hypnotic contributions: Proceedings of the Seventh Annual Conference of the British Society of Experimental and Clinical Hypnosis (BSECH). BSECH Publication, Sheffield, ch 13, p 111
Overlade D (1986) First aid for depression. In: Dowd E T, Healy J M (eds) Case studies in hypnotherapy. Guilford Press, New York

PSYCHOSEXUAL PROBLEMS
Beigel H G, Johnson W R (eds) 1980 Application of hypnosis in sex therapy. Charles C Thomas, Springfield
Degun M D, Degun G S 1991 Hypnotherapy and sexual problems. In: Heap M, Dryden W (eds) Handbook of hypnotherapy. Open University Press, Milton Keynes, ch 7, p 108
Hammond C D 1990 Handbook of hypnotic suggestions and metaphors. Norton, New York
Masters W H, Johnson V E 1970 Human sexual inadequacy. J & A Churchill, London
Misra P C 1985 Hypnosis in sexual disorders. In: Waxman D, Misra P C, Gibson M, Basker M A (eds) Modern trends in hypnosis. Proceedings of the Ninth International Congress of Hypnosis and Psychosomatic Medicine. Plenum Press, New York
Oystragh P 1980 Hypnosis in frigidity: Use of automatic writing. In: Beigel H G, Johnson W R (eds) Application of hypnosis in sex therapy. Charles C Thomas, Springfield
Wijesinghe B 1977 A case of frigidity treated by short-term hypnotherapy. International Journal of Clinical and Experimental Hypnosis 25: 63–67

EATING DISORDERS
Barabasz M 1989 Anorexia nervosa: A new hypnotic approach. In: Waxman D, Pedersen D, Wilkie I, Mellett P (eds) Hypnosis: The Fourth European Congress at Oxford. Whurr, London, ch 6, p 183
Fairburn C G 1985 Cognitive-behavioural treatment for bulimia. In: Garner D M, Garfinkel P E (eds) Handbook of psychotherapy for anorexia nervosa and bulimia. Guilford Press, New York, ch 8
Fairburn C G 1997 Eating disorders. In: Clark D M, Fairburn C G (eds) Science and practice of cognitive-behaviour therapy. Oxford University Press, Oxford, ch 9, p 209
Garner D M, Bemis K M 1985 Cognitive therapy for anorexia. In: Garner D M, Garfinkel P E (eds) Handbook of psychotherapy for anorexia nervosa and bulimia. Guilford Press, New York, ch 6
Gross M 1982 Hypnotherapy in anorexia nervosa. In: Gross M (ed) Anorexia nervosa. Collamore Press, Lexington, ch 15, p 119
Gross M 1984 Hypnosis in the therapy of anorexia nervosa. American Journal of Clinical Hypnosis 26: 175–181
Hawkins P 1991 The use of hypnosis in the treatment of bulimia. In: Heap M (ed) Hypnotic contributions: Proceedings of the Seventh Annual Conference of the British Society of Experimental and Clinical Hypnosis (BSECH). BSECH Publication, Sheffield, ch 13, p 111
Pettanati H M, Horne L R, Staats J S 1990 Hypnotisability in patients with anorexia and bulimia. Archives of General Psychiatry 147: 1014–1016
Serfaty M, Turkington D, Heap M et al 1999 A trial of cognitive therapy for anorexia nervosa. European Eating Disorders Review 7: 334–350
Torem M S 1987 Ego state hypnotherapy for dissociative eating disorders. American Journal of Clinical Hypnosis 29: 137–142. (Reprinted in Hypnos: Swedish Journal for Hypnosis in Psychotherapy and Psychosomatic Disorders 1989, 16: 52–63)
Vanderlinden J, Vandereycken W 1990a Hypnosis in the treatment of eating disorders (anorexia and bulimia). Hypnos: Swedish Journal for Hypnosis in Psychotherapy and Psychosomatic Disorders 17: 64–70

Vanderlinden J, Vandereycken W 1990b The use of hypnosis in the treatment of bulimia nervosa. International Journal of Clinical and Experimental Hypnosis 38: 101–111

SPEECH AND LANGUAGE THERAPY
Doughty P 1990 Case study: the use of hypnosis with a stammerer. British Journal of Experimental and Clinical Hypnosis 7: 65–67
Dunnet C P, Williams J E 1988 Hypnosis in speech therapy. In: Heap M (ed) Hypnosis: Current clinical, experimental and forensic practices. Croom Helm, London, ch 23, p 246
Giacalone A 1981 Hysterical dysphonia: Hypnotic treatment of a ten year old female. American Journal of Clinical Hypnosis 23: 289–293
Gibson H B, Heap M 1991 Hypnosis in therapy. Erlbaum, Chichester
Hill C S 1990 Hypnosis with an unusual case of congenital dysphonia. British Journal of Experimental and Clinical Hypnosis 7: 129–132
Horsley L A 1982 Hypnosis and self-hypnosis in the treatment of psychogenic dysphonia: A case report. American Journal of Clinical Hypnosis 24: 283–287
Kraft T 1994 Successful treatment of a case of stuttering, with a 10-year follow-up. Contemporary Hypnosis 11: 131–136
Lees R M 1990 Some thoughts on the use of hypnosis in the treatment of stuttering. British Journal of Experimental and Clinical Hypnosis 7: 109–114
Little M E 1990 Hypnosis in the treatment of a case of spastic dysphonia. British Journal of Experimental and Clinical Hypnosis 7: 181–183
Lockhart M S, Robertson A W 1977 Hypnosis and speech therapy as a combined therapeutic approach to the problem of stammering. British Journal of Disorders of Communication 12: 97–108
Morris C 1991 A case illustration of hysterical aphonia. Therapeutic success or failure? In: Heap M (ed) Hypnotic contributions: Proceedings of the Seventh Annual Conference of the British Society of Experimental and Clinical Hypnosis (BSECH). BSECH Publication, Sheffield, ch 14, p 117
Moss G J, Oakley D A 1997 Stuttering modification using hypnosis: An experimental single case study. Contemporary Hypnosis 14: 126–131
Opris V 1973 Working method in hypnotherapy of psychogenic dysphonias. Otorinolaringologie 18: 447–452

COMMON NERVOUS HABITS
Wagstaff G F, Royce C 1994 Hypnosis and the treatment of nail biting: A preliminary trial. Contemporary Hypnosis 11: 9–13

RECOMMENDED READING ON HUMAN PERFORMANCE

Below are some papers that describe the use of hypnotic procedures in sports. The chapter by Morgan (1993) also includes a review.

Krenz E W 1984 Improving competitive performance with hypnotic suggestions and modified autogenic training: Case reports. American Journal of Clinical Hypnosis 27: 58–63
Liggett D R, Hamada S 1993 Enhancing the visualization of gymnasts. American Journal of Clinical Hypnosis 35: 190–197
Lodato F J 1990 An experimental investigation of the effects of self-hypnosis, behavioral rehearsal and visualization on the improvement of athletic performance of hockey players. Hypnos: Swedish Journal for Hypnosis in Psychotherapy and Psychosomatic Disorders 17: 141–147
Lodato F J, Kosky E M, Barnett B 1991 The application of hypnosis in enhancing the performance of a youth swim team. Hypnos: Swedish Journal for Hypnosis in Psychotherapy and Psychosomatic Disorders 18: 209–216
Mairs D 1988 Hypnosis in sport. In: Heap M (ed) Hypnosis: Current clinical, experimental and forensic practices. Croom Helm, London, ch 31, p 340

Masters K S 1992 Hypnotic susceptibility, cognitive dissociation, and runner's high in a sample of marathon runners. American Journal of Clinical Hypnosis 34: 193–201

Morgan W P 1993 Hypnosis and sports psychology. In: Rhue J W, Lynn S J, Kirsch I (eds) Handbook of clinical hypnosis. American Psychological Association, Washington DC, ch 29, p 649

Naruse G 1965 The hypnotic treatment of stage fright in champion athletes. International Journal of Clinical and Experimental Hypnosis 13: 63–70

Medical and psychological problems in children and adolescents

INTRODUCTION

The methods discussed in earlier chapters for the treatment of medical and psychological problems in adults may be adapted for children and adolescents, and we have already described how this may be done in the case of common hypnotherapeutic procedures (Chs 14 and 19). In this chapter, we shall examine some specific medical and psychological problems that have commonly been reported in the clinical hypnosis literature.

GENERAL CONSIDERATIONS

The following are some guidelines for using hypnosis with the child patient. We assume, of course, that readers are already familiar with working with children with these problems and are seeking to augment their practice with hypnosis. Consequently, we shall be sparing in our general advice for working with children as we do not wish to instruct readers in matters of which they will already be knowledgeable and well versed.

Professional and legal requirements

Readers will have different requirements in terms of their professions and the law regarding the matter of obtaining informed consent (from both the child and the parents) but it is good therapeutic practice to have this, to be fully open about the methods one is using, and to reassure all concerned that these are considered to be efficacious for the problem being treated. The child must freely and willingly engage in therapy without any undue pressure from the parents.

We have discussed in Chapter 8 the matter of when one introduces one's intervention explicitly as 'hypnosis', and agreed that this is not a simple matter in the case of adult patients. Neither is it so for children, since on many occasions, therapists may find themselves using, in an informal way, the hypnotic procedures that we have described for children, blending them into the therapeutic interaction in a seamless, natural manner. On the other hand, one does not wish to be confronted by angry parents demanding to know, 'Have you just been hypnotising our child?' if, say, as very occasionally happens, they have religious scruples concerning hypnosis. We have also remarked that in some countries such as the USA, there may be possible legal repercussions concerning the use of hypnosis. We recommend that any readers who have concerns and doubts about the use of hypnosis with children in their profession should seek the advice of their governing professional body, and, where necessary, employing authority.

The presence of a chaperone (who may not necessarily be in the room itself, but nearby) is eventually determined by the therapist's professional working practices. Children under the age of 8 may well be too frightened to be left alone with the therapist. Indeed, the presence of parents may provide additional opportunity for them to understand how they themselves may play a contributory role in alleviating the child's problems. This is important when the request for the child to 'have hypnosis' may be made by parents who are denying their own responsibilities, as well as those of the family as a whole, in maintaining the child's problems.

The earlier sessions for children aged 8 to 12 may also require the presence of parents for the same reason, but if this is consistent with the therapist's normal practice, the child can be alone in later stages provided the child's parents are nearby. Depending on their level of maturity, children above 12 may be seen for treatment sessions on their own, but again this is dependent on normal professional protocol.

Developing the therapeutic relationship

Readers who work with children will have developed their own ways of establishing a relationship of trust and acceptance, both with the child and with the parent or parents. Here we list some considerations that are particularly important for hypnotherapeutic work.

The importance of building a good rapport cannot be overemphasised if the child is going to engage in the process of hypnosis. If at all possible, this should start from the time of making the appointment by communicating directly with the child about the arrangements. The relationship thus established between the child and the therapist can continue throughout the treatment. For example, at the initial visit, one may address the child first and the parents later, and obtain as much history from the child as possible, inviting the parents to assist when necessary. One should show an interest in what the child is wearing, the toys that the child may have brought, and so on. Always try to reframe in a positive way any derogatory remarks made by the parents, thus supporting the child and providing him or her with a secure therapeutic environment.

In the case of children with longstanding emotional, behavioural or educational problems, it is not unusual that they lack any set vision of their future. They feel that they have no rights or are not worthy of any ambition in life that may provide the motivation to get better. They believe nothing or nobody can change their life. Hence, when they come for treatment, they are in a state of dejection, anxiety and depression. Some of them will not have any insight into their problems, as they are so confused. It is essential to be clear about the exact nature of their problems and their implications in their life now and in the future.

It is of paramount importance to allow children to feel free to express their emotional needs. In all communications, one must strive to reflect a genuine desire to help the child, and the parents must be gently encouraged not to undermine him or her. One should not talk down to children in therapy; instead one should always make them feel that they are the most important person in that room and that they are listened to, loved and protected, in spite of all that they and others present may say during therapy. Often it may be necessary to make statements to that effect in front of their parents. Remind children of their self-worth at every opportunity, openly stating that their parents love them, whatever they may say or do in the therapy. This boosts children's egos and helps them feel that the therapist is their trusted ally.

Taking a history and assessing the problem

In taking the history of the problem, special attention may be given to the following details:

- What were the child's feelings and fears at the time of onset of the problem?
- What were the family circumstances, attitudes, and so on at the time of onset of the problem and what are they now?
- How much is the child affected by the problem in everyday life?
- What does the child want to change that might be used to set a target or targets for the therapy and thus to motivate the child?
- Does the child and the family think that he or she can achieve the targets set?

If deemed appropriate, it may be useful to introduce some form of scale at the time of taking the history to measure the severity of the problem to start with and to use this to monitor progress. The use of such a scale was discussed in Chapter 25. The scale devised should be visually appealing to the child and designed to motivate and reward the child for making progress. It should emphasise positive achievements rather than 'the problem' – for example, by recording *dry* as opposed to *wet* beds in the case of enuresis – and, in many cases, the child can be responsible for monitoring personal progress.

At the outset, one can relate to children anecdotes of cases similar to theirs and this will help them feel that they are not alone in having their problem, and that they can overcome it. This builds the child's confidence in the therapist and will help the child to be actively engaged in the therapy. It is useful that the child has an explanation of the problem that is simple and that he or she can comprehend. Hence, one should explain the dynamics of the problem using an appropriate working model in language that the child understands, and the ways in which hypnosis may help. Diagrams are very useful aids for this and the child can keep these at home.

HYPNOTIC PROCEDURES FOR FURTHER EXPLORATION OF THE PROBLEM

If the child has difficulty engaging in the initial sessions of rapport-building and identifying and assessing the problem, then the methods described in Chapter 14 and in Chapter 19 (for children) may be useful. Procedures such as 'tidying the desk (or wardrobe)' or age-progression procedures, using a crystal ball, magic mirror or time machine fantasy, allow children to begin to think about their problems and circumstances while being in full control of disclosure to the therapist. Ideas for enhancing motivation and for goal-setting may also surface. Throughout these procedures, children need encouragement to share any revelations with the therapist but there should be no demand on them to do so. It is not unusual at this level in therapy, particularly when there is a preponderance of emotional influences, for children themselves to begin to consider possible solutions and actions to be taken. During this process, the therapist's own knowledge and wisdom, indirectly conveyed through the use of metaphors, brief anecdotes and stories, may prove helpful to the child.

HYPNOTHERAPEUTIC PROCEDURES FOR SPECIFIC CONDITIONS

We shall not attempt to cover all of the complaints and conditions that are likely to be encountered by the general practitioner, paediatrician, child psychologist or child psychotherapist. However, readers should by now have a good idea of how the methods we have presented for adults can be adapted to the treatment of children and young people. Further ideas may be obtained from our consideration of several common areas in which hypnosis has been reported to be an efficacious adjunctive procedure.

Asthma

Asthma is ever increasing amongst children, along with various allergies. As we described in Chapter 25, hypnosis for asthma can focus on the release of tension and the anchoring of relaxation, ego-strengthening, self-hypnosis, and symptom-oriented suggestions (which may also be used during self-hypnosis). Where indicated, hypnosis may be used psychodynamically to resolve, or at least to minimise, any psychological influences.

It is important to explain to both the child and parents the structure of the respiratory system and how it is affected by asthma, by drawing diagrams or showing simple pictures. If the child is too young, it is still vital to educate the parents. The diagrams can be used to inform the patient and parents how the therapist is planning to alter the condition by using hypnosis as well as any other medical procedures or environmental manipulations. This gives the therapist the opportunity to introduce a working model that can provide the basis for a therapeutic metaphor.

Case example

A case seen by one of us (KKA) serves as a good illustrative example. Tim, a boy of 10, was at the stage when he required too many inhalers. He was always anxious and falling behind. However, he loved football and he wanted to be a professional footballer (the usual boy's dream). Sadly, he could only watch his friends playing from the side of the pitch because of his wheezing and his small size. During therapy, following the hypnotic induction, it was suggested that he create the fantasy that on one particular day his school team needed a substitute and he was called onto the field. He proved to be very good and was the main scorer. This idea pleased him immensely, and was anchored by the clenched fist method. Following this, his therapist asked him to imagine that every time he kicked the ball the bronchial lining (an expression with which he was familiar) became stronger and the bronchial muscles relaxed, which in turn eased his breathing. The contents of his self-hypnosis routine included all these positive features. As time progressed, he imagined taking part in all kinds of sports. He also had other forms of ego-strengthening and anxiety management training as described in earlier chapters.

Tim's lung function, as well as his sense of self-worth, progressively improved and he started visualising his own 15-year-old self and what he would be like. Eventually, he came to accept that he would always be small but nevertheless happy. He could not become a footballer so instead he decided to learn karate. His asthma became almost insignificant and eventually he was chosen to be part of the UK youth karate team for an international competition.

Nocturnal enuresis

Nocturnal enuresis in children under the age of 6 does not require treatment, as it is within normal development. If a child in that age group has been dry for some time and then has relapsed, usually it is for an obvious reason such as moving house or school, or an addition to the family. Commonsense advice to reassure the parents will usually suffice. In older children who have never been dry, a full investigation to exclude any physical causes is essential. When the enuresis is benign, hypnosis can be introduced any time after the diagnosis is made, whether or not conventional methods, such as an alarm or medication, are used.

During history-taking, the earlier guidelines for creating rapport are particularly important, as the child often comes to therapy feeling very ashamed. It is better to broach the problem only after a good therapeutic alliance has been developed. The child must be wanting help rather than be attending under pressure from the parents.

Let us assume for simplicity's sake that, as is more often the case, the patient is a boy. Explanations are given as to how the kidneys produce urine (or 'pee', 'wee', or whatever is the child's preferred word); how it is collected and stored in the bladder; and how the bladder is kept closed all the time except when it is safe to let the urine out – namely, in the toilet. It is useful to locate each of these organs on the body of the child, to draw diagrams and write down the technical words used. The drawings are for the child to take home at the end of the session. One should also ensure that the child is comfortable with the use of the technical terms, as these will be employed later during hypnosis.

Next, a working model is introduced of what happens in the control of urination during sleep, in contrast to daytime. Most children would agree that they do not wet themselves during daily activities such as watching television. At such times, they can hold on and wait for a long time without any 'leaking', before going to the toilet. The explanation for this is given that a part of the brain, the bladder itself, and the bladder neck with its sphincter or 'tap' are 'talking to each other' all the time. During the day, when the bladder gets full, it tells that special part of brain; to indicate this, you may touch a spot on the child's head and say that it lies 'somewhere under there', and point it out on the drawings. It is the job of that part to ask the other parts of the brain to check whether the child is standing in front of the toilet. When the 'other parts' assure the 'bladder part' of the brain that it is perfectly all right to let go of the urine (or open the 'tap'), only then will the child 'do a wee'. If the child is involved in something or is otherwise not able to go to the toilet, the 'bladder part' of the brain will send a message down to the bladder and its neck to 'hold on'. They will then keep the 'tap' closed and stretch the bladder like a strong balloon that can carry on stretching to hold up to 2 litres of urine. At this stage, it is useful to suggest that the child give a name to the 'bladder part' of the brain. The child may, for example, choose the name of his best friend, let's say Henry.

Now, when the child is asleep at night, the 'leak' is caused because Henry goes to sleep as well. This means that Henry is not doing his job, and so the bladder 'gets fed up'. It decides to let the 'wee' go, even though it is not the proper time or the place to do so. (The child is easily able to identify with this.) The reason that Henry goes to sleep is that too much excitement or too many upsets that happen in the child's life make the whole brain get muddled and confused, including Henry. So Henry, along with all the other parts, goes into a deep sleep.

The therapy is therefore to teach the child how to release inevitable negative feelings, to strengthen self-worth, and to rehearse the symptom-control imagery. If the child is too young to memorise the self-hypnosis, it is useful to make a tape-recording of the session. The tape may be recorded by the therapist without the child's presence and handed over at the next visit, but we recommend that, if this is practical, it is made during the actual session so that it includes spontaneous additions to the script that are appropriate for that child.

The first hypnotic session should also contain details of a typical evening's ritual of going to bed, using self-hypnosis before going to sleep, and asking Henry to stay awake all night. The therapist can 'confirm' that Henry is happy to do his job perfectly, because he 'has got rid of all the worries and upsets about using hypnosis and other ways'. Suggest that when it is really necessary, Henry will wake all parts of the brain and himself as well. Then ask him to watch as he goes to the toilet and safely passes the urine. Henry then goes back to sleep to find, with surprise and pleasure, that the bed is dry on waking up in the morning.

Still during hypnosis, the following additional suggestions may be given:

Now I shall count to 3. When I say 3, you will be aware of a feeling of fullness low down in your stomach. You will awaken, go to the toilet, empty your bladder, and return to your seat (or couch, etc.). Immediately you will sit (or lie) down, your eyes will close, and you will be asleep once more.

If the child responds to those suggestions, you next give the posthypnotic suggestion:

You will do the same thing at home while you are asleep in bed ... each night and every night ... and you will always wake up when your bladder becomes full.

At the end of the session, the parents are tactfully instructed that they should not put undue pressure on their child to do the self-hypnosis.

Should the child fail to respond to these methods, then a more psychodynamic approach may be appropriate. A session conducted with the child alone may bring new information concerning the family dynamics. This happened in a case (seen by KKA) of a 9-year-old girl. Exploratory hypnotherapeutic methods disclosed that she was caught up in the conflict between her divorced parents who were using her to get back at one another. A different approach than that described above was therefore required.

Dermatological conditions

Eczema is a common skin problem in children and not infrequently its atopic nature also predisposes them to asthma as well. The itch–scratch–itch cycle is a vicious one and children are frequently stressed twice: first, by the constant itching and second, by self-consciousness and teasing from others. This may be compounded when parents, relatives and doctors alike repeatedly nag them to 'stop scratching'. Who can refrain from scratching when the skin is itching so badly and the stress that it causes is part of the vicious cycle? One of the main aims of hypnosis treatment is therefore to ease the itching and scratching.

The basis of the working model presented to the patient is that stress is a brain function and the brain also influences and even controls the activity of the skin through chemicals as well as through nerve connections. Readers will recall from Chapter 25 the examples of mind–body communications that one uses to illustrate this simple model for the patient, namely the experience of blushing when ashamed, sweating when scared or anxious, and salivating when imagining chewing a piece of lemon. Therefore, stress management, ego-strengthening and therapeutic metaphors are, as with asthma, the ingredients for hetero- and self-hypnosis.

As we said in Chapter 25, it may be better to use metaphorical imagery chosen or created by the patient and, in the case of children, this may often have magical connotations, such as a magic cream or oil given by a wise person or kindly wizard and made from various herbs on a mythical mountain. Cool streams, rock pools, lagoons on a 'paradise island' and many similar ideas, may be elicited, with the therapist's help, from the child's creative imagination.

As eczema is one of the more immediately visible conditions, introducing the image of the 'future cured self' may be very apposite, and in eczema, all going well, this could be as soon as 3–4 weeks. Ask the child to imagine that she is looking at, for example, a 'Saturday, 8 July 2002 Sarah', 4 weeks from the current session. Suggest to her that she observe:

How confident and relaxed you are and what a lovely skin you have. This is all because *you* (the child in the present) have been using your self-hypnosis regularly. The 'Saturday, 8 July 2002 Sarah' is thanking *you* for doing self-hypnosis so well. That has made her so happy, so why don't you shake hands with each other?

This technique, of course, is only possible in older children; younger ones may respond better to storytelling.

Case example

Jonathon, a boy (seen by KKA) with severe eczema had a 15-minute story composed for him in the first session and taped. The basic structure of the story (many details are omitted here) was that he and all his pet animals had a magic carpet ride. This fantasy served the purpose of induction and deepening. They all landed on a beautiful island where there was a magic lagoon. After doing lots of paddling in the lagoon, they went inland to meet a kind and wise old donkey. The wise old donkey held a party for them and told them that the lagoon contained magic medicine. So they all went back to have a second paddle and a swim in the magic lagoon before they went to bed. Then they all fell very soundly asleep. The surprise was that they did not scratch at all before they fell asleep and during their sleep, and in fact, when they awoke, they did not need to scratch any more.

Jonathon suddenly interrupted the therapist by saying, 'Ah! That's because they had the swim and the paddle in the magic lagoon'. 'Do you know why?' asked the therapist. The child answered, without any hesitation, 'Because it's got magic medicine in it!'

The story continued. They noticed that their skin became nice and smooth. They thanked the wise old donkey, who told them that at any time, whenever they felt bad or itchy, they would listen to the tape recording, and the magic carpet would always take them to the magic lagoon. They now know how to stop the itching and to feel great again.

The child nodded and said, 'Yes' in a sure voice. He was moving about and talking through the entire story asking for clarification or bringing his own ideas into it, all the time being fully engrossed or 'in a trance'. Such *active* involvement is far superior than having the child sit passively listening to a ready-made story.

According to his mother, Jonathon treasured the tape of the story, as his mother did too, because, so it appeared, that one session had changed the life of the whole family.

Similar techniques may be created to treat allergies and other skin conditions.

Case example

One girl of 9 (seen by KKA) was allergic to dogs, and the above methods did not prove beneficial. The use of psychodynamic hypnotic procedures revealed the memory of a dog that viciously attacked her when she was only 4. She seemingly had forgotten (or possibly repressed) this incident. Her reaction was not one of a phobia but of a psycho-somatic manifestation. By talking through the incident and listening to relevant anecdotes by the therapist, she became convinced that not all dogs are the same; on the contrary, they are 'man's best friend'. She was also told how she could be wiser now and 'distinguish the good from the bad'. She was able to be with dogs from then onwards.

Finally, warts are treatable by symptom-oriented imagery used in self-hypnosis. Images include freezing them with ice or tying or clamping the blood vessel that feeds them and starving them of the blood supply (see Ch. 25).

Pain management

Hypnotic pain management methods in paediatric practice are not so different from those used with adults (see Ch. 26) except that it is essential to use child-oriented language and age-appropriate imagery. As we noted in that chapter, patients draw on a considerable range of words to express their pain and suffering – 'terrible', 'hot', 'pounding', 'flashing', 'wicked', 'cruel', etc. Choosing their words in your communications with them, and in the images you construct, will enhance rapport and the effectiveness of therapy. With children, one can agree on some sort of scale to indicate their pain or discomfort. This can incorporate pictorial expressions, such as a glum face at one extreme and a happy face at the other. This may be used to instil the expectation of change and can be a valuable tool at follow-up as evidence that the therapy is working. In younger children, the hypnotic pain management imagery may be presented indirectly in story form in the ways previously described.

Painful, uncomfortable or anxiety-provoking procedures

Some children may be so anxious about a particular procedure, such as an injection or the drawing of blood, that some preparation using formal behavioural or hypnotic techniques may be essential. However, even when children are anxious but still able to go through with the procedure in the usual way, it is well worth some extra effort to lessen their distress so that when the time comes round again for the procedure to be administered, they will feel more confident and not go through the period of trepidation as the time approaches.

It is very important to allow children to cry if they wish, and as much as they wish, and it is helpful to make comments on how clever and brave they are even when they are crying. This helps remove their fear about future procedures as well as the fear of the doctor or nurse as 'the person who hurts'. Instead they will appreciate you as their friend. Encourage them to let all that hurt or pain go and ask the parents to join with you in throwing the hurt, or whatever caused the hurt, away.

In the case of an illness that requires repeated procedures that may cause anxiety or pain, prior discussion of the mechanics of the illness itself is vital so that the benefits of the procedures may be understood. The role of hypnosis can then be explained to the patient, parents and other carers. It is essential to pick the technique that is the right choice for that patient.

Except when the child is extremely anxious, simple, informal procedures can be very effective. Very young children, say 2–4 years of age, respond well to active distraction techniques such as bubble blowing (in reality) and looking at picture books. Putting on an imaginary magic glove or imaginary numbing cream can be a simple effective method for suggesting analgesia, especially for repetitive procedures in the treatment of, say, cancer. With older children, asking them to count, and counting with them, can produce quick and instant results during, say, routine childhood vaccinations. Another ploy is to pretend that you are creating magic 'to make it all so easy' by rubbing the disinfectant swab in an unusual way. For older children, asking them to think of their favourite television programme, with or without eyes closed, is another simple distraction technique. With more anxious children, the technique of covert modelling can be very useful (see the case of 'Jack' in Ch. 20, p. 261).

Older children can be very good at producing hypnoanalgesia by 'leaving their body' for the procedure (or if they have a painful medical condition) and 'going away to somewhere nice and exciting' in a way analogous to when their parents leave their car for repair in the garage and collect it after everything has been done.

Case example

12-year-old Indira (seen by one of the authors (KKA)) attended the surgery with a badly infected and very painful in-growing toenail. She wanted to join her dancing team the same day for a public display. Accordingly, before he started attending to the nail, the doctor encouraged her to imagine watching her favourite programme on television with her eyes closed. When she signalled that she had started watching it, she was asked to commentate continuously about what was happening on her imaginary television. The programme was a football match and at one stage she indicated that she wanted to take part in it as the goalkeeper; then, she imagined saving all the goals. At that stage, the doctor told her that he was just going to clean the toe and trim the loose nail. He assured her that she would feel fine as long as she kept saving the goals, and nothing would bother her. The doctor was able to excise the offending toenail without any twitching of her leg. She was thus able to join her dancing team later as planned. Years afterwards, she told the doctor that she had been aware that he was cutting through the nail but it did not bother her at all.

ANXIETY IN CHILDREN

Many anxieties that otherwise well-adjusted children experience are concerned with school and education as well as with self-image and assertiveness in relation to their peers. Performance-related anxiety, such as exam nerves, competition anxiety (e.g. in sports) and situational fears are also common. In all of these, children may be taught relaxation techniques during hypnosis.

Irrational fears are frequent in childhood and it is not uncommon that other family members also have phobias. Specific phobias may be treated in the standard way. School phobia is a common and often very difficult problem that child psychiatrists, psychotherapists and educational psychologists encounter regularly. This should not be confused with everyday truancy, and sometimes the problem is separation anxiety rather than school phobia as such. The school phobic child may complain of a variety of fears and psychosomatic symptoms and may develop panic disorder. The problem is often, although not necessarily, associated with unsatisfactory parent–child relationships and this possibility must be thoroughly explored.

Hypnosis can be a useful adjunct to treatment. Treatment consists of full discussion and counselling with the parents, and, if possible, with the child alone. Hypnosis is aimed at anxiety reduction and ego-strengthening. Story-telling and metaphors may be more valuable than directly giving advice. Positive anchors, rehearsed covertly, form the basis of self-hypnosis which, with practice, becomes the means to deal with phobic situations in real life.

Desensitisation techniques for this and other anxieties and phobias are similar to those as indicated in the treatment of phobias for adults. The self-control procedures outlined in Chapters 12 and 14, such as positive and negative anchoring, may be incorporated into treatment. Suggestions may be given during hypnosis that the child is experiencing, step by step, the entire scenario of the anxiety-provoking situation (e.g. going to school in the case of school phobia). Everything that could possibly happen in the situation is explored, along with ways of helping the child in each case. At every stage, the child is reminded of the experience of relaxation that has been taught. The suggestions are reinforced by, for example, saying:

Whenever you use the anchor for relaxation, you will regain your sense of being calm and in control. … Because you are calm and in control, you will be confident and perform well. More and more you are finding that whenever there is any threat of becoming anxious you are automatically using this experience. Eventually, that calmness and confidence will replace completely the unpleasant feelings and get rid of your nervousness permanently. It is not possible to have anxiety at the same time that you are calm and relaxed. So you can keep this relaxation and calmness. … Carry it with you all the time and be a winner. … Always. The more you rehearse these methods, the more *easy* it will be for you. The more *certain* it will be. The more it will become a part of you to have this relaxation and calmness upfront to beat away the fear and anxiety. … Winning again and again … and always.

Case example

Andy was a child, living in the UK with his parents who had booked a holiday in Australia. Unfortunately, he had a severe flight phobia. With only 1 month to go to the holiday, he was taught self-hypnosis, incorporating his choice of safe-place imagery, namely his sitting in a steel cage so that 'nothing could touch him'. He mastered the technique by regular practice of self-hypnosis and he was able to enjoy his holiday, which lasted for 2 months and included several flights.

The objects of the patient's phobia can, by their portrayal through hypnotic imagery, become attractive, harmless or friendly. For example, spiders can be made to appear as though they are begging for the child to be kind to them as they are afraid of the child, who is so much bigger.

Case examples

Assen, a boy of 12, became phobic of dogs to the extent that he could not make the short walk to school. He was told a true story of how a friendly dog had helped save the therapist (KKA) from an attack by three dogs. The therapist then talked about how one can identify bad dogs from good ones, and how there are in fact many more good dogs. A few months later, Assen went to buy a Staffordshire bull terrier as his pet.

Another boy, Harry, who had marginal learning difficulties, developed a phobia of toilets. This reached the stage at home and school where someone had to accompany him to the toilet. It was ascertained by his therapist that he liked to fantasise 'happy faces'. Accordingly, after negotiating with him and the rest of the family, it was agreed to install his imagery of 'happy faces' in any toilet where he had to go. This was achieved during hypnosis and he was to take his fantasy with him whenever he entered any toilet. That was the end of the phobia after a single session.

Sometimes, psychodynamically oriented methods may be necessary to unravel the dynamics that are causing failure with behavioural or cognitive forms of therapy.

Case example

Anwar started with a dog phobia and later became school phobic. Previously undisclosed fears were revealed by using the jigsaw puzzle visualisation technique (see Ch. 19). It transpired that he was afraid of his stepfather's harming his mother, himself and his sister. He felt strongly that it was his responsibility to protect his younger sister and his mother from harm. Talking through these problems helped him to understand that these fears were unreal, as he himself acknowledged that his stepfather was in reality a caring and hardworking person.

FURTHER READING

Hilgard E R, LeBaron S 1984 Hypnotherapy of pain in children with cancer. William Kaufman, Los Altos

Ioannou C 1991 Hypnotherapy with children. In: Heap M, Dryden W (eds) Handbook of hypnotherapy. Open University Press, Milton Keynes, ch 10, p 164

Køhen D P, Olness K 1993 Hypnotherapy with children. In: Rhue J W, Lynn S J, Kirsch I (eds) Handbook of clinical hypnosis. American Psychological Association, Washington DC, ch 17, p 357

Kohen D, Olness K, Colwell S et al 1984 The use of relaxation-mental imagery in self-hypnosis in the management of 505 pediatric behavioral encounters. Journal of Developmental and Behavioral Pediatrics 5: 21–25

Lawlor E D 1976 Hypnotic intervention with 'school phobic' children. International Journal of Clinical and Experimental Hypnosis 24: 74–86

Mills J C, Crowley R J 1986 Therapeutic metaphors for children and the child within. Brunner/Mazel, New York

Olness K 1981 Hypnosis in pediatric practice. Current Problems in Pediatrics 12: 1–47

Olness K, Kohen D J 1996 Hypnosis and hypnotherapy with children, 3rd edn. Guilford Press, New York

Wester W C, O'Grady D J 1991 Clinical hypnosis with children. Brunner/Mazel, New York

The professional practice of hypnosis

In the final two chapters of this book we broach a number of themes that should receive the attention of the serious researcher, practitioner and teacher of hypnosis. In Chapter 33 we raise the question of whether there is any evidence that the procedures we have described in this book actually work. Our review of the existing evidence should lead the reader to conclude that there are good indications that hypnotic procedures are of significant benefit for a remarkable range of problems commonly encountered in medical, dental and psychotherapeutic practice.

We also take the opportunity in Chapter 33 to explore the evidence for the benefits of using hypnosis in forensic investigation and arrive at a more guarded and sceptical conclusion. Finally in this chapter we again return to the theme of possible adverse effects of hypnosis and do so with a consideration of inadequately trained or lay therapists, and stage hypnosis. We note that, while there are reasons to consider that adverse consequences may arise from both, there is as yet a dearth of systematic evidence and we urge the reader to take an objective and balanced perspective.

In the final chapter we impress upon the reader the importance of understanding hypnosis and its application from the standpoint of mainstream psychology, medicine and related disciplines. To this end we offer advice concerning the current academic literature on hypnosis and the existence of learned societies for professional practitioners.

33

Evidence for the benefits and the adverse effects of hypnosis

INTRODUCTION

Does hypnosis benefit people? A cynical but nonetheless valid answer is that hypnosis benefits those who practise it – the academic, the researcher, the teacher of hypnosis, the therapist, the forensic investigator and the entertainer. Using hypnosis in these roles enables these people to gain status, power and financial rewards. Does anyone else benefit? Let us first address this question with respect to hypnosis in therapy.

THE EVIDENCE FOR THE EFFECTIVENESS OF HYPNOSIS IN THERAPY

Here we attempt a very brief, and certainly not an exhaustive, review of the existing evidence. We recommend that readers who wish to take this subject further should also consult the April 2000 issue of the International Journal of Clinical and Experimental Hypnosis (vol 48 (2)). This is a special issue on 'The status of hypnosis as an empirically validated clinical intervention'. Another source of information is the handbook edited by Rhue et al (1993). Finally, an excellent source for references on hypnosis (journal articles, chapters in books, conference presentations, etc.) is the Society for Clinical and Experimental Hypnosis's interactive database that may be accessed on the Internet. The full address of this is as follows:

http://www.hypnosis-research.org/hypnosis/index.html

At the time of writing, the number of references held was 11 612.

Another useful source of references is the American Journal of Clinical Hypnosis (see next chapter), which has a section devoted to abstracts of recent papers on hypnosis.

The effectiveness of psychotherapy

If we define psychotherapy in its broadest sense, including active treatment methods such as behaviour therapy and cognitive therapy as well as 'talking therapies' and 'counselling', then we can say with confidence that 'psychotherapy works'. That is, people experiencing psychological problems, as a whole, derive significantly more benefit from undergoing some form of psychotherapy than from having no treatment at all (Lambert & Bergin 1994).

Less clear is whether there is any great advantage of one kind of therapy over another, although more prescriptive therapies, such as cognitive and behaviour therapy, appear to have the advantage over psychodynamic therapies. It is likely that different patients and different problems are more responsive to different kinds of therapy, so that a crucial issue is how to customise the therapy for the patient. Therapist qualities have been another focus of investigation (Lambert & Bergin 1994) and of particular interest here are experience and training. Surprisingly, it has not been easy to show great advantages for either. It may be that in certain cases, perhaps the more difficult ones, these attributes are more telling.

The effectiveness of hypnosis in therapy

Hypnotherapeutic interventions typically involve induction and deepening methods that usually emphasise mental and physical relaxation, and one or more of the following:

- suggestions to encourage desired changes in perception, feelings, thinking and behaviour
- the use of self-hypnosis by the client or patient to rehearse relaxation and other self-control methods
- suggestions and guided imagery techniques to explore possible problems and conflicts that underlie the presenting complaints.

Clinical studies of the effectiveness of hypnosis have usually involved the first two of the above interventions. Typically, a treatment employing hypnosis is compared with a period of time waiting for treatment, a relatively neutral kind of intervention, such as sympathetic attention, or the usual treatment without the adjunctive use of hypnosis.

There is convincing evidence that hypnotic procedures are effective in the management and relief of both acute and chronic pain for a range of conditions (see meta-analysis by Montgomery et al 2000) and that hypnotic susceptibility is a determining factor in outcome. There have also been clinical trials that attest to the effectiveness of hypnotic procedures in help-ing patients cope with medical and surgical procedures (see Blankfield 1991 for a review, Lang et al 1996 for a controlled study in radiological treatment, Lang et al 2000 for a controlled trial for percutaneous vascular and renal procedures, Walker et al 1991 for chemotherapy in cancer) and childbirth (Brann & Guzvica 1987, Freeman et al 1986, Jenkins & Pritchard 1993).

There is encouraging evidence demonstrating the beneficial effects of hypnotherapeutic compared with control procedures (or no treatment) in alleviating the symptoms of a range of complaints that fall under the head-ing 'psychosomatic illness'. These include headaches, including migraine (Alladin 1988, ter Kuile et al 1994, and review by Holroyd & Penzien 1990); asthma (Collison 1975, Ewer & Stewart 1986, Maher-Loughnan 1970, 1984, Wilkinson 1988, and review by Hackman et al 2000); gastro-intestinal com-plaints such as irritable bowel syndrome (Galovski & Blanchard 1998, Harvey et al 1989, Whorwell et al 1984, Whorwell et al 1987); warts (DuBreuil & Spanos 1993); psoriasis (Zachariae et al 1996) and eczema in children (Sokel et al 1993). Therapeutic gains as a result of hypnotic proced-ures have also been reported in groups of adult and child patients with eczema (Stewart & Thomas 1995) and tinnitus in adults (Brattberg 1983, Marks et al 1985). In hypertension, hypnosis may be a significant compon-ent in a broader course of cognitive-behavioural therapy (Tosi et al 1992).

There have been fewer studies specifically on children, but the available evidence suggests that the above conclusions on pain and medical problems may be extended to children and young people (see Milling & Costantino 2000 for a review of the evidence).

There is evidence from meta-analysis that hypnosis enhances the effect-iveness of a course of cognitive-behavioural or psychodynamic therapy (Kirsch 1996, Kirsch et al 1995), although Kirsch (1996) prefers an interpret-ation based on response expectancy (which he considers to be the basis of hypnotic responding rather than a by-product of hypnosis). Whatever the case, more clinical trials are needed to be confident that, for any given prob-lem, hypnosis may significantly augment psychotherapy. It will also be important to have a clearer idea about which patients may be more likely to benefit from the inclusion of hypnosis. At present, it seems unlikely that hypnotic susceptibility per se is a significant determinant of outcome, but one factor that may well be relevant is a positive attitude and expectation about hypnosis on the patient's part.

There are now well-structured and validated cognitive procedures for the treatment of anxiety disorders. Hypnosis and the practice of self-hypnosis may significantly reduce general anxiety, tension and stress in a manner similar to other relaxation and self-regulation procedures (see Van Dyck & Spinhoven 1997 for a study of agoraphobia with panic disorder) but it is not clear if there is any superiority for hypnosis. However, one study on public-speaking anxiety (Schoenberger et al 1997), did find an advantage for including hypnosis in cognitive-behavioural therapy. Relaxation procedures, including self-hypnosis, may assist in insomnia (Anderson et al 1979, Stanton 1989) although there may be no difference in effectiveness in comparison to stimulus control and paradoxical intention (Espie et al 1989, Turner & Ascher 1979).

Hypnotic procedures are probably at least as effective as other common methods of helping people to stop smoking, the abstinence rates being given as 23% and 36% in two meta-analytic studies (Law & Tang 1995, Viswesvaran & Schmidt 1992, respectively). Single-session interventions tend to have a lower rate of success of around 20–25% (Ahijevych et al 2000). It remains unclear if the key ingredients include those specific to hypnosis. Meta-analyses also reveal that the inclusion of hypnosis in a weight-reduction programme may significantly enhance outcome (Bolokofsky et al 1985, Kirsch et al 1995, Levitt 1993), although some consider that its mode of action is enhanced expectancy (Kirsch 1996).

Although there are plenty of scholarly papers by experienced clinicians reporting favourably on the augmentative use of hypnosis in the treatment of specific psychological disorders such as depression, sexual dysfunction and disorder, anorexia nervosa, bulimia nervosa, speech and language disorders, post-traumatic stress disorder, phobic disorders, and drug abuse, and in sports psychology, too few studies have yet been published that systematically evaluate the contribution of hypnotic procedures to the course of psychotherapy employed.

Hypnosis is not often used in the treatment of major mental illnesses such as schizophrenia, severe major depressive disorder and bipolar affective disorder. The same tends to apply when the treatment of choice is largely behavioural and reliant on in vivo exposure, as with specific phobias and obsessive–compulsive disorder.

HYPNOSIS IN FORENSIC INVESTIGATION

The pioneering British forensic psychologist, the late Professor Lionel Haward, described (Haward 1988) how he used hypnosis for a wide variety of purposes in his work. Like others, he also used hypnosis in the interviewing of eyewitnesses to crimes on the assumption that in certain cases it may facilitate recall of details of the crime.

The use of hypnosis to facilitate eyewitness recall goes back over 150 years (Gravitz 1983). More recently its application for this purpose has been called into question. The reasons for this will now be summarised.

Arguments against the investigative use of hypnosis

- The balance of evidence from experimental investigations is that hypnosis does not improve accurate recall of factual information.

- There is also evidence that more material is elicited by hypnosis, the implication being that this is 'noise' rather than 'signal'. In other words, the extra material is at risk of being confabulation.
- Hypnotic subjects may be more susceptible to leading questions, even when these are very subtle. One reason for this is that, as we explained in the introductory chapters, hypnotic subjects are very sensitive to the expectations and demands generated by the hypnotist and the context in which hypnosis is conducted.
- More serious than the last two objections, there is evidence that hypnotic subjects may be more susceptible to the radical distortion of their memories and even the implantation of false memories that they then come to accept as true (Laurence & Perry 1983).
- Hypnotised subjects may be more inclined to alter their confidence in the veracity of their existing memories. For example, before hypnosis a witness may have a vague impression that the suspect was bald. During hypnosis, the witness may create an image of the suspect as a bald man. The image may be so vivid that the certainty of this detail may be unjustifiably strengthened.
- In court, the above witness may then testify more confidently that the suspect was bald. This greater confidence, according to Loftus (1996), may make the testimony more believable to the jury (and, in the investigations leading up to the trial, the police).
- Surveys of the general public (and therefore potential jurors) reveal a widely held but erroneous belief that memories elicited by hypnosis are particularly reliable (Johnson & Hauck 1999, Wagstaff 1988a).
- Those promoting forensic hypnosis are usually the very people who are hired by the police to undertake it; they therefore have a strong investment in defending its use. What do the police themselves think? In 1985, a symposium was held at University College, London, on the forensic uses of hypnosis. Amongst the invited speakers was Chief Inspector Michael Frost of the Police Staff College in Bramshill, Hampshire. His verdict was that after long experience of watching live and videotaped hypnotic interrogations of eyewitnesses, he could cite no instance in which new and useful information had been elicited (Frost 1988).
- Whatever the final verdict on the utility or otherwise of using hypnosis for eyewitness interrogation, there is enough concern around to provide ammunition for an opposing barrister to compromise the credibility of a witness in court if the witness has been hypnotised.

Counterarguments

The above assumptions are not held by everyone (see the extensive review by Brown et al 1998). In addition, the following arguments have been given in support of the investigative use of hypnosis.

- Investigators such as Loftus (1996) have shown that the whole process of interrogating eyewitnesses is fraught with problems. Unwittingly, it is easy to affect a witness's memory and recall of events by one's choice of words, phraseology, non-verbal mannerisms, and so on. A skilled interrogator will be cognisant of these problems and conduct the interview accordingly. The same may apply for an interview in which hypnosis is used.
- Experimental studies of hypnosis and recall have been conducted in psychological laboratories or artificially contrived situations that lack the ingredients of surprise, fear and frenzied activity that are present in many scenes of crime.
- Even if hypnosis does not offer anything unique to the interrogation of eyewitnesses, the ingredients of rapport, absorption and relaxation may be conducive to better recall. Perhaps also the known high level of motivation of the hypnotic subject to meet the role requirements may be exploited by the insistence on accuracy.
- Even if a great deal of redundant or false material is elicited by hypnotic recall, some new and useful leads may still emerge. In the ordinary processes of conducting their investigations, the police are accustomed to having to sift through a considerable amount of 'chaff' in order to get at the bits of 'wheat' that may provide real leads.
- Some of the problems of memory distortion have been exaggerated and may be applicable to other procedures such as guided imagery or the cognitive interview (Scheflin & Frischholz 1999). For example, McCann & Sheehan (1988) consider that the successful implantation of false memories is much more exceptional than some suppose and studies have failed to follow up the subjects to ascertain if there is any retraction of the memory. Also, false memories may require quite blatant and conscious manipulation on the hypnotist's part, something that an expert interrogator would avoid doing. The 'false memory' controversy in therapy may have led to an over-concern with the same phenomenon in the forensic context.
- Where a witness has been frightened or traumatised by the crime, hypnotic procedures may enhance recollection by enabling the witness to recall the event without the distress that may impede their memory.

The attitude of the criminal justice system

In the USA, in contrast to the 'open admissibility' rule that prevailed until 1980, some states have adopted the rule of per se exclusion of testimony elicited from a witness during or following hypnosis. This resulted from the case of State vs Mack in Minnesota. In contrast, 'a third way' was adopted in 1981 by the New Jersey Supreme Court, namely a 'totality of the circumstances' test. This ruling accepts 'hypnotically refreshed' testimony in court if certain guidelines have been adhered to or if the judge considers it appropriate on consideration of the full facts of the matter. This test now applies to all federal courts (Scheflin & Frischholz 1999).

In Britain, in 1987, the Home Office introduced a set of draft guidelines on the use of hypnosis by the police for interviewing purposes (Home Office 1987). Regarding procedures, the guidelines state that, if hypnosis is employed, it should be conducted by a suitably qualified psychiatrist or clinical psychologist, and the whole interview must be videotaped. Subsequently, the Home Office issued a circular stating more definitively that, because of the risks attached to its use, hypnosis should be discouraged as a tool in police investigations (Home Office 1988).

In Britain, unfortunate consequences of using investigative hypnosis have been recorded in two cases, namely R. vs Coster and Others (Wagstaff 1988b) and R. vs Browning (Gibson 1995, Wagstaff 1996). In the former case, a witness had been interviewed by a lay hypnotist who was unfamiliar with the Home Office Guidelines. In the latter case, a videotape of a hypnotic session with a prosecution witness revealed no evidence to incriminate the defendant and was not disclosed until the guilty verdict went to appeal.

Our recommendations concerning investigative hypnosis

Training and experience in hypnosis do not in themselves make a person an expert in human memory or in the interrogation of eyewitnesses to crime. There are, however, people who do have knowledge and experience in these areas. These include qualified psychologists and, in the case of eyewitness interrogation, police officers trained in memory facilitation techniques (Fisher & Geiselman 1992). It is they who should be called upon to aid police investigations when witnesses need assistance in recalling events. They are not likely to be impeded in their work by declining to use hypnosis. One possible exception to this is with a traumatised witness, in which case a skilled clinical practitioner of hypnosis, qualified in a mental health profession, may be able to assist such a witness in giving an account of what happened in a way which is also therapeutic for that person.

THE POSSIBILITY OF RISKS INTRINSIC TO HYPNOSIS

In Chapter 23, we were concerned with the question of potential adverse effects of hypnosis in general and in the treatment of specific problems. Guidelines for good practice were outlined in that chapter and in Chapters 5–8. Ethical matters are also raised in Chapter 34. Our position is that hypnosis is on the whole a benign procedure and adverse effects tend to arise from the way it is used.

Let us for the moment consider further the question of harmful effects by examining the use of hypnosis for the purposes of entertainment.

STAGE HYPNOSIS

People who use hypnosis for clinical purposes are almost universal in their condemnation of stage hypnosis. If nothing else, this form of entertainment gives the public (spectators and participants) a totally false impression of what hypnosis is like when it is used for therapeutic purposes. In addition, many people have the impression that the participants are being coerced into making fools of themselves for the delight of others.

The alleged adverse effects of stage hypnosis

For many years, opponents of stage hypnosis (e.g. Crawford et al 1992, Echterling & Emmerling 1987, Kleinhauz & Beran 1981, 1984, Kleinhauz et al 1979, MacHovec 1986, 1988, Waxman 1988, 1989) have avowed that it can have unpleasant psychological and physical consequences and may even be dangerous (say by causing longer lasting psychological problems). For that reason, they argue that it should be prohibited by law or, at least, strictly regulated. Some authorities base their concerns on the contention that there are special risks attached to hypnosis (see Ch. 23), as well as the argument that the context itself and the activities and experiences demanded of the participants may expose them to certain adverse consequences, particularly in vulnerable individuals. For example, a stage hypnotist does not know whether imagining being a jockey at the Grand National is a pleasant experience for a participant or whether it may be upsetting if, for example, the person has a phobia of horses owing to a riding accident. In addition, there may be great pressure on the participants to please the audience. It is not unreasonable to suppose that some may find it difficult to disengage from the performance if they so wish, and afterwards some may be upset at the thought that they have been held to ridicule. These potential adverse effects are discussed in greater detail by Heap (2000a).

Some writers have alleged that even more serious problems may follow stage hypnosis, and there are claims that some participants have actually suffered from diagnosable medical and psychological disorders (see above references). For example, Finer (1998, p 219) states that participation in stage hypnosis may result in the following complications:

... headaches, anxiety, irritability, fatigue, depression, unexpected weeping, dizziness, disturbed sleep or dreams, fear of panic attacks, lowered stress threshold, poor coping skills, depersonalisation, derealisation, disorientation, obsessive rumination delusions, psychomotor retardation, impaired or distorted memory, attention deficit disorder, psychotic decompression (*sic:* presumably this is intended to be 'decompensation'), concentration difficulties, sexual problems, antisocial behaviour, symptom exaggeration, post-traumatic stress disorder, and, at the extreme, death.

Astute readers may experience some unease as they peruse this catalogue of symptoms and disorders, but not because of the havoc that this form of public entertainment appears to be wreaking. Can a procedure that principally involves one person in verbal communication with another, and that appears on the face of it to be a harmless way for people to enjoy themselves, really have the ability to cause such an astonishing array of medical and psychological problems, including major psychiatric disorders and death? Is there any symptom or disorder that it *cannot* cause? What other comparable activity results in such mayhem? Do readers have any suspicions that some people may have reason to exaggerate the risks of stage hypnosis?

In this day and age, one needs no reminder that it is notoriously difficult to demonstrate that something that is popular in everyday life is harmful when it is not obviously so. Without the back-up of extensive and carefully controlled research, is it not irresponsible to proclaim that something that is in the public domain is so dangerous?

Stage hypnosis and the law in Britain

In Britain, as in many other countries, stage hypnosis is not prohibited by law. Indeed, lawmakers here need a great deal of persuading before placing prohibitions on any popular form of entertainment that also provides a livelihood for the entertainer. However, claims that stage hypnosis is potentially harmful, or indeed has actually caused harm to people, have been taken very seriously. In 1952, the Hypnotism Act stipulated rules for the licensing of public stage hypnosis shows. In the early 1980s, Dr David Waxman (Waxman 1989) and others were involved in consultations with the Home Office about regulating the practice of hypnosis. However, the point was made that there was little evidence of public concern. The only consequence of these consultations was the establishment of a voluntary body called the Federation of Ethical Stage Hypnotists with a code of conduct that was later developed into the 1988 Home Office Model Conditions on the Conduct of Stage Hypnosis, to be attached to licences for stage hypnosis shows (Home Office 1988).

Recent developments in Britain

In Britain in the 1990s, there was a spate of legal claims involving stage hypnotists. In 1995, a young man sued a stage hypnotist when he injured himself while running away from an imaginary army of giant mice. He claimed to have a phobia of mice. His case was unsuccessful. About the same time, a woman successfully sued Glasgow's Pavilion Theatre after breaking her leg when she fell off the stage during a stage hypnosis show. Also in the 1990s, one claimant sued a stage hypnotist, alleging that he had suffered years of mental illness after participating in the stage show. His initial problem was that for several nights he was overwhelmed with the uncontrollable urge to have sexual intercourse with his furniture and domestic appliances.

Incredibly, this case reached the courts and it was only on the fifth day of the trial, after great public expense, that the case collapsed, purely on a technicality (Heap 2000b).

The case with the highest profile was that of Gates vs McKenna. Here the claimant alleged that he had suffered a schizophrenic illness as a result of taking part in the defendant's stage hypnosis show. The case was heard at the High Court and was resolved in the defendant's favour (see Gruzelier 2000, Wagstaff 2000a, 2000b).

These cases were part of a series of events beginning in 1993 when a healthy young woman tragically died during the night after taking part in stage hypnosis. The verdict of the inquest was death by natural causes and hypnosis was not implicated (Heap 1995a). The mother of the deceased understandably felt that stage hypnosis was a necessary factor in accounting for her daughter's death. She and others mounted a campaign to have stage hypnosis prohibited. She was eventually granted leave to appeal against the coroner's verdict on her daughter's death and her lawyers presented a mass of documents to the Royal Courts. However, the judge considered that hypnosis was probably not a cause of her death and the original verdict was upheld.

An early contributor to this debate was the MP Colin Pickthall. He raised the matter in Parliament (Hansard 1994), warning, amongst other things, that 'This is plainly a highly dangerous business with potentially, perhaps actually, huge consequences for the National Health Service'.

But where is the evidence for this? Early in 1995, one of us (MH) distributed to all general medical practitioners in the city of Sheffield a questionnaire asking them if in the whole of their medical careers they had seen a patient who had complained of ill-effects owing to stage hypnosis. A total of 53 (16.6%) replied, none of whom had ever seen such a patient. To the question 'Do you think stage hypnosis carries significant psychological and/or medical risks?' around 28% responded 'Yes', while 66% ticked 'Don't know'. Only 6% indicated that stage hypnosis should be *prohibited* by law, while 70% believed it should be *regulated* by law.

Also in 1995, the Home Office set up a Panel of Experts to study evidence for the alleged dangers of stage hypnosis. The report and recommendations of this panel were announced in October 1995 (Home Office 1995). It concluded that stage hypnosis does not pose a significant mental health risk that would warrant its prohibition. After consulting a wide range of people, the Panel of Experts brought out a revised set of Model Conditions (Home Office 1996).

We shall summarise our own opinions on these matters at the end of this chapter. Let us stress here that it cannot be said that the safety or otherwise of stage hypnosis has not been taken seriously in Britain. Newspapers, magazines and television programmes have shown no reluctance to allow claimants, professionals and stage hypnotists to present their side of the story. Experts and would-be experts have engaged in discussions on this matter. And claimants and appellants in nearly all of the above civil actions, not to mention their lawyers, have received the generous benefits of the legal aid system.

POSSIBLE RISKS OF HYPNOSIS FROM INADEQUATELY TRAINED THERAPISTS

In certain countries, including Israel, Austria, Norway and, at the time of writing (though deregulation may be in the offing), South Africa and certain states of Australia, there are statutory regulations concerning who should employ hypnosis with members of the public, and who should offer psychotherapy generally. In Britain, as in some other countries, there are no such restrictions. Indeed, the number of individuals offering private services as 'hypnotherapists' in relation to those designating themselves as 'psychotherapists' or 'counsellors' appears to be disproportionately high. This does not correspond to any need in the population for 'hypnotherapy' as opposed to any other form of treatment. Rather it is a product of a number of factors – historical, cultural, sociological and socio-economic. We may therefore ask, 'Can hypnosis cause harm during therapy if the therapist is inadequately trained, both in hypnosis and in psychological therapies generally? If so, how great is this risk?'

There is no doubt that great harm and suffering will be caused if a layperson were to attempt to perform *surgery* on a patient. Even qualified surgeons cause harm when they attempt operations for which they have not received the required specialised training. Can we make equivalent statements about psychotherapy and the use of hypnosis in therapy?

There is certainly evidence that great harm can be caused by psychotherapists, as victims (families, if not the patients themselves) of 'recovered' false memories of sexual abuse have testified over the last 10 years. There are also other reports in the media and in the learned literature of people who have suffered at the hands of psychotherapists or counsellors. Sometimes it is clear that therapists have deliberately taken advantage of their patient or client. Examples are those people who have been indecently assaulted by their therapist, hypnosis being used in some of these cases (Gibson 1992, Heap 1995b, Hoëncamp 1989).

Other patients have suffered because of a lack of consideration by the therapist or from incompetence, or because the procedures that the therapist was using exposed the patient to adverse influences. Such a case was described by Heap (1984) and presented in Chapter 11. Other casualties are exemplified by victims of 'recovered' false memories as noted earlier. The therapists concerned may be guilty of a lack of care and concern, but others may be genuine and dedicated to their patients and believe that what they are doing is in their best interests.

An extreme example is that of 'Carol' whose case was reported by Heap (1996). She went to a lay hypnotist complaining of longstanding emotional problems. This practitioner had undertaken his training by a correspondence course. The methods promoted on this course include asking the client to imagine a series of horrific scenes – for example, as a child, being engulfed in flames, being held under water, and being surrounded by hostile faces – and strong intimations that the client had been sexually molested as a child. (Readers may recall our comments at the beginning of Chapter 1 concerning the 'extraordinary and bizarre ideas and practices' that people are willing to advocate in the name of healing.) The net effect of all of this was that at the end of treatment Carol had acquired a further psychological problem, namely post-traumatic stress.

Is all of this harm predominantly done by practitioners who have insufficient training or who do not belong to established professions such as medicine and clinical and educational psychology? The answer is 'No'. Malevolence, lack of care, and ill-conceived methods are not restricted to those practitioners outside of the aforementioned professional groups. Moreover, whereas untrained would-be surgeons cannot help but harm a patient if they were minded to 'have a go', such cannot be stated with due certainty about a sincere, insightful and sympathetic person, who, though lacking any formal qualifications, endeavours to provide some form of structured counselling to people in distress. Indeed, such therapists may even provide significant benefits to their clientele.

Unless they are doctors, professional psychologists or well-qualified psychotherapists, we generally call such individuals 'lay practitioners', though in practice, this is a very ill-defined term. There are many privately organised courses in hypnosis in Britain for people with no prior experience or qualifications in working with patients, although professional people such as doctors and clinical psychologists also register for these courses. They vary considerably in their length, scope and level of sophistication.

There are some doctors and psychologists in Britain who would dearly like Parliament to emulate governments in countries mentioned earlier and to pass laws prohibiting the use of hypnosis by anyone other than, say, medically qualified doctors, psychologists and dentists (and people supervised by them). One of the main reasons that people give for this is the claim that lay therapists do a great deal of harm or take their clients' money in exchange for ineffective therapy, or that they behave unethically. Another reason given is that practitioners from the above professions, if they are negligent or misbehave, can be struck off their professional registers, with dire consequences. Lay therapists do have their own registers but it is not such a big deal for *them* if they are 'struck off'.

As we stated earlier, in Britain at least, lawmakers are reluctant to be involved in preventing people from earning a living where there is an obvious public demand for their services and when these are offered with good intention; more likely any preference to the status quo would be voluntary regulation. At least Parliament would need good evidence that people are being harmed. But where is the evidence? Recall our earlier reference to Dr Waxman's unsuccessful attempts by him and others to persuade the government that such laws are necessary.

The only evidence we have about the harm done by lay hypnotherapists is anecdotal and single case examples. But what about the stories that lay practitioners hear from *their* clients about how badly they have been treated by their doctors, psychiatrists and psychologists? As the saying goes, 'People who live in glass houses …'.

In reality, we have no reason to suppose that lay practitioners are not as a rule sincere, ethical and insightful people who do their best for their clients. And, as for their effectiveness, as we have noted earlier, it has proved difficult to gather convincing evidence that the extent of the therapist's training makes a substantial difference to the outcome of psychotherapy.

CONCLUSIONS CONCERNING THE BENEFITS AND THE ADVERSE EFFECTS OF HYPNOSIS

Benefits

We believe that hypnosis is an interesting and valid subject for scientific investigation and the result of these investigations enhances our understanding of the human mind and psychophysiological processes.

We consider that there is good evidence that hypnosis is an effective therapeutic medium with adults and children, notably for pain relief, psychosomatic problems, anxiety, insomnia, smoking, weight loss and childbirth. It may enhance the efficacy of broader therapeutic approaches such as cognitive-behavioural and psychodynamic therapy. It may thus also be an effective adjunct in the treatment of other psychological problems such as depression, eating and sexual disorders, post-traumatic stress disorder and speech and language problems, but as yet this claim is made with insufficient systematic evidence, likewise in sports psychology. In some cases, the effectiveness of hypnosis may be more related to non-specific factors, such as enhanced expectancy and general relaxation, but in the treatment of problems with a significant somatic component, including pain of organic origin, there may be effects specific to hypnosis.

We acknowledge that stage hypnosis is a popular form of entertainment that some people enjoy both as participants and spectators.

Non-beneficial, or possible adverse, effects

We ourselves do not consider that there is good evidence that hypnosis per se has any harmful properties. We believe that it is reasonable to assert that the way hypnosis is used, particularly when due care is not exercised, may have adverse consequences. Some people may have anxieties relating, for example, to loss of control. We consider that allegations that subjects are at risk of inadequate wakening from their trance or from uncancelled suggestions are made on weak theoretical grounds. However, as Heap (2000a) has indicated, there may be a non-hypnotic rationale for adverse consequences in both cases (e.g. drowsiness or failure to fully orientate one's thoughts to the immediate present in the case of 'inadequate termination of the trance', and obsessive–compulsive tendencies in the case of 'uncancelled suggestions').

We are not convinced that the investigation of hypnosis in the laboratory is associated with more reports by participants of unpleasant after-effects than for other ethically approved experiments.

Like any effective psychotherapeutic procedure, hypnosis may also have unpleasant or adverse consequences for the patient. We are unsure if hypnosis is associated with more adverse effects than other active therapeutic techniques, with the possible exception of the distortion of memory and the creation of false memories.

We are not sure that there is good systematic evidence as yet to indicate that patients are significantly more at risk from lay practitioners of clinical hypnosis. We are not presently in favour of legal restrictions on who should use hypnosis. Different therapists provide people with different ways of understanding their problems; accordingly, it is an important freedom that people should be allowed some choice as to what kind of person to consult. The government should be economical with any restrictions it imposes on people's freedom in this respect. We have laws that punish therapists who are engaged in any criminal activity, or who are criminally negligent with their patient or client, and civil action is available to anyone whose therapist has failed in a duty of care. Perhaps with regard to the latter, there should be a legal requirement for all therapists to have professional insurance. (The model conditions for stage hypnosis stipulate this for the entertainer.)

We consider that there are risks inherent in the use of hypnosis as a forensic investigative tool that outweigh any benefits, except possibly in the interrogation of the traumatised witness. In our opinion, there are better established procedures, such as the cognitive interview. At all times, the use of psychological procedures to interview witnesses should only be undertaken by professionals who are trained in this kind of work. If hypnosis is to be used, the 1987 Home Office Draft Guidelines should be adopted for the interview.

We agree that the risks of hypnosis that we have acknowledged above also apply to stage hypnosis, and there may be additional negative side effects that result from having to perform convincingly in front of an audience. We are unsure by what degree these adverse effects are more pronounced or prevalent than with other comparable activities. We do not consider that there is evidence that participants in stage hypnosis are at significant risk from subsequently developing a psychiatric disorder, although we do not rule out this possibility in certain vulnerable individuals.

REFERENCES

THE EVIDENCE FOR THE EFFECTIVENESS OF HYPNOSIS IN THERAPY
Ahijevych K, Yerardi R, Nedilsky N 2000 Descriptive outcomes of the American Lung Association of Ohio hypnotherapy smoking cessation programme. International Journal of Clinical and Experimental Hypnosis 48: 374–387
Alladin A 1988 Hypnosis in the treatment of head pain. In: Heap M (ed) Hypnosis: Current clinical, experimental and forensic practices. Croom Helm, London, ch 15, p 159
Anderson J A D, Dalton E R, Basker M A 1979 Insomnia and hypnotherapy. Journal of the Royal Society of Medicine 72: 734–739
Blankfield R P 1991 Suggestion, relaxation, and hypnosis as adjuncts to the care of surgery patients: A review of the literature. American Journal of Clinical Hypnosis 33: 172–186
Bolokofsky D N, Spinler D, Coulthard-Morris L 1985 Effectiveness of hypnosis as an adjunct to behavioral weight management. Journal of Clinical Psychology 41: 35–41
Brann L R, Guzvica S A 1987 Comparison of hypnosis and conventional relaxation for antenatal and intrapartum use: A feasibility study in general practice. Journal of the Royal College of General Practitioners 37: 437–440
Brattberg G 1983 An alternative method of treating tinnitus: Relaxation therapy primarily through the home use of a recorded audio cassette. International Journal of Clinical and Experimental Hypnosis 31: 90–97
Collison D R 1975 Which asthmatic patients should be treated by hypnotherapy? Medical Journal of Australia 1: 776–781
DuBreuil S, Spanos N P 1993 Psychological treatment of warts. In: Rhue J W, Lynn S J, Kirsch I (eds) Handbook of clinical hypnosis. American Psychological Association, Washington DC, ch 28, p 623
Espie C, Lindsay W R, Brooks D N et al 1989 A controlled comparative investigation of psychological treatments for chronic sleep-onset insomnia. Behaviour Research and Therapy 27: 79–88
Ewer T C, Stewart D E 1986 Improvement in the bronchial hyper-responsiveness in patients with moderate asthma after treatment with a hypnotic technique: A randomised control trial. British Medical Journal 293: 1129–1132
Freeman R M, MacCauley A J, Eve L et al 1986 Randomised trial for analgesia in labour. British Medical Journal 292: 657–658
Galovski T E, Blanchard E B 1998 The treatment of irritable bowel syndrome with hypnotherapy. Applied Physiology and Biofeedback 23: 219–232
Hackman R M, Stern J S, Gershwin M E 2000 Hypnosis and asthma: A critical review. Journal of Asthma 37: 1–15
Harvey R F, Hinton R A, Gunary R et al 1989 Individual and group hypnotherapy in the treatment of refractory irritable bowel syndrome. Lancet 1: 424–425
Holroyd K A, Penzien D B 1990 Pharmacological versus non-pharmacological prophylaxis of recurrent migraine headache: A meta-analytic review of clinical trials. Pain 42: 1–13
Jenkins M W, Pritchard M H 1993 Hypnosis: Practical applications and theoretical considerations in normal labour. British Journal of Obstetrics and Gynaecology 100: 221–226
Kirsch I 1996 Hypnosis in psychotherapy: Efficacy and mechanisms. Contemporary Hypnosis 13: 109–114
Kirsch I, Montgomery G, Sapirstein G 1995 Hypnosis as an adjunct to cognitive-behavioral psychotherapy: A meta-analysis. Journal of Consulting and Clinical Psychology 63: 214–220
Lambert M, Bergin A E 1994 The effectiveness of psychotherapy. In: Bergin A E, Garfield S L (eds) Handbook of psychotherapy and behavior change, 4th edn. Wiley, New York, p 143–189

Lang E, Joyce J S, Spiegel D et al 1996 Self-hypnotic relaxation during interventional radiological procedures: Effects on pain perception and intravenous drug use. International Journal of Clinical and Experimental Hypnosis 44: 106–119

Lang E V, Benotsch E G, Fick L J et al 2000 Adjunctive nonpharmacological analgesia for invasive medical procedures: A randomised trial. Lancet 355: 1486–1490

Law M, Tang J L 1995 An analysis of the effectiveness of interventions intended to help people stop smoking. Archives of Internal Medicine 155: 1933–1941

Levitt E E 1993 Hypnosis in the treatment of obesity. In: Rhue J W, Lynn S J, Kirsch I (eds) Handbook of clinical hypnosis. American Psychological Association, Washington DC, ch 25, p 533

Maher-Loughnan G P 1970 Hypnosis and autohypnosis for the treatment of asthma. International Journal of Clinical and Experimental Hypnosis 18: 1–14

Maher-Loughnan G P 1984 Timing of clinical response to hypnotherapy. Proceedings of the British Society of Medical and Dental Hypnosis. 5: 1–16

Marks N, Karle H W A, Onisiphorou C 1985 A controlled trial of hypnotherapy in tinnitus arium. Clinical Otolaryngology 10: 43–46

Milling L S, Costantino C A 2000 Clinical hypnosis with children: First steps toward empirical support. International Journal of Clinical and Experimental Hypnosis 48: 113–137

Montgomery G H, DuHamel K N, Redd W H 2000 A meta-analysis of hypnotically induced analgesia: How effective is hypnosis? International Journal of Clinical and Experimental Hypnosis 48: 138–153

Rhue J W, Lynn S J, Kirsch I (eds) 1993 Handbook of clinical hypnosis. American Psychological Association, Washington DC

Schoenberger N E, Kirsch I, Gearan P et al 1997 Hypnotic enhancement of a cognitive behavioral treatment for public speaking anxiety. Behavior Therapy 28: 127–140

Sokel B, Christie D, Kent A et al 1993 A comparison of hypnotherapy and biofeedback in the treatment of childhood atopic eczema. Contemporary Hypnosis 10: 145–154

Stanton H E 1989 Hypnotic relaxation and insomnia: A simple solution? Hypnos: Swedish Journal for Hypnosis in Psychotherapy and Psychosomatic Disorders 16: 98–103

Stewart A, Thomas S E 1995 Hypnotherapy as a treatment for atopic eczema in adults and children. British Journal of Dermatology 132: 778–783

ter Kuile E G, Spinhoven P, Linssen A C G et al 1994 Autogenic training and cognitive self-hypnosis for the treatment of recurrent headaches in three different subject groups. Pain 58: 331–340

Tosi D J, Rudy D R, Lewis J et al 1992 The psychobiological effects of cognitive experiential therapy, hypnosis, cognitive restructuring, and attention placebo control in the treatment of essential hypertension. Psychotherapy 29: 274–284

Turner R M, Ascher L M 1979 Controlled comparison of progressive relaxation, stimulus control and paradoxical intention therapies for insomnia. Journal of Consulting and Clinical Psychology 47: 500–508

Van Dyck R, Spinhoven P 1997 Does preference for type of treatment matter? A study of exposure in vivo with or without hypnosis in the treatment of panic disorder with agoraphobia. Behavior Modification 21: 172–186

Viswesvaran C, Schmidt F 1992 A meta-analytic comparison of the effectiveness of smoking cessation methods. Journal of Applied Psychology 77: 554–561

Walker L G, Lolley J, Dawson A A et al 1991 Hypnotherapy for chemotherapy side-effects: Further developments. In: Heap M (ed) Hypnotic contributions: Proceedings of the Seventh Annual Conference of the British Society of Experimental and Clinical Hypnosis (BSECH). BSECH Publication, Sheffield, ch 6, p 63

Whorwell P J, Prior A, Faragher E B 1984 Controlled trial of hypnotherapy in the treatment of severe refractory irritable bowel syndrome. Lancet 2: 1232–1234

Whorwell P J, Prior A, Colgan S M 1987 Hypnotherapy in severe irritable bowel syndrome: Further experience. Gut 28: 423–425

Wilkinson J B 1988 Hypnosis in the treatment of asthma. In: Heap M (ed) Hypnosis: Current clinical, experimental and forensic practices. Croom Helm, London, ch 14, p 146

Zachariae R, Øster H, Bjerring P et al 1996 Effects of psychological interventions on psoriasis: A preliminary report. Journal of the American Academy of Dermatology 34: 1008–1015

HYPNOSIS IN FORENSIC INVESTIGATION
Brown D P, Scheflin A W, Hammond DC 1998 Memory, trauma, treatment, and the law. Norton, New York
Fisher R P, Geiselman R E 1992 Memory enhancing techniques for investigative interviewing: The cognitive interview. Charles C Thomas, Springfield
Frost M J 1988 Forensic hypnosis: A police perspective. In: Heap M (ed) Hypnosis: Current clinical, experimental and forensic practices. Croom Helm, London, ch 35, p 376
Gibson H B 1995 A further case of the misuse of hypnosis in a police investigation. Contemporary Hypnosis 12: 81–86
Gravitz M A 1983 An early case of hypnosis used in the investigation of a crime. International Journal of Clinical and Experimental Hypnosis 31: 224–226
Haward L R C 1988: Hypnosis by the police. In: Heap M (ed) Hypnosis: Current clinical, experimental and forensic practices. Croom Helm, London, ch 33, p 357
Home Office 1987 Draft circular: The use of hypnosis by the police in the investigation of crime. British Journal of Experimental and Clinical Hypnosis 4: 189–191
Home Office 1988 Circular No. 66/1988: The use of hypnosis by the police in the investigation of crime. Home Office, London
Johnson M E, Hauck C 1999 Beliefs and opinions about hypnosis held by the general public: A systematic evaluation. American Journal of Clinical Hypnosis 49: 10–21
Laurence J-R, Perry C 1983 Hypnotically created memory amongst highly hypnotizable subjects. Science 222: 523–524
Loftus E F 1996 Eyewitness testimony. Harvard University Press, Cambridge, Mass
McCann T, Sheehan P W 1988 Hypnotically induced pseudomemories: Sampling their conditions among hypnotizable subjects. Journal of Personality and Social Psychology 54: 339–346
Scheflin A W, Frischholz E D 1999 Significant dates in the history of forensic hypnosis. American Journal of Clinical Hypnosis 42: 84–107
Wagstaff G F 1988a Public conceptions of forensic hypnosis: Implications for education and practice. In: Heap M (ed) Hypnosis: Current clinical, experimental and forensic practices. Croom Helm London, ch 37, p 395
Wagstaff G F 1988b Comments on the 1987 Home Office Draft Circular: A response to comments of Gibson, Haward and Orne. British Journal of Experimental and Clinical Hypnosis 5: 145–149
Wagstaff G F 1996 Should hypnotized witnesses be banned from testifying in court? The role of hypnosis in the M50 murder case. Contemporary Hypnosis 13: 141–146

STAGE HYPNOSIS
Crawford H J, Kitner-Triolo M, Clarke S W et al 1992 Transient positive and negative experiences accompanying stage hypnosis. Journal of Abnormal Psychology 101: 663–667
Echterling L G, Emmerling D A 1987 Impact of stage hypnosis. American Journal of Clinical Hypnosis 29: 149–154
Finer B 1998 Book review. Hypnos: Swedish Journal for Hypnosis in Psychotherapy and Psychosomatic Disorders 25: 219–220
Gruzelier J 2000 Unwanted effects of hypnosis: A review of the evidence and its implications. Contemporary Hypnosis 17: 163–193
Hansard 1994 12.12.94, p 748
Heap M 1995a A case of death following stage hypnosis: Analysis and implications. Contemporary Hypnosis 12: 99–110
Heap M 2000a The alleged dangers of stage hypnosis. Contemporary Hypnosis 17: 117–126
Heap M 2000b A legal case of a man complaining of an extraordinary sexual disorder following stage hypnosis. Contemporary Hypnosis 17: 143–149
Home Office 1988 Hypnotism Act 1952: Regulation of exhibitions, demonstrations or performances of hypnotism. Annex to Home Office Circular No. 42/1989. Home Office, London
Home Office 1995 Report of the expert panel appointed to consider the effects of participation in performances of stage hypnosis. Home Office, London
Home Office 1996 Model conditions to be attached to licences for the performance of stage hypnotism. Annex to Home Office Circular No. 39/1996. Home Office, London

Kleinhauz M, Beran B 1981 Misuses of hypnosis: A medical emergency and its treatment. International Journal of Clinical and Experimental Hypnosis 29: 148–161

Kleinhauz M, Beran B 1984 Misuse of hypnosis: A factor in psychopathology. American Journal of Clinical Hypnosis 26: 283–290

Kleinhauz M, Dreyfuss D A, Beran B et al 1979 Some after-effects of stage hypnosis: A case study of psychopathological manifestations. International Journal of Clinical and Experimental Hypnosis 27: 219–226

MacHovec F J 1986 Hypnosis complications: Prevention and risk management. Charles C Thomas, Springfield

MacHovec F J 1988 Hypnosis complications: Risk factors and prevention. American Journal of Clinical Hypnosis 31: 40–49

Wagstaff G F 2000a Can hypnosis cause madness? Contemporary Hypnosis 17: 97–111

Wagstaff G F 2000b Hypnosis and madness: Identifying the issues. Contemporary Hypnosis 17: 135–142

Waxman D 1988 The problems of stage hypnotism. In: Heap M (ed) Hypnosis: Current clinical, experimental and forensic practices. Croom Helm, London, ch 40, p 426

Waxman D 1989 Hartland's medical and dental hypnosis, 3rd edn. Baillière Tindall, London

POSSIBLE RISKS OF HYPNOSIS FROM INADEQUATELY TRAINED OR REGULATED THERAPISTS

Gibson H B 1992 A recent British case of a man charged with rape and other sexual offences. Contemporary Hypnosis 9: 139–148 (followed by several discussion papers)

Heap M 1984 Four victims. British Journal of Experimental and Clinical Hypnosis 2: 60–62

Heap M 1995b Another case of indecent assault by a lay hypnotherapist. Contemporary Hypnosis 12: 92–98

Heap M 1996 The case of a woman claiming damages from a therapist trained in hypnosis by a correspondence course. Contemporary Hypnosis 13: 89–93

Hoëncamp E 1989 Sexual coercion and the role of hypnosis in the abused therapeutic relationship. In: Waxman D, Pedersen D, Wilkie I, Mellett P (eds) Hypnosis: The Fourth European Congress at Oxford. Whurr, London, ch 6, p 160

See also MacHovec (1986, 1988) under references for stage hypnosis.

34

Issues in professional practice

INTRODUCTION

We begin this, our final chapter, by asking readers a question: 'What sort of hypnosis do you want?' It is our contention that this is the most relevant question that academics and clinicians should be now debating. It does involve ethical matters and it does impinge on the discussion of the problems that arise from the substantial presence of the lay sector. However, approaching the question from a purely ethical standpoint misses one crucial issue that many clinicians, who are otherwise very vocal on these matters, fail to address.

THE NEED FOR SCIENTIFIC ORTHODOXY

The main problem as we see it with what we have loosely called the 'lay' sector can be gleaned from the following description of a workshop on 'psychoneuroimmunology' by one of the lay hypnotherapy organisations.

In the trance state, the whole body–mind system comes under the control of right-brain functioning and its imagery. Both scientists and mystics agree that this can enable people suffering from illness, both physical and psychosomatic, to lower cholesterol levels, speed up the healing of wounds, reduce dependence on insulin, minimise pain, and in some cases extend life expectancy beyond previously projected levels.

(LCCH News Autumn/Winter 2000/2001, 16)

This is about as good as it gets. Unfortunately, it can get a whole deal worse. For example, a well-known lay hypnotherapist in Britain claims that when he is hypnotising his patients he matches the frequency of his voice to the patient's brain waves (Gibson & Heap 1991, p 197), a remarkable achievement by therapist and patient alike.

We could give dozens of examples. The lesson is this: the most important question that the professionals should be addressing is not 'Who should use hypnosis?' but 'What sort of hypnosis should we be using?' or, metaphorically speaking, 'On which mast are we going to nail the colours of hypnosis?' Can we not all commit ourselves to establishing an orthodoxy of hypnosis that is grounded in mainstream psychology and psychophysiology and that informs its application in the areas covered in the previous chapters? Likewise, should we not be cognisant of what the evidence of clinical trials tells us about the effectiveness, or otherwise, of hypnosis as a therapeutic medium? Clearly, the lay practitioners do not have these commitments, and it is not the intention of the authors to suggest that they should do so. They have not contributed to the scientific research on the nature of hypnosis, or to the systematic investigation of its clinical effectiveness. Let them go their separate way.

The establishment of so many private organisations, colleges, and institutes of hypnosis creates for them a problem: which ones are 'the authentic representatives of hypnosis' and which ones are the 'cowboys'. Just as with unorthodox health practices so in the hypnosis industry the trend is for lay organisations and the people they train to assume all the trappings of the orthodox professions and to endeavour to give every semblance that they are really 'part of the establishment'. For example, it is not uncommon now for their promotional literature to contain carefully worded claims of 'accreditation' by such bodies as the British Medical Association and meaningless claims that their courses are 'recognised for health service funding'.

Another ploy is to hold their training events in suites of rooms rented in hospitals, universities and postgraduate medical centres. So long as nobody asks too many questions, graduates of these courses may legitimately claim that they have 'trained in hypnosis at X Hospital' or 'the University of Y'. (Indeed, we know of lay therapists and trainers who hire rooms at universities to give lectures and then boast that they have 'lectured at the University of A, B, C, D etc.') Occasionally, the certificates issued by these organisations actually display the name of the hospital or university whose rooms they have hired. For instance, Jane (not her real name) understood that her hypnotherapist had trained at a centre for complementary medicine in a London hospital, notwithstanding the fact that he also managed to hold down a full-time job as a plumber, and would turn up at her house in his van. Therapy was conducted as Jane lay in front of her hearth, with the therapist crouched over her. One thing led to another and a charge of indecent assault ensued. We fear that we shall merely irritate readers by referring yet again to the fact that there are no boundaries on what therapists and their patients will get up to in the name of healing.

WHO ARE THE 'EXPERTS'?

Nowhere is the need for a commitment to science and orthodoxy more telling than in the provision of expert advice and assistance in matters of concern to the government, the legal professions, and the public at large. Who should advise the government, for example, on matters relating to the forensic use of hypnosis, or the supposed dangers of hypnosis for entertainment? Who should act as an expert witness in a criminal case in which the accused is alleged to have used hypnosis? Someone who has magical beliefs about how the human brain (or at least half of it) functions? Someone whose speech pattern resembles an electroencephalograph (or so he believes)? Consider the following two examples.

Some years ago, one of us (Heap 1995) was asked to examine depositions in a case of alleged indecent assault by a lay hypnotist. The police had already obtained a statement from a person, whose opinion was that the complainant was not hypnotised but was in a 'trance of terror' or 'fugue'. This person claimed to be recognised as 'the country's leading authority on hypnosis'. He was in fact a stage hypnotist with no qualifications at all.

In 1996, a programme was broadcast on British television (The Cook Report, Central Television) featuring the case of a man who had been accused of a notorious murder, but whose trial had collapsed because of the extraordinary lengths taken by the police in attempting to secure a confession. On the programme, the man agreed to undertake a polygraph 'lie-detector' test, which he duly passed, and to be hypnotised, on the understanding that he would thus be compelled to tell the truth. In the event, he changed his mind about this, or as the programme had it, 'He resisted all attempts to be hypnotised'. The hypnotist in question was a man with no training or qualifications in any relevant scientific, therapeutic or forensic profession, but who gave his professional title in the business telephone directory as a 'hypnotherapist and expert in past-life regression'. A complaint to the programme's producers by the British Society of Experimental and Clinical Hypnosis went unacknowledged, but the campaigning journalist Paul Foot did a damning exposé of the programme in the satirical magazine *Private Eye* (13 December 1996).

We also noted in the last chapter that a trial at Maidstone collapsed when it was discovered that the 'expert witness' on hypnosis had no qualifications. We could detain readers for some time with more of these stories. Some, we are sorry to say, would include opinions in the press given by professional people who have strayed outside their disciplines when commenting, say, on hypnosis and memory enhancement. The lessons of this should be apparent in the examples given. Yet all this is taking place at the same time that the lay sector, as we noted earlier, is frantically assuming the style, if not the substance, of the orthodox health care establishment.

Unfortunately, the commitment to mainstream science is far from universal amongst those in the professions. One of us (MH) while attending training workshops at two separate international conferences was given the advice that it is better to sit on the left-hand side of the subject while doing hypnosis so that one can communicate with his or her right brain. On both occasions, the workshop leaders were well known in the field and had degrees in medicine.

Clearly, those in the professions should be careful to distance themselves from the lay sector but not primarily on ethical grounds. The 'clear blue water' that separates the two should reflect the commitment of the former to mainstream knowledge and disciplines and the commitment of the latter to alternative ideas about the human mind and body, just as we see with orthodox and alternative medical practitioners.

SOME FURTHER PROFESSIONAL AND ETHICAL GUIDELINES

In Chapter 1, we mentioned that there are various national societies throughout the world that reserve their membership for doctors, psychologists, dentists and other mainstream health care professionals. We do not necessarily advocate that readers join one of these; this will depend on the extent to which they use hypnosis in clinical practice. Many practitioners limit their use of hypnosis to relaxation procedures and will find it unnecessary to belong to a hypnosis organisation. However, if you are using hypnosis for a wider range of applications, then it may be helpful to register with a national society. The societies that we are referring to are those that are affiliated to the International Society of Hypnosis (ISH). The ISH Central Office is currently in Australia and its website is:

www.ish.unimelb.edu.au

It holds a tri-annual, weeklong congress split into scientific papers and workshops.

Societies of hypnosis

In Britain, there are three societies affiliated to the ISH. These are The British Society of Medical and Dental Hypnosis (BSMDH), BSMDH (Scotland), and The British Society of Experimental and Clinical Hypnosis (BSECH). The BSMDH website is:

www.bsmdh.org

and the BSECH website is:

www.bsech.com

Each of these societies holds training workshops at different levels. (The BSMDH has a category of 'accredited member' for those who have completed its course of training.) They each have a newsletter and have several branches that hold academic meetings. The BSMDH and the BSECH hold a joint annual conference, which consists of training workshops and a scientific programme. By joining any of these societies, you will also be able to enlist on an international email network and thus communicate with many international colleagues, including well-known authorities. You may also receive a discount on attendance fees for any meeting held by a society affili-ated to the ISH.

These societies are also affiliated to the European Society of Hypnosis, which holds a tri-annual congress with workshops and scientific papers.

In Britain, there is also the Hypnosis and Psychosomatic Medicine Section of the Royal Society of Medicine (RSM) which holds meetings at the RSM in London.

It is also possible to join the ISH as an individual member if you belong to an ISH affiliated society. (This requirement is waived if there is no such society in your country.). For this you receive a very well-presented quarterly newsletter, discount on the registration fees for the ISH congresses, and a CD-ROM membership directory. The ESH does not have individual members.

Hypnosis journals

There are several journals to which readers may be interested in subscribing. The most prestigious of these is the quarterly *International Journal of Clinical and Experimental Hypnosis* (IJCEH):

www.sunsite.utk.edu/IJCEH

Papers tend to be experimental and theoretical or they discuss clinical issues. The *American Journal of Clinical Hypnosis* (AJCH) is also quarterly and has a greater clinical emphasis, but is perhaps less scientific than the IJCEH. The IJCEH is sponsored by the Society for Clinical and Experimental Hypnosis in the USA and the Dutch Society of Hypnosis:

www.sunsite.utk.edu/IJCEH/scehframe.htm

The AJCH is the journal of the American Society of Clinical Hypnosis:

www.asch.net

The BSECH also publishes a highly regarded quarterly journal, formerly the *British Journal of Experimental and Clinical Hypnosis*, now (since 1991) called *Contemporary Hypnosis*. BSECH members receive this journal automatically at discount.

Other countries have their own ISH-affiliated societies and publish their own journals. *Hypnos*, the journal of the Swedish Society for Clinical and

Experimental Hypnosis, is designated as the official journal of the ESH. It is very useful for clinicians (there is little experimental reporting) but the quality is often indifferent and idiosyncratic by the standards of a learned journal.

Ethical guidelines

For the professional practitioner (medical doctor, dentist, psychologist, psychotherapist, etc.), the most appropriate set of ethical guidelines on the practice of hypnosis are those provided by the ISH. In Britain, the ethical codes of the BSMDH and the BSECH are based on the ISH rules. The ISH Ethical Code is contained in Appendix 2 of this book.

The golden rule in the above ethical codes is that practitioners using hypnosis for clinical or therapeutic purposes should confine its application to those problems that they are professionally qualified to treat. It follows from this that where practitioners use hypnosis to augment a broader course of counselling or psychotherapy, they should already be qualified to undertake that form of counselling or psychotherapy.

A good guideline for anyone to follow is only to use hypnosis for the treatment of those problems that one would be treating anyway, without the use of hypnosis. Practitioners should resist the temptation to treat problems that are the province of qualified specialists, unless the patient has already consulted such a person without sufficient benefit. For example, general practitioners should not offer hypnosis to their patients where it would be more appropriate to refer them to a psychiatrist, and psychologists should not treat speech problems if the patient has not yet had the opportunity to be seen by a speech and language therapist.

Ethical and professional matters concerning training

A discussion of training in hypnosis for the professional will be influenced by the country in which the professional is working. In countries where there are laws that restrict the use of hypnosis to certain professional groups, there are well-structured training schemes for these people. Other countries have no such laws and, as well as courses for the above professional groups, there are organisations that offer training to a wider range of people including those who often have no experience or qualifications whatever in any health profession. The question facing medical doctors, dentists, psychologists or other health service professionals who may wish to use hypnosis in their work is 'What training course is appropriate?'

It is important to bear in mind that while one can study and learn all the available hypnotic procedures in clinical practice, one will still know nothing about the nature of any of the problems and disorders that hypnosis may be used to treat. This is because hypnosis itself does not provide any account of why people have these problems. This is where hypnosis contrasts with other clinical disciplines such as medicine and its specialties, and certain major schools of psychotherapy such as behaviour therapy, cognitive therapy and psychoanalysis. All of these attempt to provide an understanding of the aetiology, pathology or psychopathology, and clinical characteristics of the problems treated, in addition to treatment itself.

It is not within the scope of this book to present a structure and syllabus that we recommend for a clinical hypnosis course (although we have already done this for two university-based courses in Britain). However, as a guide for the person seeking training, we make the following recommendations.

1. The training course should adhere to the professional and ethical rules listed in this section, including a code of ethics based upon the ISH Guidelines. In particular, the aim of the course should be to enable trainees to apply hypnosis competently, at the level they wish, to problems that fall strictly within their existing professional work and which they are already qualified to treat.
2. Where a hypnosis course has the objective of training people to use hypnosis within the framework of counselling or psychotherapy, trainees should already possess or be undertaking a substantive standalone qualification in that form of counselling or psychotherapy.
3. The training offered should be sufficiently flexible to cater for the requirements and objectives of the various professionals who register for the course(s).
4. The content of the syllabus and the ideas and practices taught should be compatible with current scientific knowledge of human psychology and physiology.

In Britain, the BSMDH and the BSECH collectively offer training that endeavours to adhere to these guidelines. Also, from 1990 to 2000, the University of Sheffield ran Certificate, Diploma and Masters' courses in clinical hypnosis on the above basis. These courses ended when the Director (MH) left and his post was not re-advertised. Since 1993, almost identical Diploma and Masters' courses have been running at University College, London, and these continue at the time of writing. Also at the time of writing, a Diploma course is being set up at the Caledonian University of Glasgow. This is the initiative of the BSMDH (Scotland).

In addition to these are literally dozens of what are loosely described as lay hypnosis courses run by various private organisations. These vary in duration and scope and include some correspondence courses. Our knowledge of these is limited, but we know of none that adheres to the above guidelines.

In Britain, therefore, as in many other countries, professional people have a wide choice of training courses. In our country, many do register with what we have described as lay organisations, rather than with the BSMDH or the BSECH. Indeed, some are actively involved in running such courses.

In our experience, many professionals only wish to learn relaxation and ego-strengthening methods that they can use with their patients. Others wish to apply hypnosis within a specialised field, such as pain management or educational problems in schoolchildren. Yet others are keen to apply hypnosis to a broad range of medical and psychological problems that fall within their professional remit.

Ultimately, therefore, in the absence of any enforceable regulations, the responsibility lies with the professionals in satisfying themselves that the training undertaken is sufficient for the purposes for which they intend to use hypnosis. They must not be tempted to use hypnosis in ways that require training that they have not yet undertaken.

The importance of maintaining peer contact and support

It is not possible in this book to deal with every eventuality that has a safety or ethical implication, but in many cases these issues also arise in one's non-hypnotic clinical work, and one's use of hypnosis must always be consistent with the rules of conduct of one's profession. It is always a good idea to keep in touch with colleagues who are also using hypnosis so that you can discuss and seek their advice on matters that concern ethics and safety, as well as clinical practice in general. This is one of the advantages of subscribing to an ISH-affiliated society, and indeed the electronic mail system now allows one to communicate internationally with groups of colleagues in the form of email networks.

REFERENCES

Gibson H B, Heap M 1991 Hypnosis in therapy. Erlbaum, Chichester
Heap M 1995 Another case of indecent assault by a lay hypnotherapist. Contemporary Hypnosis 12: 92–98

Appendices

APPENDICES CONTENTS

Appendix 1

Clinical hypnosis and memory

The following statements and guidelines for members of the British Society of Experimental and Clinical Hypnosis (BSECH) are based primarily on Brown (1995), Williams (1995), the American Society of Clinical Hypnosis Guidelines on Clinical Hypnosis and Memory (Hammond et al 1995), the British Psychological Society Report on Recovered Memories (1995) and the collection of papers published in Conway (1997).

ON MEMORY

There is a generally accepted view in cognitive psychology that there is more than one memory system in humans, that memory is reconstructive rather than reproductive and is generally better for central events rather than peripheral details. Whatever the methods used in the process of retrieving material from memory, some of the information retrieved will be accurate and some will be inaccurate. The only certain way of distinguishing between the two is independent corroboration of the original events. Suggestion, expectancy and post-event misinformation can lead to the creation of false memories (pseudomemories), especially in individuals who are high in hypnotisability or interrogative suggestibility, where there is uncertainty about detail, and in conditions of anxiety and stress. Most of the relevant work on memory and pseudomemory has involved laboratory or experimental situations which may not reflect accurately the processes involved in memory for traumatic events. There is growing evidence that 'traumatic memory' is processed differently from narrative memory (memory for non-traumatic everyday events). There is also evidence that traumatic events may be experienced as partially or wholly forgotten by the individual and then recalled very much later. Though further research is needed, there are reports which suggest that in some cases these so-called 'recovered memories' reflect events which actually happened and for which corroborative evidence exists, whilst in other instances there may be no such corroborative evidence. Whenever a clinician asks about a client's history, the situation is created for possible false memory production and the beliefs of therapists may set the scene for pseudomemories. This is a most significant consideration perhaps when, as in victims of trauma or abuse, the events subject to recall may be considered central to the client's presenting problem.

ON HYPNOSIS AND MEMORY

Hypnosis by itself should not be assumed to make memory retrieval either more accurate or less accurate. Hypnosis is an adjunctive procedure which, through processes such as enhanced absorption and imaginal involvement, might be expected to facilitate established procedures, such as repeated retrieval and contextual reinstatement, which are held to improve recall. Hypnotic procedures may also facilitate access to painful or traumatic memories and assist in their integration by providing a safe context for recall. On the other hand, if an individual is highly hypnotisable, whether or not formal hypnotic procedures are used, suggestion and post-event misinformation may lead to inaccurate or distorted memories. The hypnotist's and the subject's expectations and beliefs about the effects of hypnosis on memory may also influence the process of recall. In particular, a hypnotic context may increase confidence in the validity of material which is recalled whether or not it is objectively accurate, though research has shown that this effect is reduced or even eliminated if prior warning is given that it might occur. Hypnotic procedures are relevant to the question of memory recovery following a period of apparent memory loss. For example, hypnosis can be employed in experimental settings to create temporary amnesia which can later be followed by accurate recall of some or all of the 'forgotten' material. The latter does not prove, however, that material recovered in this way in other contexts is necessarily accurate or that similar memory recovery effects would be seen in the case of trauma. Considerable experimental research has shown that hypnotic age regression is not a literal return to an earlier physiological or psychological stage of development and the apparently recalled material which forms the basis for the regression experience may be both accurate and inaccurate in an historical sense.

GUIDELINES FOR CLINICAL PRACTICE: STANDARDS OF CARE WITH POSSIBLY TRAUMATISED CLIENTS

The following guidelines are intended to apply to all clinicians whose work brings them into contact with survivors of trauma and abuse. Because hypnosis may be expected to facilitate both good and bad practices in therapy, and in light of views which have been widely expressed about the role of hypnosis in creating false memories, those therapists who employ hypnosis in their work should be especially mindful of good clinical practice.

Concerning the nature of therapy

Classic abreaction and the use of memory recovery techniques as a *main* focus of treatment are contraindicated.

What is preferred is a *phase-oriented treatment* approach with three main stages:

1. *Stabilisation:* management of intrusive re-experiencing symptoms, developing coping strategies and skills.
2. *Systematic uncovering:* a graduated process of integrating memories and associated affect related to the trauma into current biographical memory and awareness, using primarily free recall and memory integration methods.
3. *Postintegrative support:* developing new social competencies and self-esteem.

Concerning the dangers of false memory production in therapy

The likelihood of creating false memories is *reduced* if:

a. the client gives informed consent following discussion of what is known from current research about the nature of human memory and an explicit statement that not all memories recovered in treatment are accurate.
b. the therapist recognises a duty to both the client and the community. Clients should not be encouraged to cut off from family or friends or sue as part of therapy, even when abuse memories are corroborated, as this is rarely beneficial therapeutically and is arguably not part of the therapist's role.
c. the risks are assessed, especially with clients with post-traumatic stress symptoms but no identifiable stressor or memories of abuse. Risks which are commonly identified include:
   - high hypnotisability
   - high interrogative suggestibility (where interpersonal pressure is added to post-event suggestion (Gudjonsson 1984))
   - deep involvement with self-help trauma groups or their literature.
d. the therapist assesses personal beliefs and biases about possible trauma and its treatment, especially when assessing new patients. The belief that trauma is the primary cause of most psychological problems and that memory uncovering is the primary treatment is likely to create conditions conducive to the development of false memories

by the client. Uncritical acceptance that trauma did not occur is as unjustifiable as lightly accepting statements of trauma as fact. After a thorough assessment, the therapist should treat the condition presenting and not the condition suspected.

e. the therapist is informed about current memory research and its relevance to clinical settings.

f. the therapist is aware of the role of suggestion in memory distortion and does not use persuasive techniques or interrogative methods, but adopts a more egalitarian and permissive approach.

g. free-recall strategies are adopted (not structured enquiry or leading questions).

h. anxiety, distress and uncertainty about the course of therapy are kept to a minimum.

i. the client is assisted in tolerating ambiguity and uncertainty about the past and not pushed towards 'disambiguation' or to 'remember more'.

REFERENCES

British Psychological Society (BPS) 1995 Recovered memories: The report of the working party of the British Psychological Society. BPS Publications, Leicester

Brown D 1995 Pseudomemories: The standard of science and the standard of care in trauma treatment. American Journal of Clinical Hypnosis 37: 1–24

Conway M A (ed) 1997 Recovered memories and false memories. Oxford University Press, Oxford

Gudjonsson G H 1984 A new scale of interrogative suggestibility. Personality and Individual Differences 5: 303–314

Hammond D C, Garver R B, Mutter C B et al 1995 Clinical hypnosis and memory: Guidelines for clinicians and for forensic hypnosis. American Society of Clinical Hypnosis, Des Plaines

Williams L M 1995 Recovered memories of abuse by women with documented child sexual victimization histories. Journal of Traumatic Stress 8: 649–674

Acknowledgement

This document has been prepared by Dr David Oakley and Mrs Marcia Degun-Mather of the British Society of Experimental Hypnosis (BSECH) with the advice of members and Council officials of the BSECH. It is reprinted here with the permission of the BSECH.

Ethical guidelines of the International Society of Hypnosis (Ratified August 1979 – currently under revision)

The International Society of Hypnosis (ISH) is dedicated to the scientific investigation and clinical utilisation of hypnosis at the highest professional level. Ethical guidelines to which a member must subscribe are stated to allow for the multidisciplinary nature of the membership. There is implied a personal commitment to behave according to high standards of personal and professional conduct.

GUIDELINE 1

1. A member of ISH shall always place first the welfare of the patient or the experimental subject when using hypnosis or hypnotic techniques in clinical practice or in experimentation.

a. The standards of professional relationships which guide the physician, dentist, psychologist (with doctoral degree), or other defined professional worker, within the appropriate professional or scientific field, shall prevail in his or her use of all hypnotic techniques.
b. Proper safeguards shall be maintained whenever a patient or subject is exposed to unusual stress or other form of risk. If stress or risk is involved, the person or subject should be informed and give consent. Estimation of risk is a difficult matter, and when in doubt the practitioner should consult with professional colleagues.

GUIDELINE 2

2. Hypnosis is considered an adjuvant to other forms of scientific or clinical endeavours, so that competence in hypnotic techniques alone is not acceptable as a basis for professional service or research.

a. In view of the dependence of hypnotic practice upon other qualifications, the membership requirements of ISH require proper standing in the recognised national organisations, whether clinical or scientific, appropriate to the field of competence not represented by hypnosis. That is, a medical doctor is expected to belong to the appropriate medical association, a dentist to the appropriate dental association, a psychologist to the appropriate psychological associations, and so on.
b. Item 2a requires acceptance of the ethical and scientific standards of a responsible professional organisation. It does not imply endorsement by ISH of the particular policies or practices of any particular organisation.

GUIDELINE 3

3. Each member of ISH shall limit the clinical and scientific use of hypnosis to the area of competence as defined by the professional standards of his or her field.

GUIDELINE 4

4. Hypnosis should not be used as a form of entertainment.

a. No member of ISH shall offer services for the purposes of public entertainment or collaborate with any person or agency engaged in public entertainment.

GUIDELINE 5

5. A member of ISH shall not support the practice of hypnosis by lay persons.

a. A lay person is defined here as one who is not a member in good standing of a therapeutic or scientific profession; that is, he or she is not a physician, dentist, psychologist, or member of another recognised therapeutic or scientific profession with credentials in addition to competence as a hypnotic practitioner.
b. A member of ISH shall not give courses involving the teaching of hypnotic techniques to lay individuals who lack training in a relevant science or profession. Lectures informing lay individuals about

hypnosis are of course admissible providing they do not include demonstrations or didactic material involving inducting of hypnosis.

c. Exceptions are made to students, in training in the appropriate sciences or professions. While ISH explicitly recognises that hypnosis is not an independent science or art, the technique may appropriately be utilised by nurses or paramedical assistants under the immediate and direct supervision of an individual whose credentials and training would permit membership in ISH and who has an agreed commitment to this Code of Ethics either directly or through a National Constituent Society. Special arrangements can be made for the training of such nurses or paramedical personnel provided that arrangements have been made for such individuals to work directly under the supervision of an ISH member or the equivalently trained professional as outlined.

d. Consultations with lay representatives of the press or other media of communication are permitted to minimise distortions or misrepresentations of hypnosis. Talks with lay representatives of the press and radio or TV appearances are welcomed so long as these benefit the Society from wise and informed views on issues in hypnosis.

GUIDELINE 6

6. It is recognised that an ethical code cannot by its very nature specify all of the practices that are considered ethical and mention all of those considered unethical. Hence, behaviour in accordance with the ethical norms of the nations in which the professional worker or scientist lives are taken for granted, and violation of these norms (e.g. through illegal behaviour, or discordant behaviour that brings disrepute upon others who practise hypnosis) may be the occasion for adverse action by the ISH, even though not specified in this code.

Acknowledgement

From the International Society of Hypnosis Membership Directory 1997 International Society of Hypnosis, West Heidelberg, Australia, p 75–76. Reprinted with the permission of the International Society of Hypnosis.

Index